PEASANT IN PARADISE

- FOUR SEASONS ECO-LIVING

by Alanna Moore

PYTHON PRESS

Alanna Moore is the author of:

Divining Earth Spirit - 1994, 2nd ed. 2004
Backyard Poultry – Naturally - 1998, 3rd ed. 2014
Stone Age Farming - 2001, 2nd ed. 2013
The Wisdom of Water - 2007
Water Spirits of the World - 2008, 2nd ed. 2012
Sensitive Permaculture - 2009
Touchstones for Today - 2013
Plant Spirit Gardener - 2016

PEASANT IN PARADISE - FOUR SEASONS ECO-LIVING

ISBN - 978-0-6452854-0-6

Published by Python Press,
Ireland and Australia.
www.pythonpress.com

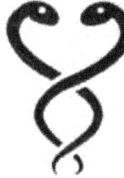 Alanna Moore © 2021

Text, diagrams, design and most of the photos by Alanna Moore.

All rights reserved. No reproduction, copy or transmission of this publication may be made without written permission of the publisher. No person should rely on this book as a substitute for specific advice and the author disclaims any liability in connection with the use or misuse of the information herein.

Printed globally by Ingram Spark.

INTRODUCTION

The year 2020 was looming with a lead-up of dark warnings from astrologers. Planets would be aligning in significant ways and we were in for some kind of shift, though I couldn't imagine what the big shake-up, or re-set, could be from. It felt appropriate to offer some courses in eco-living and I put together a programme. But it wasn't meant to be. A global pandemic and economic mayhem were coming. Things would be changing in a big way indeed!

The pandemic lockdowns of 2020 allowed me greater focus on eco-living and saw me grow more food than I'd ever imagined. And I wasn't alone, people were emptying the supermarket shelves of veggie seed packs and bicycles sales went exponential. It was the great gift of time.

I could experiment with new crops and recipes, nurture nature and get more in tune with my locale. No more jet-setting off for teaching weekends. Travelling generally made me sick anyhow, due to being electro-sensitive. No, this was a year to enjoy health, harmony and the riches of simple living.

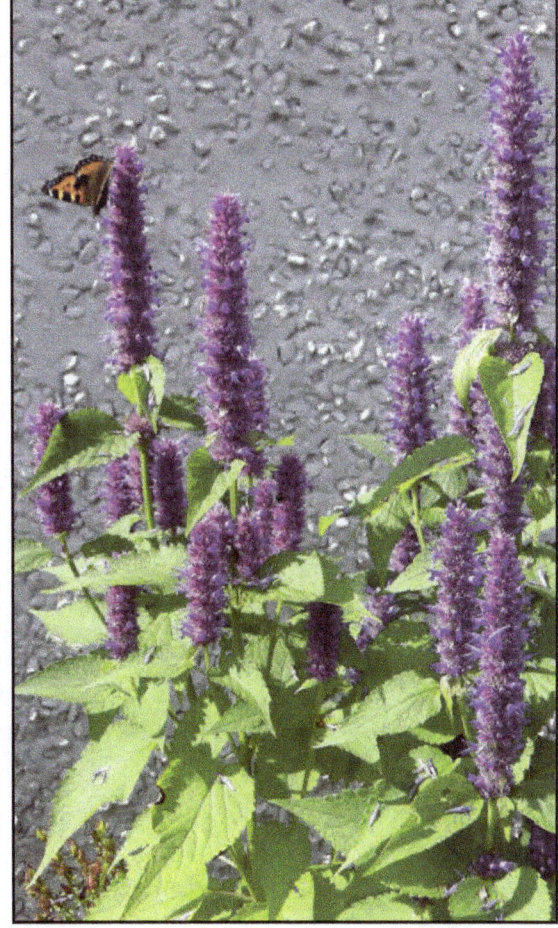

So I embraced the eco-peasant life, aiming for as much self-sufficiency as possible. Free from wage slavery. Growing a big variety of plant foods for husband Peter Cowman and self, plus gifts for friends and neighbours. Not growing for selling, which diminishes it's true cost and value.

I found out that peasanthood was something to be proud of. Not to be confused with the feudal serfdom that continued in Ireland longer than anywhere else. No, I owned my old Irish cottage and a hectare of lovely land with no debts. It was my sovereign domain and despite a diminished income, by living the Good Life frugally I could still pay the bills, follow my heart and pursue wholesomeness. I was loving it!

2020 turned out to be a perfect time for realising the frugal splendour of being a peasant in paradise.

CONTENTS

1. LIVING WITH LESS

The Imperative for Eco-Living - 8. Reasons for Environmental Alarm - 9. Pale and unhealthy green - 9. Food Security - 11. Value of home grown food - 11. Recipe for Healthy Eco-Living - 12. Irish Eco-Homestead - 14. Eco-Living in a standard house - 15. Low cost, low-Carbon life - 17. Powering the low-Carbon life - 18. Do we really need so much electricity? - 19. Power for the Internet - 20.

2. THE NEW PEASANTRY

The Peasantry - 22. Peasant economy today - 24. To sell produce or not to sell? - 24. Four seasons of life - 25. Peasant kitchen - 26. Before the refrigerator - 27. Sugar free fruit 'jams' - 28. Low Carbon diet - 29. Evolution of my eco-healthy diet - 29. Conscious Diet - 30. Wholefood Diet - 31. Whole grain pancakes: Mung bean and Buckwheat pancakes - 32. Idlis - 33. The Best Yoghurt - 34. Kitchen cookware - 35. Peasant bathroom - 36. The Power of Pee poem - 37. Shower vs Mandi, Traditional Bathhouse - 38. The modern Fire Bath - 39. Peasant Clothing, Peasant Chic - 41. Cotton blues - 43. Khadi - a Revolution in Home made Clothing - 43. Frugal fabrication the Boro way - 44.

3. THEY CALL THIS 'POOR LAND'

Design for sustainability with Permaculture - 50. Windbreaks - 51. Getting help to start with - 51. Making soil in Leitrim - 53. Soil dreaming - 54. Making compost - 55. Seedy stuff - 55. Seven types of composting: Hot compost, Worm compost - 56. Bokashi compost, Humanure compost - 57. Sheet compost, Rough compost - 58. Hugel Mounds. Raised garden beds - 60. Remineralising with rockdust - 62. Cover crops - 62. Living mulch - 63. Weeds - 63. Slug problems and solutions - 64. Miracles of mulching - from lawn to Potato patch - 65. Making an Oca bed - 66. Microbe power, Bokashi microbes - 67. Indigenous microorganisms in Korea - 68. Garbage Enzymes, Food growing and climate change - 69. Polytunnel Food Forest - 71. Fruit for the polytunnel, Annuals for the polytunnel - 72. Perennials for the polytunnel - 73. Wicking Beds and Bucket Gardening - 73. Making water wick, Wicking Bucket gardens - 75. Strawberry buckets - 77. Improved Wicking Gardening - 78. Gardening for biodiversity - 78. Flower meadows, Native trees, Hedgerows - 79. Wildlife values - 80. Wild foraging, Forest Gardens - 81. Origins of Food Forestry, Developing a Food Forest - 82. Ideal trees and plants for temperate Food Forests, Tall trees, Smaller trees - 85. Shrub layer, Perennial herbs and vegetables - 86. Rhizosphere root crops, Climbers - 87. Trees for Food Forests profiled: Alder, Apples - 88. Ash, Beech - 89. Bullace, Cherry, Wild and Bird Cherry - 90. Cornelian Cherry, Crab Apple, Damson plum - 91. Elderberry, Eucalyptus gunni / Cider Gum - 92. Guelder Rose, Hawthorn/Whitethorn - 93. Hazel - 94. Holly, Monkey Puzzle Pine, Oak - 95. Pears,

CONTENTS

Pines, Plum - 96. Rowan, Silver Birch - 97. Sloe - 98. Spruce, Strawberry tree, Profile references - 99. Fruit tree varieties recommended for the wet west of Ireland - 100. The value of wetlands and bounty of bogs - 101. Peat medicines - 102. Peat Moss protection - 103. Waste water treatment wetlands - 103. Useful plants for constructed wetlands: Common Reed - 104. Greater Reed Mace, Yellow Flag, Water Mint - 105. Watercress, Non-European Wetland Plants, Phormium tenax - 106. Cordyline australis - 107. Plants for Percolation Areas, Willows - 108.

4. PLANTS AND ANIMALS

Staple Crops, Potatoes - 110. Broad Beans - 112. Kale, Onions and Garlic - 113. Apples - 114. Useful Garden Plants Profiled: Angelica, Aronia - 115. Barberry, Bamboo, Bay - 116. Beetroot, Bergamot, Blackcurrant - 117. Blueberry, Burdock, Cardoon, Celery Leaf - 118. Chickweed, Chicory, Chinese Artichoke - 119. Chives, Clovers, Comfrey - 120. Cowslip, Dandelion, Day Lilly, Elaeagnus - 122. Elecampane, Evening Primrose - 123. Fennel, Fuchsia, Garlic - 124. Globe Artichoke, Goji, Golden Berry - 125. Good King Henry, Grape - 126. Horseradish, Horsetail, Hops - 127. Ivy - 128. Kale, Japanese Knotweed, Jerusalem Artichoke - 129. Korean Mint, Kohl rabi, Lavender, Leef Beet and Chard - 130. Lemon Balm, Lovage, Mallows - 131. Marigold, Marshmallow - 132. Mashua, Meadowsweet, Mint 133. Mitsuba - 134. Mugwort, Nasturtium, Nettles - 135. Ocas - 136. Onions - 137. Plantain, Potatoes, Raspberry - 138. Rhubarb - 139. Rose, Rosemary, Salad Burnett, Seabuckthorn - 140. Shepherd's Purse, Shungiku - 141. Soapwort, Sorrel, Strawberries, Wild Strawberry - 142. Alpine Strawberry, Sumac, Sunflower - 143. Maximilian Sunflower, Sweet Cicely, Sweet Woodruff, Tetragonia, Violet - 144. Thyme, Watercress, Wild Garlic - 145. Winter Savory - 146. Growing Grains: Oats - 147. Quinoa - 149. Corn/Maize - 150. Foxtail Millet - 151. Buckwheat - 153. Rye, Barley, Plant profile references - 154. "Are you going to have animals?" - 155. Homegrown animal feeds, Fodder crops for poultry - 156. Potatoes, Jerusalem Artichokes, Plantain, Oats, Other Grains, Sunflowers, Comfrey - 157. Nettles, Korean Natural Farming approach to poultry feed - 158. Kune Kune Pigs - perfect Permaculture pets - 159. Why choose Kune Kunes? - 160. To Bee or not to Bee?, Big Bee - 162. Which Bee is best? - 163. Therapeutic honeys, Keeping Bees healthy naturally - 164. Animal references - 165.

5. WINTERTIME

Wintertime - 168. Winter activities - 169. Sacred hearth of the home - 171. Winter harvest - 173. Winter Composting - 175. Seed Sprouting, Micro-Greens - 177. What can be sprouted: Alfalfa, Almonds - 178. Beans, Buckwheat, Cabbage family - 179. Clovers, Corn, Cress, Garlic Chives, Lettuce, Linseed, Millet, Mitsuba - 180. Oats, Onion, Peas, Perilla, Plantain, Pumpkins and Squash, Quinoa, Radish, Rice, Rye - 181. Shungiku, Sunflower, Watercress, Wheat - 182. References, Winter recipes: Catalan Soup - 183. Pink and Green Hummus, Leek, Potato and Sunroot Soup - 184. Fermented Green Bean Salad; Polish Peasant Soup; Wine Dark Sea Soup - 185. Broad Bean Soup Sicilian style, Recipe references - 186.

6. SPRINGTIME

Springtime - 188. Spring activities - 188. Tree planting time, Seed sowing - 189. Spring Foraging, Spring Wild Foods - 192. Silver Birch, Beech, Hawthorn - 193. Lime / Linden, Nettles, Spruce trees, Wild Garlic, Foraging recipes - 194. Spring Leaves, Stems, Bulbs and Shoots - 195. Edible spring garden flowers, crop staples and fruit - 196. Spring recipes: Angelica - 196. Broad Bean and Potato Mash; Garlic Pickles - 197. Mint Chutney; Mint Pesto; Mint and Parsley Tabouli Salad - 198. Mint Yogurt Salad Dressing, Nettles and Potatoes (Sag Aloo style) - 199. Nettle Pie; Watercress and Seaweed Soup; Wild Garlic and Seed/Nut Pesto - 200. Spring recipes references - 201.

7. SUMMERTIME

Summertime, Midsummer Dancing at the Crossroads - 204. Summer activities, Summer Fruits - 206. Summer Wildflower Recipes: Meadowsweet; Lime / Linden - 207. Elderflower Fritters; Elderflower Cordial; Dandelion Flower Bud Salad; Dandelion Flower Tempura - 208. Summer's edible garden flowers - 209. Summer's edible leaves and shoots - 210. Summer harvest in the polytunnel - 211. Summer Recipes: Fermented Green Beans; Blackcurrant and Honey spread; Blackcurrant Syrup - 212. Potato Cakes; Tomato Sauce, fermented - 213. Summertime references - 214.

8. AUTUMN

Autumn harvest, Autumn activities - 216. Autumn's edible leaves and shoots, Autumn's edible flowers, Autumn's edible berries, seeds and nuts - 218. Autumn's edible roots, Ditching the refrigerator - 219. Traditional ways to preserve food: Cellars and clamps - 220. Dehydration, Fermenting - 221. Benefits of home made preserves. Types of fermentation: Lactic acid fermentation, Yeast fermenting, Vinegar based pickles, Moulds - 222. The one pickle jar revolution - 223. Root veggies pickled in vinegar - 224. Autumn foraging: Beechnuts, Elderberries, Elderberry Juice, Elderberry Syrup - 225. Hazelnuts, Hawthorn berries, Hawthorn berry leather, Hawthorn berry syrup, Oak acorns - 226. Rosehips, Rosehip Vinegar, Rosehip Syrup, Fermented Rosehip Puree, Rowan berries - 227. Sloe Syrup, Pickled Sloes, Dandelion drink, Dandelion root stir fry - 228. Autumn crops recipes: Fruity Carrageen Fool; Stir-fried Fava Bean Sprouts - 229. Sweet Squash Pie - 230. Quinoa Patties; Horseradish Sauce and Syrup; Beetroot, Apple and Horseradish Relish - 231. Sauerkraut - 232. Apple Cider Vinegar, Recipe references - 233.

THANKS, PHOTO CREDITS, NOTES, ABOUT THE AUTHOR - 234

INDEX 235 - 240

ALANNA MOORE'S BOOKS - 241

CHAPTER ONE:

LIVING WITH LESS

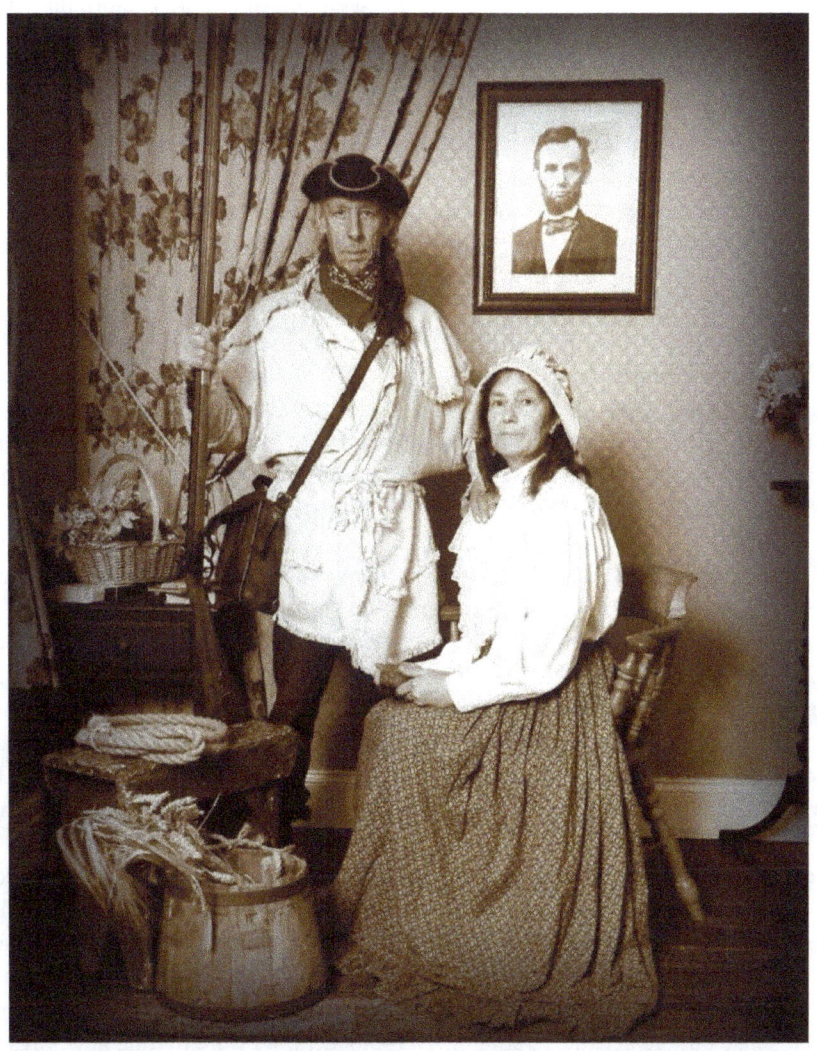

Our peasant ancestors hailed from Ireland, England and Cornwall.
Many emigrated to America and Australia. Peter and I have
also spent many past-lifes together. As peasants, no doubt.

THE IMPERATIVE FOR ECO-LIVING

Worrying prospects of climate change, wildlife extinctions, famine and the like are finally waking humanity up. We agree the need to adapt to a polluted and resource depleted world, to tread more lightly on the planet, to let go of convenient luxuries. To reduce our polluting ways, we must confront the elephants in the room and use less energy, chemicals, oil and plastics. It's easy to be lost in gloom seeing dire environmental decline, but we can't keep sticking our heads in the sand, especially as there's a global shortage of the stuff! It does spur many on to actively reduce their Carbon footprint. But can the average person make much difference? Yes! and when the power of one to lessen consumption is multiplied, the power of many will usher in mass change. It's high time!

People started to wake up to the crises in the 1960's, when Rachel Carson's alarm-ringing book Silent Spring came out. My parents had a copy and I remember reading some of it as a child. It was the sad indictment of a planet being systematically poisoned. Then, in the heady, gas guzzling 70's there was the shock of the Oil Crisis and energy efficient technologies were rapidly developed in response. Small cars became the norm. (But things went backwards and now big cars are the norm and nobody questions this.)

In the late '70's I had my own environmental epiphany as I watched Australian anti-nuclear activist Helen Caldecott's film If You Love This Planet. To me, Caldecott was the embodiment of sacred feminine power in defence of a peaceful world without nuclear war. She helped spearhead a new way to respond to the fears of the world and it was heartfelt and nourishing, inspiring positive action. She gave value to the realm of emotional intelligence, in a time before it was acceptable.

It led to a decision to devote my life to caring for Mother Earth in whatever way I could do best and exercising all of my creative powers in that objective. In the 1980's I put in years of voluntary work - as an activist for Greenpeace Sydney, as a bush regenerator with local bush care groups, and then, in the 90's working with the production team of the Permaculture International Journal. We may not have saved the planet, but we were successfully raising awareness. Small scale, eco-responsible food gardening, that is the crux of Permaculture design for sustainable food production (- 'permanent agriculture'), can be an answer to many of the world's ills. In fact, Permaculture can be seen as a revolution disguised as gardening!

As a teenager in Sydney I was an avid reader of Grass Roots magazines, where the wholesome Good Life in the countryside was celebrated. Stories about making home-made pickles and clothing, keeping hens happy and the like, were a real inspiration. It had me dreaming of living amidst the Gum trees, crochet hook in hand. Eventually I made the move and got to relish the eco-life, living in land sharing communities, so down-to-earth that we were grinding Wheat to make our bread at the beginning. Neo-pioneers, we were finding new ways to relate with the Earth and each other, forging a bold new society. Hundreds of such communities sprang up. But the back-to-the-land movement never went fully mainstream, except for some aspects. We were always on the fringe. Meanwhile, the business of wrecking the planet stubbornly continued on as usual, sometimes in disguise.

> ### REASONS FOR ENVIRONMENTAL ALARM
>
> * Extreme weather events from Climate Change, plus a coming Ice Age.
> * Human urban over-population, rural de-population and loss of Earth caring skills.
> * Peak Oil and Peak Gas - leading to wars, harmful gas fracking and windfarming.
> * Drastic animal biodiversity and forest loss.
> * Chemicals and plastics polluting air, soil, food crops, oceans, water and us.
> * Unsustainable levels of meat consumption, causing inequity of food access for all.
> * Nuclear weapons, technologies and power stations, plus radioactive waste.
> * Toxic high-tech electromagnetic radiation blanketing Earth and Magnetosphere.

PALE AND UNHEALTHY GREEN

> "Green consumerism is a dangerous mirage"   De-growth in the Suburbs

These days the green movement has diverged greatly from the wholesome path of health and wellbeing for people and planet (as espoused by the Permaculture movement). In the name of engaging with mainstream society, it adopted the industrial mode of thinking and now advocates for unhealthy products and technologies, such as 'smart' meters. A plethora of new industries have sprung up to cater for the modern eco-consumer. But the Carbon footprint of new, supposedly green technologies can be embarrassingly high. You have to be careful of greenwashing, it's rampant! Better to keep the old things going, than to rush out and buy new 'green' versions, such as light bulbs with Mercury in them, that, when dropped, are a toxic environmental hazard! 'Techno-optimists' may hold sway today, but their vision is usually only very pale green.

Do-it-yourself eco-living, on the other hand, takes the simple, frugal, slow approach. We forage and innovate, re-purpose and re-create to avoid new purchases. There's no need for plastic bottles of water, when there's rain; or bottles of 'green' cleaning products, when a bit of hot water and soap, white vinegar or bicarbonate of soda, will do the job. No need for plastic bottles of hair and skin goo, when a few drops of Olive or Coconut Oil can do wonders.

As for energy efficiency, many of today's rules don't make good sense and can even sicken us. Like the highly insulated homes that, without vents or window openings, have no ability to 'breathe'. This goes against the tenets of Building Biology, developed in Germany in the 1970s, that advises lots of air exchange in rooms for optimum health. I studied Bau Biologie when it had just been translated from into English, in 1989. Unfortunately, it's wisdom has not become mainstream either.

During the pandemic, vacuum-tight new houses didn't suit the lockdown rules, where we are told to stay home, open windows and ventilate to discourage co-infection between people. Older houses that are draughty are perfect now! The old ways of living often prove to be the healthiest and most sensible. When windows were made to be opened, our ancestors didn't need engineers to design ridiculously complex ventilation systems! It's easier to lead a healthy eco-life in an old home that can be retrofitted in harmony with good Building Biology.

The belief that wind turbines will save the planet is another unhealthy greenwash concept. In fact it's a bit of a con. Only turbines in the windiest of places might make a return of more energy than the huge amount used to make and run them. They do make people and animals downwind from them very sick and many have to abandon their homes. With new turbines reaching 185m tall, installation may involve cutting down trees or whole forests, while views and underground hydrology can be ruined. Wind company propaganda says otherwise, of course. Do your own research, don't believe what the business wants you to think, they only relate best-case scenarios for output, for example. It has been said that the only money made from wind farming is in government start-up subsidies. This technology just doesn't deliver on the green promise. From my experience, only small scale household wind power systems, ones that are easily taken down for servicing, have any merit.

Are community wind farms okay? Potential investors might want to find out if they actually deliver a return on investment, before losing their money. Certainly turbines are very expensive to dispose of in landfills when worn out, which doesn't take long to happen, what with all their moving parts, like gigantic gearboxes. The enormous PVC plastic blades cannot be recycled either. One thing that they do very effectively is to divide communities, such as where I lived in Victoria, Australia. A lot of bad feeling was generated when local farmers opposed a wind farm proposal. I did the research and backed the farmers, becoming a pariah to the greenies. But I'm still friends with the farmers! Wind farms are definately destructive from a social perspective, leaving fragmented communities in their wake.

Really, there is no magic bullet for the environment. We all have to reduce consumption, as happened in the USA when, in 2020, there was a 10% drop in greenhouse gases generated as people stopped globe trotting and stayed home in lockdowns. Ireland was said to have had a 6% drop in greenhouse gas production over 2020, lesser perhaps because of the big pharmaceutical factories etc that continued producing stuff here in the low tax environment.

1. De-Growth in the Suburbs - a radical urban imaginary, Samuel Alexander and Brendan Gleeson, Palgrave Macmillan, Australia, 2019.

FOOD SECURITY

So what are the parameters of an eco-life? Food consumption patterns is the big one. Food production is mostly high in energy cost, plus a source of toxins and environmental destruction, unless you buy local and organic, or grow it yourself. Large scale organic food production is not always perfect either, especially monoculture farming. Soil can be destroyed almost as much as on conventional farms. Usually we don't see the effects of monoculture farming because our food is imported, the problem is elsewhere, out of sight.

With a high level of imported food, countries make themselves vulnerable in terms of food security. The UK, for example, only produces 70% of its food needs and 30% is imported. In Ireland, I was astonished to learn that around 70-80% of potatoes are imported! These are no doubt in the form of processed chips. And while grains are grown here, there are no flour mills to grind them and they are sent off to UK mills. With a possible no-trade-deal Brexit looming in January 2021, when Britain left the European Union, there was the potential for flour to be in very short supply in Irish shops. Disruptions to the food supply chain did happen and there was panic buying too. With borders opening and closing erratically, and Brexit's regime change, the pandemic shone a sharp light on food security.

Aiming for national food security is a no-brainer, but it wouldn't suit multinational companies that dictate the food business. Ireland is a fertile country, well able to produce enough plant foods. Only an estimated 8% of agricultural land is currently used for plant food production. Cows dominate the rest. To provide vegetables for five million people, organic farmer Klaus Laitenberg has reckoned that Ireland would only need some 50,000 hectares of farm land, while currently 13,600 hectares are under Potatoes and other vegetables [1]. So, it is possible.

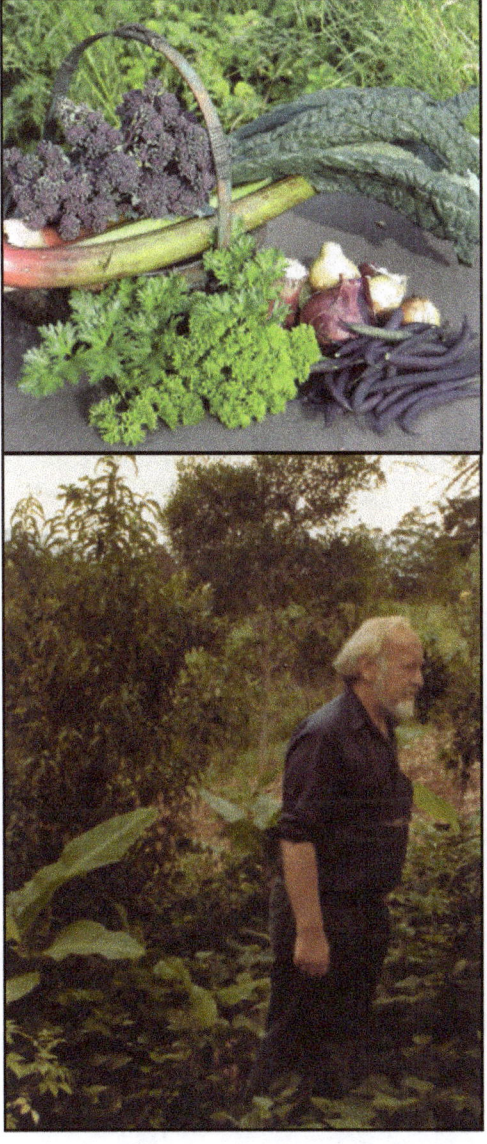

VALUE OF HOME GROWN FOOD

We are accustomed to buying ridiculously cheap food, mass produced on huge mega-farms that are not sustainably run. The costs of environmental degradation caused by farming are not factored into prices. But people only want to spend relatively little money on food, preferring to blow it on frivolities instead perhaps. 'Cheap and nasty' is what they go for. Even the Italians, who value quality food greatly, only spend around 18% of their average income on food. On the other end of the scale, Americans spend a puny 6.4% of income, while Irish people spend less than 10%. [1] It's obvious that most people don't value food, especially best quality fresh food, highly enough.

In producing home grown food oneself, you get a whole new perspective. People may well be put off by the time and effort required. The time needed depends on what your expectations are. Bill Mollison, the co-originator of Permaculture, pictured on the left in his garden, used to tell his students that he only needed twenty minutes per week to grow vegetables. This I recently found out to have a surprising rider - Bill only grew Potatoes, they were the only vegetable that he ate! He didn't want to put people off, I suppose. I got to know Bill when working at the Permaculture International Journal. He would also sometimes cheekily make up 'facts' to justify his cause, knowing the urgent imperative to get his message across. But he was a genius and he won prestigious awards.

To fully appreciate the benefits of home grown food, the time spent producing, harvesting, storing and preparing food crops is a lifestyle choice that delivers fresh air, exercise and the joy of immersion in nature's magic. Extra nutrients in high quality organic produce are well documented and boost our health and immunity greatly. It's pointless to compare homegrown with commercially grown veggies on a monetary basis. The price of quality is intangible and inestimable. It's far nicer to barter surplus produce in a Gift Economy.

Nature is a great beneficiary too, when our backyards become homes for wildlife, like mini Noah's Arks, with welcoming insect hotels, frog ponds, and scraggly grassed corners sporting seeds for birds to feast on. In our own backyards, we can address the loss of biodiversity as well as reduce food miles as we harvest our precious crops. We can limit consumption and use less fossil fuels. But starting new ways of living could well be a daunting, new frontier for many. At least it doesn't have to be rocket science.

1. The Self-Sufficient Garden, Klaus Laitenberg, 2021, Ireland.

RECIPE FOR HEALTHY ECO-LIVING

1. Take eco-responsibility for one's lifestyle, for the resilience of planet Earth.

2. Take self-responsibility for one's health, with a wholefood diet
rich in fresh and fermented, organically produced plant foods.
Take plenty of exercise and fresh air, and avoid sickening environments,
technologies and belief systems.

3. Minimise dependence on fossil fuels and their products, such as plastic.

4. Minimise imported foods in the diet
and learn to love eating locally produced foods.

5. Plant trees and food plants wherever possible,
and develop a plant-based diet,
eating what grows well around you.

6. Nourish one's spirit with the peace and satisfaction gained from
delightful interactions with nature in one's gardens and locality;
love your life and follow your heart.
Give gratitude for the harvest of joy, sustenance and all of one's blessings.

7. Maintain a solutions based approach to problems both big and small, personal
and planetary. And the simplest, least high-tech solutions, the better!

8. Contribute positively to the local economy and community.

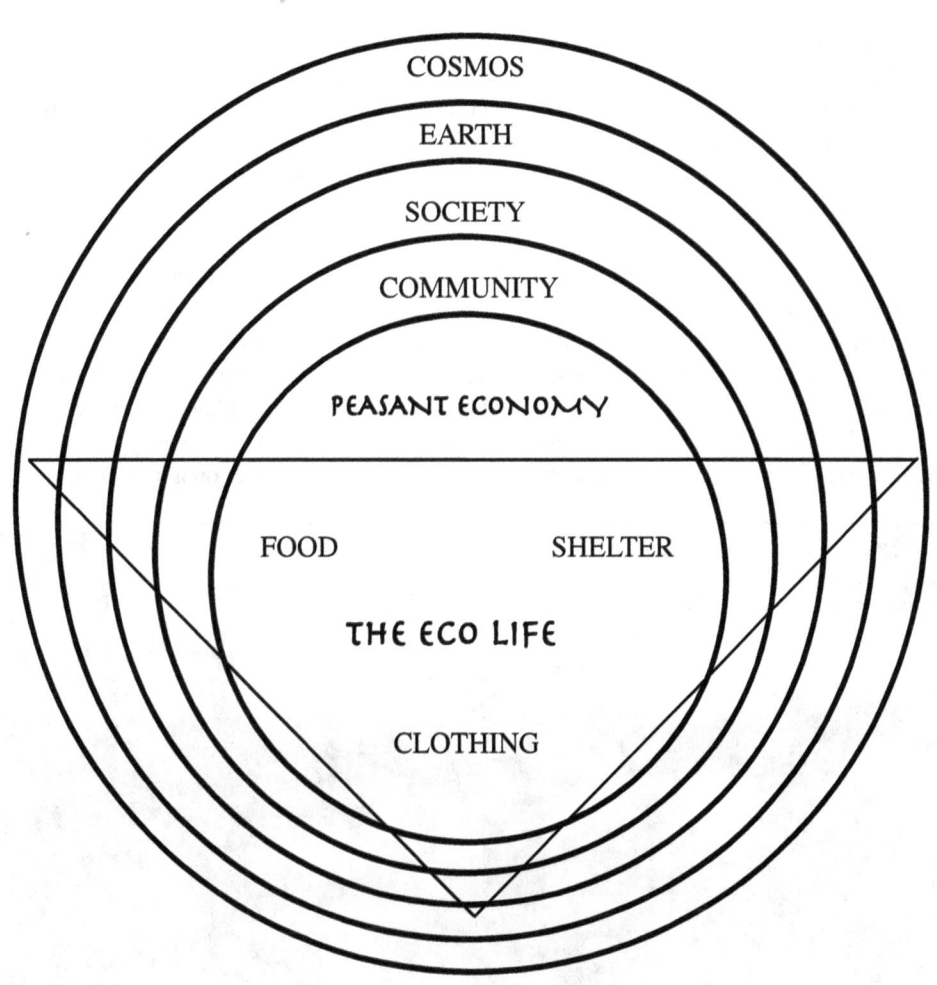

IRISH ECO-HOMESTEAD

"Why would you move from Australia to Ireland?" I'm often asked this question by puzzled Irish people, who all dream of living in Australia. Well, husband Peter is Irish and he prefers it here. And my last Australian dream of making a dry, rocky landscape into a place of fertile food growing had been beset with pests, frost, heatwaves and drought, making it way too hard. I could let that dream go.

I visited Ireland on a regular basis, spending half the year at Peter's place in County Leitrim, and then, like a migratory bird that dashes south at the first touch of frost, spending a second summer in the southern hemisphere. But I finally saw the greater wisdom in settling down to live in Ireland. By this time I was fully enchanted by the largely unspoilt rural landscapes of Ireland's north west, so quietly peaceful, shimmering green and richly steeped in fascinating history and mythos.

Finding a cottage to buy was easy, eventually. I had searched all over the local area by bicycle for a place to buy, only to find a suitable one that was literally under our noses, across the road from Peter's place. A traditional cottage on about a hectare (two acres) of flat to gently sloping land, divided into three fields, these were enclosed by wildly overgrown hedges of trees and shrubs that had been shooting skywards freely for years. The almost blank slate to work with was perfect, I could start a Permaculture landscape design from scratch! Now our migrations were local. We alternated living at each other's places, changing over on a weekly basis.

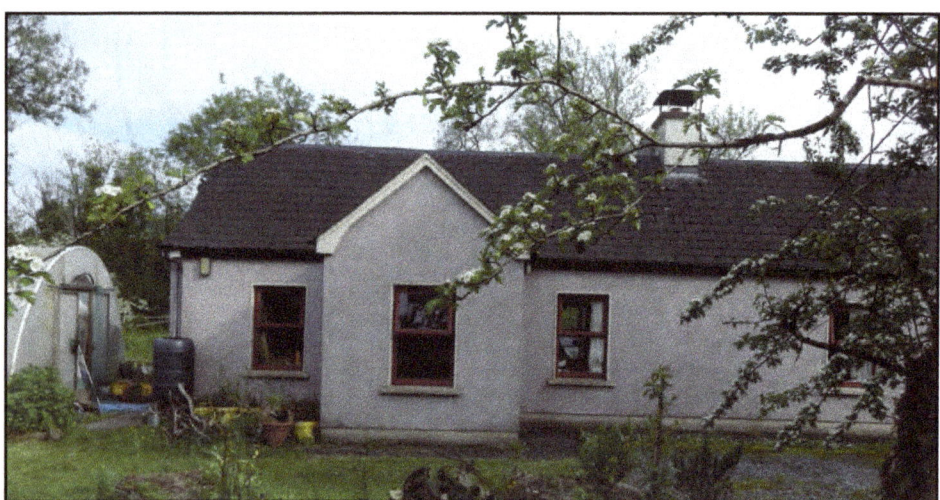

A succession of For Sale signs had been languishing at the road entrance for over eight years, waiting for me to discover the place. This was a de-populated county with few job prospects, following the global recession of 2008. Many people have traditionally migrated permanently to America and Australia to find work, and people are said to be Leitrim's best export. The farmers left behind with a handful of Cows scratch a living from rough, soggy landscapes, surviving on European Union subsidies and off-farm jobs. Heavy clay soils and a wet climate mean that the locale has always been considered poor land, often unfit for livestock. But the way that I saw the land here was quite different. As someone on a plant based diet, the endless opportunities to grow staple food crops here with guaranteed rain was like being guardian of a secret treasure. I already knew the potential from gardening at Peter's place and reaping abundance. I could see value in those wet, rushy fields.

You know you've made a good decision when all your plans and dreams fall into place effortlessly. This is how it quickly unfolded. The first to see would buy my farm in Australia, after only thirty minutes inspection. I had to move fast to keep up, life was spinning me on a wonderful trajectory and I'd soon be free of the regular anxieties of life there, with its more-extreme-than-ever climate and the frequent and terrifying bush fires of this century.

Now I had a wonderful project that has kept me engaged and engrossed. On the day of settlement in late spring of 2015, I wheeled Peter's home made hand cart the 250 metres up the road with a bulging bag of bare rooted fruit trees, their buds near to bursting and needing urgent planting. A Permaculture plan developed as I mapped out the landscape, looking for where the soggy areas, solar hotspots and protected corners, etc, were located. It was such a great excitement to begin painting a brand new canvas, to experiment with new ways of gardening and work with old ways that had worked for me in Australia too.

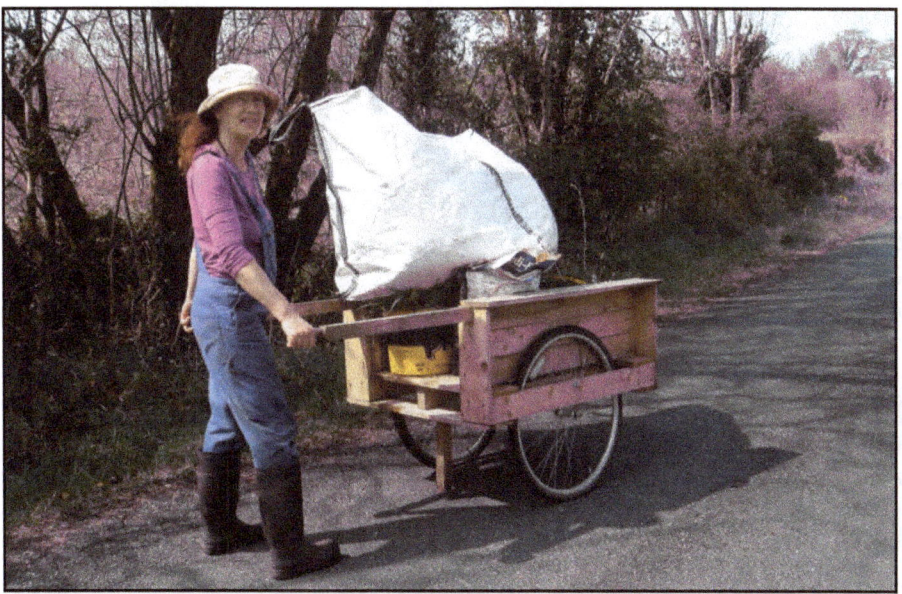

ECO-LIVING IN A STANDARD HOUSE

Previously, as an owner-builder in Australia, I had designed and built three homes. But now I was living in an old stone cottage with a concrete block kitchen and bathroom extension added when the house was renovated in the 1980s. Typical of Irish farm houses, it's cold and damp unless managed carefully, and it doesn't have many eco-friendly features. The oppposite to my last house, with it's solar electric system, council-approved worm compost toilet, well insulated roof, floor and walls, plus stand-alone rain water collection and use.

Could I still pursue the eco-life here, in this traditional Irish home? Of course! You don't need a specially built 'eco-home' to start making lifestyle changes. Living eco in our normal homes is what the planet needs us to do!

My cottage is off the road and does not face onto it, for there was no road when it was built. Instead, like most old cottages, it faces south, to maximise solar exposure. Low windows catch the winter sun that streams in through to the back wall, lighting up the house on a bright day; while summer sun, at a higher angle, doesn't much enter. Some of the rooms are cool enough to keep perishables foods in and selling the standard refrigerator that came with the house was one of the first things I did. I rarely need one, but when I do, I use a little chest 'fridge (from a camping shop) on hot days.

As for waste management, all organic matter is composted. Kitchen scraps mostly go into the Bokashi closed composting system. Garden waste is used for mulch or fire lighting. In the bathroom, a small wee bucket is stationed near the standard septic toilet, while an outside compost toilet building gives another alternative to the flush toilet, the humanure being composted in a dedicated heap. More on that later. With the existing standard toilet in place, I don't need a license for the other system! A normal 'water-closet' may be the preference for a visiting granny, but this way I'm saving the waterways from potential effluent leaching of the majority of valuable nutrients. I can have it both ways.

In my low Carbon kitchen, the wood burning heater warms the house sustainably and is perfect for self-reliance. The local firewood and turf I burn make a cosy glow, plus it heats water in the tank, which also feeds into the radiators around the house. (Only when there's a power cut stopping the pump is there a hiccup in the system.) When the forest trees I planted are bigger, I can burn my own fuel. Already I've had loads of burning from unwanted trees here. A few sickly Ash trees that shaded the orchard were professionally cut down and their trunks cut to the right lengths to fit in the heater. Over two winters I've had the job of splitting the logs, which is good exercise.

The turf that fuels the wood heater comes from a local farmer's bog. We felt proud of our efforts at 'footing the turf', after strict supervision from Fred Gill the village elder! On top of the heater there's just enough space to sit a pot or two of beans, grains or stew to cook or keep warm. A cast Iron teapot left to stay warm on top has hot tea on hand for when I come in from the cold. Not all teas taste good when over-brewed, I found, you have to experiment. But it does work well for Rooibos tea and Nettles.

Clothes hang above the heater to dry and we keep a couple of hot rocks on top. These are thrown into the bed on cold nights for pre-warming it. They retain heat very well and never leak, unlike hot water bottles. Absolutely no need for unhealthy electric blankets. And since adding a second layer of insulation batts to the ceiling of the entire cottage, we really notice the extra warmth. I have no expectations of having a hot house. In winter I contract into using mainly the kitchen only, where the heat is. Having a mostly cool house means I can keep food in another room and rarely need to use the small portable refrigerator.

We enjoy drinking the rainwater that blows in, relatively clean, from the Atlantic or Arctic and is collected from the garage roof, to avoid smoke contamination from the house roof.

Ireland is incredibly fortunate to have such a well moistened location and is said to be well positioned to survive and thrive in a Climate Changed world. I drank rainwater for decades in rural Australia, where it was the ony water available, holding it in 5000 litre potable quality tanks. Rainwater is soft for washing, lathering up so well. In Leitrim our reticulated water comes from the River Shannon and, while treated to the usual standards, is hard water heavy with minerals, plus traces of herbicides from farming. I try to avoid watering garden plants with hose water because the chlorine in it can harm friendly bacteria in the soil.

Trying to be eco-friendly without a car proved rather exhausting, when Peter and I did the weekly shop, a 25km round trip, by bicycle. We needed the rest of the day to recover. So I bought a relatively cheap, second hand Nissan Leaf electric car and I love it! Silent, cheap to run, no dirty exhaust fumes. The range may be small now that it's ten years old, but it still suits our lifestyle, and we always can park it at the train station for longer trips. In winter we never use the car heater, but travel dressed for the weather and keep warm rugs in the car.

I don't kid myself that my electric car might be 'Carbon Neutral'. Loads of Carbon/energy was used to make it and to generate the electricity that it uses. In a Peak Oil scenario, how would they be able to make such cars, or any cars at all? And what about the rare metals needed for the batteries?... Looking through all the hype is a grim reality.

> **"It is highly questionable whether electric vehicles should receive the high praise they so often do as an eco-product. They are arguably problems disguised as solutions, deepening an already catastrophic path dependency."** [1]

>> 1. De-Growth in the Suburbs - a radical urban imaginary, Samuel Alexander and Brendan Gleeson, Palgrave Macmillan, Australia, 2019.

LOW COST, LOW-CARBON LIFE

The climate here is often cool and damp, and winter nights are long, so one can spend a lot of time indoors in winter. The electric car is mostly charged from a normal household power point and doesn't use much electricity. We don't go out much, we self-entertain. I do have a washing machine and wet clothes are hung to dry in the polytunnel or around the wood heater. Sometimes even outside, if weather permits. I have website based businesses and they seem to thrive well enough on neglect. There's no television and not many standby switches are left on. So my power bill has never been over €14 a week, which is much less than the average Irish household expenditure of €1200 per year, that was quoted on the radio (RTE) mid 2021.

I buy high-quality organic food from as close a source as possible, there's free tap water, and household rates are low. The landline telephone (I've never had a mobile phone), seems a costly indulgence, but keeps me connected. Land lines are much more sustainable and largely disaster proof, compared to mobile phones.

Then there's the garbage fee, paid by weight. It's very low because we don't have much to throw away. We avoid waste, in the form of packaging and plastics, such as single use plastic water bottles, as much as possible. The recycling bin is not put out often. All the talk about recycling plastics can disguise the fact that not much plastic gets to be recycled these days, since China stopped taking it. Rather than putting the onus on the customer to send it off properly for recycling, if indeed it can be - the producers should not be producing it!

As for glass, which is not collected but is recycled, we rarely buy in bottled drinks and don't drink alcohol, so there's very little of that too. Glass jars are re-used over and over, or recycled via the bottle bank. Waste paper and cardboard gets used for fire lighting and mulching in the garden. My kitchen scraps are spoken for. So the garbage collection by weight costs very little. Other expenses include household insurance and gas for cooking. Added to the average food bill, it all comes to only about €100 per week total living expenses - certainly an affordable lifestyle.

To grow plenty of food, I do need to spend twenty hours per week, or more, working in the garden. But that's usually fun, good exercise and there's no need to pay for a gym. With a low cost of living, I don't have to chase much money. With less stress and greater health, it's a winning lifestyle for sure. And very low Carbon and generally eco-friendly too.

POWERING THE LOW CARBON LIFE

While coal, oil and gas burning has been demonised, electricity often escapes notice, with the Carbon emissions of nuclear power being low. But the mining, processing and cleaning of radioactive material is a filthy, polluting and dangerous industry that impacts strongly on Aboriginal land and sacred sites in Australia, and elsewhere. 'Alternative' power supplies haven't proven to be a worthwhile option. They are usually reliant on subsidies and fossil fuel back up. There are no really easy, clean options for power generation, distribution and storage (unless you live in Iceland, with it's glut of geothermal power and ugly giant pipes sprawling across the landscape.) The best thing for the planet is for everyone to reduce power consumption.

Before 'greenwash' took sway, we were always being encouraged to reduce power consumption. But then Big Business moved in and we were led to believe that all electrical desires could be fulfilled by technology, if we just had enough solar panels or wind turbines. In the process we contaminate our homes with 'dirty electricity' from the solar invertors that change the direct current to an alternating current. The oil embargo of 1973 and resulting energy crisis, when the energy efficient appliance industry came into being, inadvertently ushered in the era of 'dirty electricity', an invisible threat to our health.

I have lived in various low power households, in rural shacks and 12 volt powered bush homes, or in mains connected homes where I have always strived to use minimal power from the grid and gas. I switch things off at the power point when not in use and I don't need more technology to help me reduce my consumption. But there are gadgets available and 'smart' electricity meters supposedly facilitate reduced power use - that's a joke! They are more likely looking to find your preferred times of use, so that they can charge the highest tariff then! Plus they on-sell all your data for advertising purposes. This has all come to pass since 'smart' meters were introduced to Victoria in 2009, with zero benefit to the consumer, a report found. Even worse, these wireless radiation broadcasting meters also make many people horribly sick.

Fortunately in Ireland one can register with the ESB that you don't consent to having a 'smart' meter replace your old, perfectly good one.

Stand alone power generation used solely for 12 (or 24) volt appliances is the most economical and the healthiest way to go, if serious about reducing one's electricity footprint. The amount of power required for a purely 12 volt home is a fraction of that from higher voltages. If you have the luxury of designing and building your own home from scratch, a 12 volt wired home could be the most low-Carbon option. It's also the healthiest, with far less electro-smog.

I would never connect a solar photovoltaic power system to the grid again, as I did in Australia. You lose control over it, don't have power in a black out, plus 'smart' meters are involved. The 'smart' meter installed while I was overseas contaminated my home with electro-smog and 'dirty electricity'. Returning there, I felt so uncomfortable that it made me sell up and move to Ireland, which was a good thing in the end, I suppose.

DO WE REALLY NEED SO MUCH ELECTRICITY?

People are consuming ever higher amounts of power. How can it be justified to have unlimited everything, when our unique and precious planet has limits? Cutting down one's power consumption can involve a huge shift for people, as we are well and truly addicted.

What is the true value of electricity? How was life possible before it came in? Is it even necessary? Reading the memoirs of a local man from my part of Ireland, electricity at first wasn't much valued by people at all. They all led low-Carbon lifestyles that were generally happy and fulfilling. Why would they want electricity?

When rural electrification came to his area in the 1950s, O'Suilleabhain's father declined getting "the light", as it was referred to in those days, as did 20% of other households around them. "The possibility that the 'lectric' could work other gadgets never entered into it," he wrote. "People had never heard of an electric cooker, a 'fridge, a dishwasher, a washing machine or an electric blanket. It was strictly the 'light versus the lamp'."[1] They couldn't see the point of changing and took some convincing of the need for it. There was fierce debate for years. A big worry was - how would they be able to afford the 'lectric bills?

"It was eight years later, in April 1964, before we got connected. We did get a Tilley lamp sometime in the intervening period but, while it was an improvement on the oil lamp, it was nowhere nearly as good as the electric light…. Before long people wondered how they had ever lived without it….Sixty years later, we take it for granted. The light is only a minute part of our electricity consumption now. Still, it is probably the item we would find it hardest to do without."

1. Under the Thatch - Memories of a Longford Childhood,
Sean O'Suilleabhain, Ireland 2018.

POWER FOR THE INTERNET

- THE ELEPHANT IN THE ROOM!

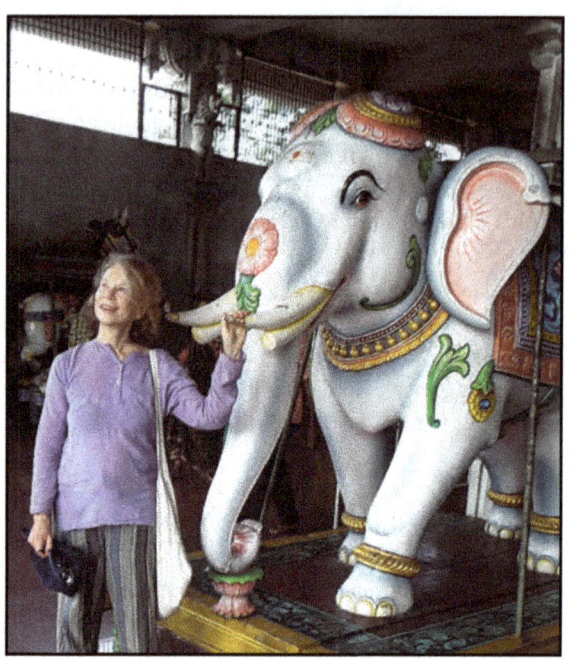

I've heard it said that a quick google search uses enough electricity to boil a jug of water. That was in the past. Today it's an even worse guzzler with consumers constantly offered ever more unlimited everything. For example, the Australian Broadcasting Commission reported in 2019 that:

"Every year the amount of internet data Australians consume increases by between 20 and 30 per cent. Last year, the average home had seventeen devices connected to the internet and that number is expected to more than double in the next three years." [1]

This type of hype is just sales talk, but I subsequently read in July '21 of a survey by Deloitte that found the average American home currently has twenty five different wireless devices! Talk about Microwave soup! Actually, most household devices have wireless functions these days and it's hard to avoid. But do we really need fridges that talk?

As for the 5G network, with higher radiation to frizzle us faster, I have heard from a good source that the telecommunications industry is not too happy about it. Why? Because it is such a high energy user and that this affects their profits. Already the extractive effects of having lots of data centres in Ireland is starting to strain the electrical system badly, with blackouts common and, in times of drought these places might be using around one million litres of water daily! Telling us to conserve water by turning off the tap when brushing teeth is like saving a drop in the sea that's wasted by our internet habits.

So, how sustainable is it to have unlimited downloading 24/7 of films and the like from the web currently? Not at all! This is partly why I always try to minimise time spent online, rarely download films or watch You Tube and never participate in social media. I don't sell big downloads from my website, mainly just real books, CDs and DVDs. Not being online very often, I avoid electro-smog and eye strain, enjoying life the better for it! If I do get a bad electro-smog exposure I suffer brain fog, headache or vomiting all the next day or more and often a break-down of my immune system follows. I can't do any work then. But if I avoid or protect myself from exposures, I'm generally happy, healthy and productive. Fortunately I live far enough from neighbours' wifi and transmission towers, while neighbouring farmers won't have a bar of 5G either!

1. https://www.abc.net.au/news/2019-04-23/what-happened-to-superfast-nbn/11037620

CHAPTER TWO

THE NEW PEASANTRY

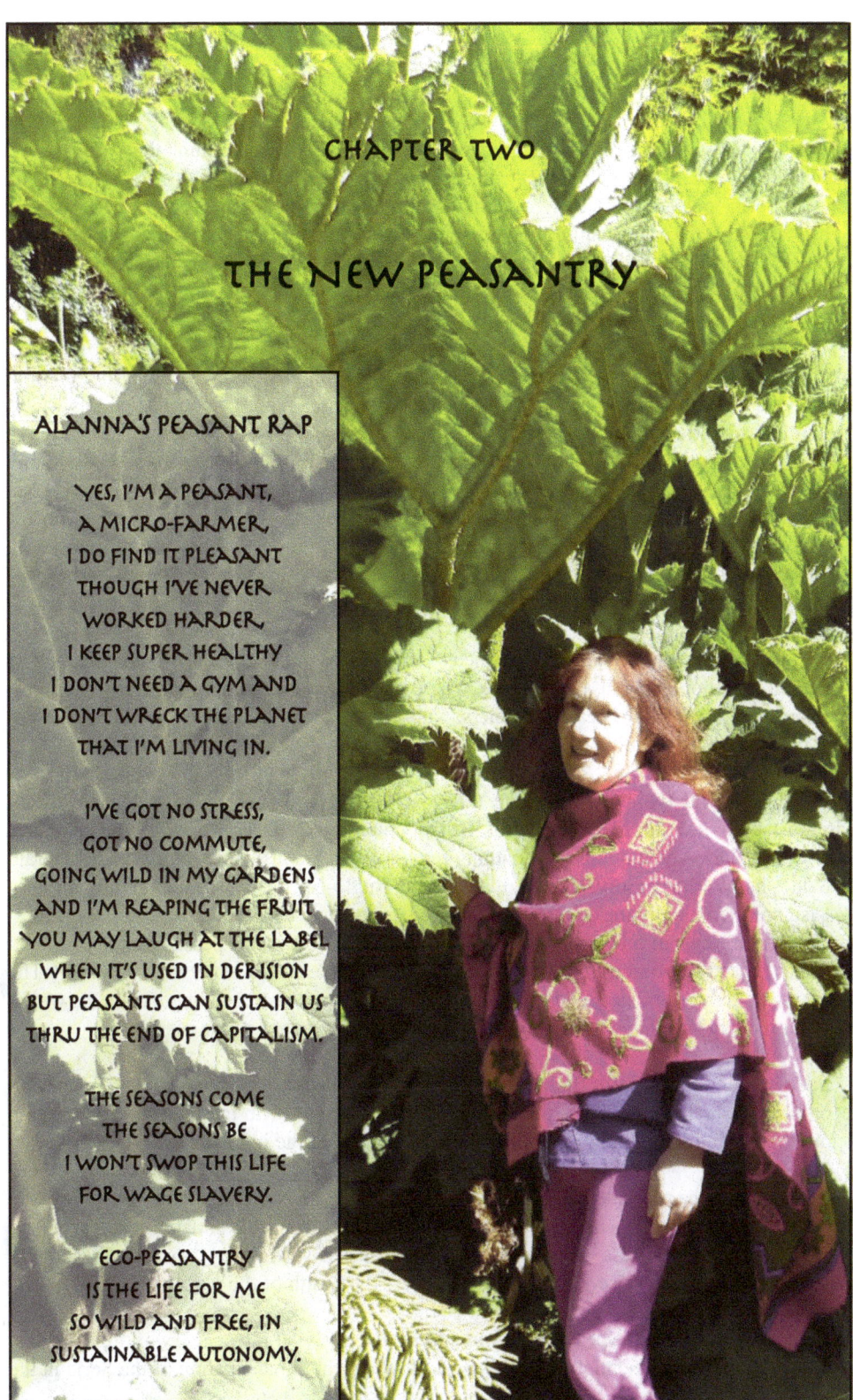

ALANNA'S PEASANT RAP

YES, I'M A PEASANT,
A MICRO-FARMER,
I DO FIND IT PLEASANT
THOUGH I'VE NEVER
WORKED HARDER,
I KEEP SUPER HEALTHY
I DON'T NEED A GYM AND
I DON'T WRECK THE PLANET
THAT I'M LIVING IN.

I'VE GOT NO STRESS,
GOT NO COMMUTE,
GOING WILD IN MY GARDENS
AND I'M REAPING THE FRUIT
YOU MAY LAUGH AT THE LABEL
WHEN IT'S USED IN DERISION
BUT PEASANTS CAN SUSTAIN US
THRU THE END OF CAPITALISM.

THE SEASONS COME
THE SEASONS BE
I WON'T SWOP THIS LIFE
FOR WAGE SLAVERY.

ECO-PEASANTRY
IS THE LIFE FOR ME
SO WILD AND FREE, IN
SUSTAINABLE AUTONOMY.

THE PEASANTRY

With 70% of the world's foodstuffs produced by peasants, one would think they were valued members of society worldwide.[1] But this isn't the case in over-developed countries. The English term 'peasant' is usually a derogatory one. A dictionary calls the peasant a 'poor subsistence farmer or agricultural labourer of low social status' usually inhabiting 'poorer countries', or worse - 'an ignorant, rude, or unsophisticated person'. The French word 'paisent' simply means 'country dweller'. Surely these essential workers who ensure the survival of mankind ought to be more highly thought of?

Western, elitist notions of peasantry show a poverty of understanding. Comparing them to ourselves, we denounce them as 'poor', when the peasantry cannot be quantified this way if they are outside the money economy. The peasant economy has wealth of a more intangible kind and is an antithesis to capitalism. So, rather than labelling them as deprived or needing of foreign 'development', these are just people getting on with their traditional lifestyles and capitalism can gain little foothold with them. What they do is a danger to capitalism, an impediment to the seeking of new markets. Thus, at the time of writing, the neo-liberal government of India is trying to take away protection for traditional small farmers and expose them to the mercy of global markets.

So-called 'third-world development projects' are used as vehicles of neo-colonialism. The 'Green Revolution' is a classic example, where costly fertilisers, unproven seeds and agro-poisons were foisted onto peasant farmers, whose livelihoods were often ruined as a result. The harvests never even lived up to the hype. It's the new face of an old painful story.

Colonisers would typically denigrate their victims first, or take advantage of difficult circumstances, in order to seize control. British colonisers of Ireland deemed the peasantry stupid, lazy, ignorant and inferior. Scathing remarks were published by propagandist Gerald of Wales in the 12th century. He was related to the Anglo-Normans who sent in their military 'assistance', stole away the country from its true owners and ushered in a new order of rules, social mores, weapons and technologies. They went on to destroy the peasants' autonomy and drained the land's resources (timber in particular) via all the roads and railways they built. The peasants were thrust into a feudal economy, one of the longest lasting to linger on in the world. Colonisers may have had clever engineers, but they were never benign overlords.

What's so dangerous about the peasant economy? It has been defined as an agricultural economy in which the family is the basic unit of production, with the Industrial Revolution supposedly bringing an end to it. Well, that was the wish of the industrialists!

To ethnologists, the peasantry are "those for whom agriculture is a livelihood and a way of life, not a business for profit... to be a peasant is not a socio-economic situation and carries no pejorative baggage. These days...the rural idyll of self-sufficiency...(is)...a thoroughly desirable vocation for those whose main concern is the health of the planet." [2]

Karl Marx thought that the peasant life was ending and evolving into a new working class that used modern farming techniques. In Russia, following The Emancipation of the Serfs in the

1861 and the work of land reforms, there were intense studies made of the peasant economy there, resulting in the richest body of analytical literature on the subject in the world. The greatest Russian agricultural economic theorist was Aleksandr V. Chayanov, who became a leading authority on peasant economics in Russia between 1919 and 1930. In Chayanov's book, On the Theory of Non-Capitalistic Economic Systems, he asserted that "at the national or macro level, peasant economy ought to be treated as an economic system in its own right, as a non-capitalistic system of national economy". He put it on a par with the other three major economic systems in the world: capitalism, slavery/feudalism and communism. [3]

Chayanov argued that, with 90% of Russian family farms at the time having no hired labour, standard economics could not be used for analysing the economic behaviour of peasant farms that relied on family labour alone. Capitalism is defined as commodity production for profit, based on the use of wage labor. On these family farms not only labour wages, but also land rent, interest on capital borrowings and business profits, were not a feature.

Peasants did occasionally sell their produce and labour, arts and crafts. Their strength was the family unit. Chayanov concluded that "in conditions where capitalist farms would go bankrupt, peasant families could work longer hours, sell at lower prices, obtain no net surplus, and yet manage to carry on with their farming, year after year. ...[thus] the competitive power of peasant family farms versus large-scale capitalist farms was much greater than had been foreseen in the writings of Marx, Kautsky, Lenin and their successors". Chayanov had set himself against mainstream Marxist and Western thought. In 1930 he and a number of colleagues were arrested and the research ended. He was silenced, but thirty years later Chayanov's theories started to become influential again.

So how did pre-industrial-era Irish farmers cope in times of peak labour need, when more hands were needed and they had no money for wages? When the hay needed gathering before rain? When the corn was ripe for harvest? They organised a meitheal (pronounced meh-hul), a working bee with friends, family and neighbours attending. Afterwards, a party and dancing! Harvest was looked forwards to eagerly as a very joyful season, with everyone helping each other in turn, as needs arose. And when a Pig was killed annually, a family would share the best bits amongst their extended family and neighbours. Neighbours would do the same, in a co-ordinated way. No-one had refrigeration, so they all shared the fresh pork around at regular intervals. Community was family and the clan provided solidarity and social strength to individuals. Further back, in Celtic times, high ranking people maintained their popular status through acts of generosity and the giving of community feasts.

It's no wonder then that in the late 1700s English agriculturalist Arthur Young, writing of his observations of farming in Ireland, reported that families with a field of Potatoes and a Cow foraging on the Commons were better off than the landless peasants who were subject to changing food prices on the open market. [4]

1. Foodies Guide to Capitalism, Eric Holt-Giménez, Dev, India, 2018.
2. European Peasant Cookery, Elisabeth Luard, Grub St, London, 2004.
3. A Post-Marxian Theory of Peasant Economy - the School of A V Chayanov, Daniel Thorner, The Economic Weekly, India, February 1965.
4. Arthur Young's Tour in Ireland 1776 - 1779, G. Bell and sons, 1892, UK.

PEASANT ECONOMY TODAY

"People know the price of everything and the value of nothing" Oscar Wilde.

With modern agriculture accounting for up to one-third of greenhouse gas emissions globally and causing mass degradation of farm soils, we need a huge re-set of more sustainable alternatives. In my own lifetime the situation has become dire as "a third of arable land globally has disappeared because of erosion, exacerbated by the rise of industrial agriculture and artificial contaminants in the soil," say French eco-farmers Perrine and Charles Herve-Gruyer [1]. It is the peasant farmers who are more likely to conserve the soil for their future generations, in the timeless tradition. And being naturally more energy efficient, they don't "use land to convert petroleum into food".

The Herve-Gruyers worked hard to set up an organic market garden. They were eventually so successful that they were able to verify the findings of grower guru John Jeavons, who asserted in the late 1970's that, with his Bio-Intensive growing methods used on a small scale -

"it is possible for an experienced market gardener, working by hand, to produce, in an equal of work time, as many vegetables as a farmer equipped with a tractor." [1]

TO SELL PRODUCE OR NOT TO SELL?

But is the selling of one's produce a good idea? The Herve-Gruyers present a heroic case of 'self-exploitation', to use Chayanov's term. A huge amount of work was involved to make a living for their family. On the other hand, Bill Mollison, founder of the Permaculture movement, suggested we should simply give away surplus produce. To barter or gift it, rather than sell it. This fits better with the peasant economy approach.

Assigning a cash price to food is demeaning to it. The low prices of commercial produce do not reflect their true cost - the degradation of farm land and the health and wellbeing of farmers. There are plenty of good reasons to detach the notion of monetary value from one's own garden produce, unless you do value-adding to it. It's way too precious and priceless to be sold. Better to swop your produce for someone else's. To produce enough food just to live on oneself, with a small surplus to trade, is a more dignified lifestyle.

You don't need a large amount of land to do this. With just 370m^2 / a quarter acre of cultivated land, one has sufficient space to grow all of a vegetarian person's needs for a year, including space to grow the biomass to make sufficient compost for fertiliser. Forty years of research with Bio-intensive Micro Agriculture techniques led John Jeavons to this conclusion [1].

Embracing the life of the eco-peasant, free to sell produce or not, well fed and able to do part-time paid work, art, craftwork, or business that generates income to cover money expenses - one can enjoy great self-satisfaction and be firmly grounded. Others may be green with envy!

1. Miraculous Abundance - one quarter acre, two French farmers and enough food to feed the world, Perrine and Charles Herve-Gruyer, Chelsea Green, USA, 2016.

FOUR SEASONS OF LIFE

All life runs in cycles. We Earthlings dance in the microcosmic cycles of the whole cosmos. Human life cycles can equate to the classic four seasons of the year in temperate zones. Good Permaculture planning incorporates these seasons into one's homeplace design. On the Russian family farms Chayanov's researchers observed the multi-generational activities and noted how the fortunes of families ebbed and flowed cyclically. Fortunes were seasonal.

When my son Sky was a child, in the springtime of his life, I stayed close to the family domain in Sydney. He could play with cousins and grandparents, aunts and uncles, who all helped to raise him. The Chinese say that it takes a whole village to raise a child and I'm sure this is the ideal situation. Later, just before the start of school, we went to live in the countryside on land sharing communities, where neighbours kids could play together in bushland and learn about nature first hand. In the past, country kids would get to practise the skills required for animal and crop care by helping out on the farm. It was a natural part of the education system, whereas today this is considered exploitation and only adults can be employed and they must be paid. Worse still, machines are replacing many workers.

As teenagers and young adults, Sky and his friends craved more choices and town life beckoned. They needed more stimulation, more company. So, like other families with teens, we left the bush community and went to live on the edge of a nearby town and he later went back to live in Sydney, where we'd started, going full circle! Young adults in the summer of their lives need to express their energy at this peak activity time, but if they want to live off the land, as I did, rarely do they own their own places to do this. So unless there is a family farm to be shared, a cheap land sharing community, or a 'kin domain' of some kind, it's not usually until middle age or later when people finally get a chance to sink their roots into the Good Earth and start to harvest the fruits of their labour, in the autumn of their lives. By this time they've slowed down enough to savour the rewards.

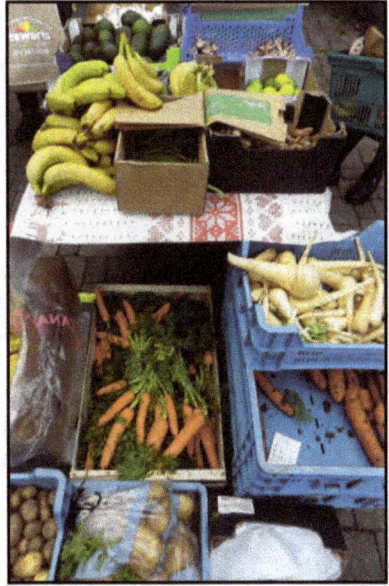

The organic producer at my local Farmer's Market one day didn't offer to remove the green tops from a carrot bunch I was buying, while her young helper would have. I twisted them off myself. She never offers to do this, she told me, because, after a lifetime of intensive gardening, her wrists are worn out and painful. She hopes to retire early. I commiserated, knowing the wear and tear on hands, wrists and arms that comes from years of digging, weeding, pruning, harvesting etc. These days, for self-preservation, I have to limit my time spent in daily gardening and I only work when I feel like it. I wouldn't want to grow food for sale, to compete with supermarket, industrial scale prices. I am not a machine. I want to stay alive and well until I die.

In the 'golden age', the winter of one's life, a full harvest of wisdom and economic stability is usually gained, with mortgages and debts paid off and stress reduced. Perennial gardens will have matured and home grown food abundant. There's time to slow down and reflect, and other such luxuries that busy young parents would only dream about. Life becomes simplified. We adapt to changed or reduced abilities. To lessen the wear and tear of gardening, work times are reduced, tools and buckets are smaller and lighter. Jobs are broken down into smaller parts, so that a sense of achievement can still be had, incrementally. There's more time to pickle veggies in the kitchen, winnow grain, mend clothes and do fiddly jobs that younger people might not have the time or patience for.

A peasant family unit with several generations living close by will have a complimentary suite of abilities and work preferences suited to each age group. Everyone plays a valuable part, whether it's childcare, cooking, cleaning, working off-farm, working the land, or telling the stories of the land and the people of the past. The elders getting the 'plum jobs.' Such are the seasons of life.

PEASANT KITCHEN

Pre-industrial era diets were confined to local produce with a bit of exotic imported spices like Ginger occasionally available. Over millennia the peasantry bred tasty vegetable varieties from wild plants, developed delicious, nutritionally balanced meals with them and spent a lot of time in the kitchen preparing and cooking them. The industrial era ushered in fast and convenience foods for the new working class. It was a nutrient poorer, inferior diet that they purchased with money earned.

Peasant dishes came to be looked down on as primitive, a legacy of deprivation. Workers aspired to the foods associated with the elite, such as beef and costly imports. Wheaten bread became a symbol of wealth and attainment. It was an emblem for the 'upper crust' of society, so the working classes demanded bread as well. They yearned to 'earn a crust'. Potatoes were shunned as food, fit only for the 'miserable poor', who they were closely associated with. Things have changed nowdays, a bit. But still the majority of Potatoes eaten in Ireland are imported, despite benign conditions for growing them. They must still be low status here.

The old peasant diet was simple but sound, wholefood based and with a lifestyle that kept them healthy and fit. This was in contrast to the elite, who didn't lead healthy lifestyles. In England's feudal times the peasantry, those who survived childhood, went on to live longer and healthier lives than did their overlords, who stuffed themselves to illness and death with meat, white bread and rich tidbits.[1]

A peasant diet revolves around the cycle of seasons, the micro-climate, the soil, the weather. It is the wholesome and creative combination of seasonal and stored produce. Eating seasonal fare is fundamental to the Japanese culinary philosophy called Macrobiotics. Rather than seeing it merely as a restriction of dietary intake, the seasonal foods available are said to match peoples' needs at that time. Root crops enjoyed in winter, for example, provide us with bulk carbohydrates to sustain us in the cold, while fresh spring greens cleanse our sluggish systems and the salads of summer cool us down.

1. European Peasant Cookery, Elisabeth Luard, Grub St, London, 2004.

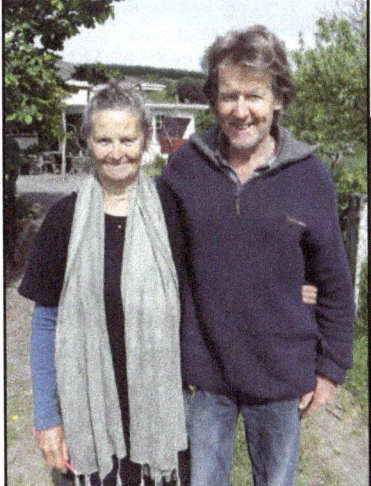
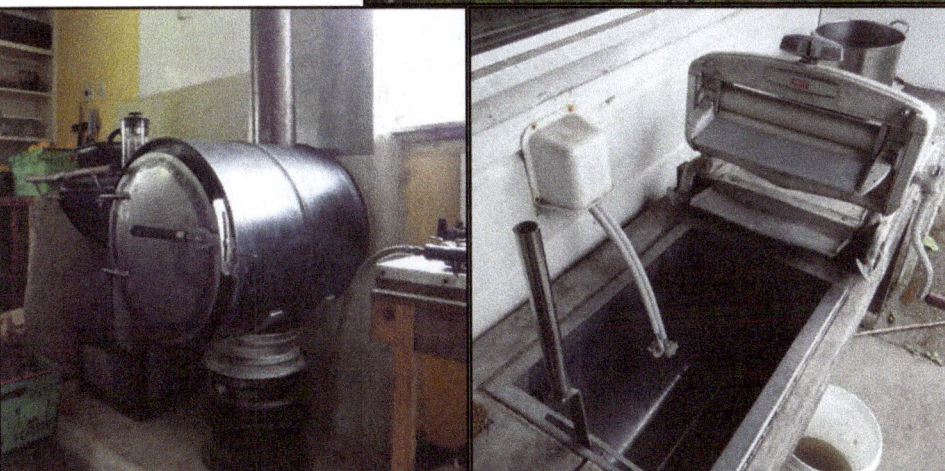

Left: Kay Baxter and Bob Corker - premier Permaculture peasant pioneers of New Zealand at their teaching centre - the Koanga Institute, Wairoa, November 2019.
Below: Kay and Bob's tiny home and Solar Oven.

Below: Homemade wood stove at the Koanga Institute.

Below right: Original hand washing 'machine' in the old house at Koanga.

BEFORE THE REFRIGERATOR

When refrigeration was originally invented it was not for the kitchen, but to facilitate the business of shipping meat from the far reaches of New Zealand to Europe without it spoiling. When the 'fridge was then marketed to householders, this heralded a shift away from time-consuming preserving methods for food, freeing up peoples' time and thus facilitating the labour market. But it took away the nutritional advantage that many preserving methods give us. Fermented foods faded out, but fortunately now they're making a comeback.

Across pre-modern Europe people survived and thrived without any refrigeration. Over the long cold winters they relied on stocks of stored foods in the larder. Root veggies and Apples were kept in the cellar, or buried in the ground, or kept in above ground outdoor clamps. Beans were dried, while Garlic, Onions, Rye bread and ham was hung from kitchen rafters, and rounds of hard cheese and earthenware pots full of fermented staples such as Sauerkraut filled the shelves, along with pots of beer and wine. Even fish, that most perishable of items, was made to last through the long winters.

Fish were preserved with various techniques - by drying in the wind, by hot and cold smoking, by pickling with vinegar, by fermenting and dry salting. In Scotland the Haddock was traditionally smoked dry over a peat fire. In Italy Anchovies were dry salted in barrels, where they made their own brine, becoming submerged after three days, and were then left to ferment over six months inside caves and cellars. In Arctic areas, people fermented Salmon heads, sea birds and Seal flippers.

Salted dried Cod was long a staple of the European diet, where the Church encouraged it to be eaten on fast days. The dry salted Cod trade in Norway, exporting to Catholic communities across Europe, was a huge industry based in Bergen. With its excellent keeping ability and nutritional value, Cod was one of the few things that peasants would be happy to buy or barter for. Cod fish dried in the wind kept well, with or without added salt. People on the coast availed of the sea breezes for drying, while inland people mainly used grav, the Norwegian burial method to preserve the Cod.

In Scandinavia ground is frozen half the year and since ancient times, foods such as fish, meat and cheese were buried in the ground for natural refrigeration. In inland areas salt for preserving wasn't always available either. The grav method was a hole dug in the ground with fish layered inside surrounded by Birch bark and Fir branches, with stones weighing them down on top. Buried Salmon, called gravlaks, were eaten after a week of burial, or left longer for up to twelve weeks. When ready, they were usually eaten raw. [1]

SUGAR FREE FRUIT 'JAMS'

Long before foodies shunned sugar for its detrimental health effects, our ancestors were making delicious 'jams' without it. (It's technically incorrect to call them jam, if sugar is not present.) Sugar was just not available. Across Europe, the art of making these thick syrups, Pomme/Apple Jelly and Poiree/Pear Jelly, was perfected, especially in Belgium and Germany. Likewise Raisine, the Grape Jelly famous around Perigord in south west France.

The method is basically to cut and crush the fruit, then cook it over a very low heat for a very long time in its own liquid. Acid fruits such as Red Currants can be cooked this way too, but are better with a little honey added to them. Long cooking evaporates all the water and concentrates the natural sugars. The pot must be stirred often, until the time when the 'jam' forms beads, and it can then be decanted into sterilised jars for longtime storability. [1]

1. European Peasant Cookery, Elisabeth Luard, Grub St, London, 2004.

LOW CARBON DIET

Patterns of consumption are a big driver of planetary resource depletion and, in terms of greenhouse gases, the food that we eat is one of the biggest offenders, producing up to a third of emissions globally. It doesn't have to be that way.

For most of my life I've been vegetarian, for all the usual reasons. Looking at it in terms of Climate Change and Carbon emissions, it's a much lower Carbon diet, compared to that of the carnivore. The ground truth shows other enormous footprints produced by livestock - various pollutants, intensive use of fossil fuel and water, over-use of antibiotics, etc. Finally the mainstream talks about such things and even Irish school kids are being encouraged to consume less meat and dairy. But industry is not happy, so there is always the usual flack and denials. However there are undeniable statistics that show the unsustainability of eating meat.

In his influential 1987 book Diet for a New America, John Robbins compared the amounts of land required to feed one person for one year. A vegan only needed one-sixth of an acre (approximately 700m^2), he said, a vegetarian three times as much, while a meat eater needs eighteen times as much land as the vegan.[1]

Meat eating used to be more of a luxury and as populations increase in financial prosperity, so too does their meat consumption. But the huge footprints to produce meat can no longer be accepted. There are too many humans and not enough land to justify a meat based diet for everyone. A scientist on the radio explained how two thirds of the world's agricultural land is considered marginal and only good for livestock. The remaining third is considered arable and good for tillage crops. Of this arable land, one third of it is devoted to producing food for livestock. So - vast amounts of good, arable land being used for animal feed. It can't go on like this!

Irish farmers are the biggest beef producers in the EU and they pride themselves on being 'efficient' at it. But others say that beef (and dairy) production in Ireland is the biggest greenhouse gas emitter, not just high in energy use and Carbon Dioxide emissions, but also Nitrate and Methane gas emissions. Beef farmers counter the argument to reduce the national herd size to help combat Climate Change by saying that 'less efficient' farmers will only fill the gap that's left and destructive farming in the Amazon will result, to supply demand. Whatever the case, we must reduce demand. Humans of this world and their pets need to eat less meat. And a shift by Irish farmers to more plant food production will not only reduce the Carbon footprint, but also enhance food sovereignty and improve our health.

1. Diet for a New America, John Robbins, StillPoint Publishing, 1987, USA.

EVOLUTION OF MY ECO-HEALTHY DIET

In the early days of convenience and fast food in the 1960's my mother found liberation from the kitchen in the form of new types of processed food that became available. Tins of cooked, sliced Beetroot and the like come to mind. Fortunately, in 1970's Sydney there was an explosion of interest in alternative ideas about diet and I was introduced to Zen Macrobiotic food at the Zen Inn restaurant in Bondi Junction. Of Japanese origin, it's all about simple and hearty wholefood meals, balanced in their yin and yang qualities, and it is seasonal.

Later, I started my first part time job at Sydney's very first health food restaurant, run by communist and health radical Jimmy Mitsos. The food was interesting, but rather clunky at times, in comparison to modern tastes. But it inspired and informed me how to become a vegetarian. And so I started to cook the recipes at home, like the hearty 'Hunza Pies', with their thick layers of brown Rice, Spinach and cheese on top - heavy duty fuel! I haven't eaten much meat since those days and the Macrobiotic philosphy still holds good today. Most of my diet is local produce that's seasonally available and naturally processed. In this book I'll be sharing some of the recipes that I've developed, often based on traditional recipes from around the world. The recipes focus on using the veggies that are easiest to grow, especially staple crops such as Potatoes and Broad Beans. Most are gluten free and have vegan options.

I grow food naturally, without chemical inputs, the organic way. And I always buy organic wherever possible, to support organic farmers. English foodie Daphne Lambert tells us also to be sure of getting a wide range of phytonutrients by always having a rainbow of colours on one's plate. She assures us of the wisdom of such choices, saying that:

"Organically produced foods are higher in phytonutrients than conventional foods and these phytonutrients are associated with the prevention of at least three of the leading causes of death in the West - cancer, diabetes, and cardiovascular diseases." [1]

1. Living Foods, Daphne Lambert, Unbound, UK, 2016.

CONSCIOUS DIET

Devising a diet that recognises our environmental impacts and avoids toxic elements like chemicals and sugar can be confronting and daunting. We have to navigate all sorts of propaganda and enticements thrown up by capitalism's peddlars of poor health. And there are intangible aspects of our food to be considered. Processed foods can deliver much more than meets the eye. The stress sustained by animals before slaughtering, for one, is deeply imbued into the meat. And an angry chef can contaminate food with emotional poisons too.

However when we cook meat-free wholefoods in a spirit of abundant love, we get far more than a mere tally of nutrients would suggest. Love adds a hidden dimension to flavour and quality that is not normally quantified, but is always something to aspire to bring to one's cooking. We can cultivate compassionate loving-kindness not just in our kitchens, but in our food gardens as well. This would normally be quite the opposite to mass produced food.

"Agriculture, agriculture slavery and capitalism are all tied together"

Mark Bittman, The Guardian, 25th April 2021.

So many foodstuffs and plant products are produced under near slavery conditions. From the old American Cotton fields, to the caging of hens today, cruelty has been inherent to industrial agriculture. In modern Australia, the expectation of fruit pickers is so high that their arms can become crippled in the race to pick enough fruit, slaving in orchards drenched in chemical sprays. No wonder that farmers typically rely on unsuspecting backpackers passing through to do these jobs, locals won't do this. I once had a young WWOOFer woman, fresh from a stint of fruit picking, come to my Australian farm for a work stay. Her arms were so painful from industrial scale fruit picking that she couldn't do anything.

Fortunately the Fair Trade movement is cultivating a kinder approach to the food business and very successfully too. Helping to assuage the human cost of food production, we can put our money where our heart is and buy the many Fair Trade products available.

The Biodynamic (BD) food movement incorporates deep insights into subtle energies and qualities, as observed by clairvoyant researcher Rudolph Steiner a century ago. You might call it the pinnacle of conscious food growing, as it considers the influence of the cosmos while sensitively nurturing the health and wellbeing of the soil. This is in contrast with typical organic growing regimes, where just an absence of chemical use is the usual minimum requirement and soil may still be abused.

I find the BD calendar invaluable. Considering the planetary influences, it maps out the times most suitable for growing, tending and harvesting different crops. Using it's guidance I'm able to spread the jobs around, rather than planting things all at the same time, or at unfavourable times. Thus it eases my work load, while I follow the cosmic flow of life. [1]

    1. The Maria Thun Biodynamic Calendar, Maria and Matthias Thun, Floris Books, UK.

WHOLEFOODS DIET

> **"[Near to] 50% of the food that's available [in the US] is in the form of ultra processed food. ...what I call junk food...[and this] Cheap food has had a terrible impact on public health. As every country switches from a traditional diet to a more American diet, their rates of chronic disease go up".**
>
> **Mark Bittman (author of Animal, Vegetable, Junk)**
> **The Guardian, UK, 25th Apr 2021.**

The concept of natural eating could be summed up in the word 'Wholefoods'. No processing, or minimal only, and the inherent nutrition is kept more intact with no contaminants introduced to degrade it. But we may need to do our own processing to make some foods more digestible. Unpolished varieties of cereals, for example, are more nutritious than polished versions, but also harder to digest and so pre-soaking is recommended. Soaking is the beginning of fermentation and soaked grains give enhanced quality, digestibility and flavour, plus storage ability. The opposite story is that of the flour we buy - heated, ground and degraded by the processing. I will never forget the taste of freshly ground organic flour made into pancakes, from a farm in the Mallee, western Victoria. So vibrant and delicious! Nutritional factors decline after milling and oils can go rancid, so flours don't stay fresh like that for long.

A few years back, a diagnosis of gluten intolerance for Peter meant a big shake-up in our diet. Commercial bread was out, because gluten-free bread in the supermarket tasted like cardboard and no organic gluten-free product was available. Peter had to bake his own. But the gluten-free flours available were limited, not always organic and were also rather tasteless.

In the lead-up to Brexit in 2020, when Great Britain left the European Union without a well-thought-out trade deal, food shortages began. People were worried that flour could be hugely affected, because, although grains are grown in Ireland, there are no grain mills here. It's all sent to the UK for processing. A flour shortage could be imminent because of this reliance and it was flying off the supermarket shelves as a result of panic buying.

What to do? Well it's good to have a hand operated grain grinder on hand. You buy the whole grain, keep it in an airtight container and grind it to flour only when needed. In my own kitchen there is no suitable bench to fix my small, but heavy, stone grain grinder to. I need a proper peasant kitchen that caters for various food preparation activities and storage needs. In the meantime, I've found alternative recipes and developed new staple meals in our diet. For example - flour-free, gluten-free pancakes that are made from whole organic grains and pulses. Making them is simplicity itself, but you do need to plan ahead.

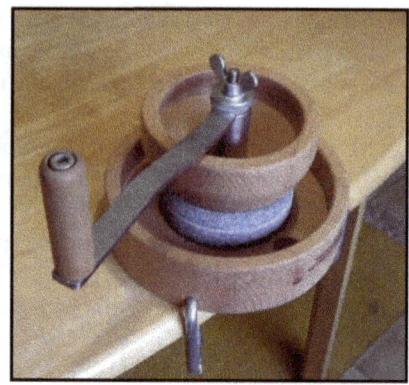

WHOLE GRAIN PANCAKES

MUNG BEAN PANCAKES

Popular in India and Asia, these pancakes are usually made as a tasty savoury dish, but can also be plain or sweet. The nutritional value of the beans is enhanced by first soaking them overnight, a period of ferment. After soaking, beans are liquidised in a blender, together with spices, if desired, to become a smooth paste. A lightly beaten egg or two (optional) is then beaten into the batter, which should have good pouring consistency. The batter keeps well for several days. Fry as per a normal pancake.

An Indian version has no eggs and adds chopped Chillies, Ginger, salt and Garlic to taste, plus some yoghurt. Fry as per a normal pancake.

A Korean recipe has various things added to the batter after the beans are blended. Along with beaten eggs, shredded Chinese Cabbage, sliced Spring Onions, as well as Chilli powder, salt and chopped Garlic are mixed into it, the carnivores adding some diced ham too. These are fried like a normal pancake and served with Soy sauce or dips.[1]

BUCKWHEAT PANCAKES

These are always a delicacy, but when I discovered Daphne Lambert's recipe for a fermented wholefood version, then it all went up a notch![2] Solid and wholesome, they can be made vegan or use eggs, which makes them hold together better, but is not essential.

Soak a large cupful of Buckwheat groats overnight and then give them several rinses in the morning. Blend until smooth with a teaspoon of salt and a couple of tablespoons of Sauerkraut juice or Kefir, plus just enough water to make a smooth batter. This is covered over and left to ferment in a warm place for twelve to eighteen hours. After this I like to add a couple of beaten eggs, mix them well into the batter and fry as per normal pancakes.

IRISH IDLI PANCAKES

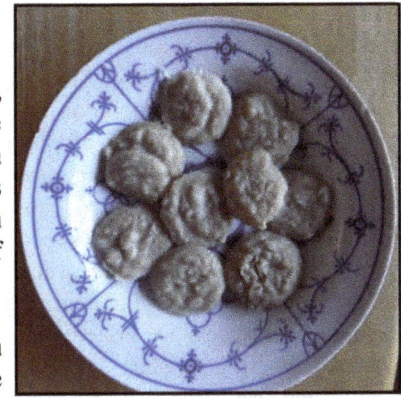

A popular food featuring in southern Indian cuisine, Idlis are a fermented legume/grain combination, the batter being steamed as small cakes, or fried as a thin pancake to make the famous Indian Dosa. This is definitely slow food - it takes days to prepare! But then the batter keeps well over several days and is of excellent nutritional value.

Enjoying Idlis and Dosas at a southern Indian restaurant in Malaysia, I was informed that they're great for digestion. I was hooked, so on returning to Ireland we bought an Idli steamer online (seen below) and it was sent over from India. After practising the art of Idli making, the great sourdough flavour of a light, fluffy Idli proved delicious combined with pickles, soup or curried veggies. But there was a downside - it's a drag to clean the fiddly Idli steamers. Surely there's an easier way, I mused.

So I came up with a new way to steam Idli batter that is easier, more versatile, the utensils more commonplace, and thus anyone can make this nutritious food, for good guts sake!

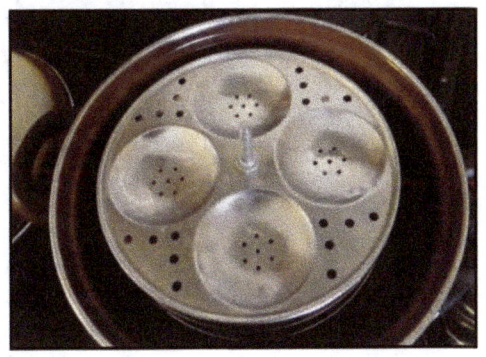

1 small cup Lentils
3 small cups Rice
Salt
Tomato leather (optional)
Parchment baking paper smeared with oil

Rinse Rice and Lentils separately then put them into separate bowls to soak in plenty of good water overnight. In the morning drain them, then liquidise to a creamy constituency in a blender/food processor, with a minimum of water plus a teaspoon or two of salt, to make the batter just pourable. Combine the two batters, then whisk them together for a few minutes by hand, cover over and set the Idli mix aside in a warm place to ferment a further 24 hours. When it's ready it will have risen and have a light crust over it. Whisk it up again and use, or if not risen enough, whisk and leave for another day. It takes longer in cooler weather.

For two meal sized Idli Cakes I have a medium sized saucepan with two metal steamers at the ready, the water boiling away. I also have two circles of parchment baking paper, cut a bit smaller than the size of the steamer bottoms. These have a light smearing of Olive oil put over them. After whisking the batter for a bit, I pour a couple of large spoonfuls onto the middle of the steamer paper and spread it evenly around it with the back of the spoon. The thicker it is, the longer the steaming takes. For a pizza like effect, at this stage I sometimes cover the surface of the Idli Cake with a 'crazy paving' of spicy Tomato leather pieces. (There's plenty of room for more experimentation in this area!)

The steamers are then put over briskly boiling water for five to ten minutes, depending on thickness. I swop the two steamers over several times and check to see how cooked the Idlis are. When firm and dry looking, they should be ready. If still a bit soggy, I flip them over to cook the top for another minute. When ready, I peel off the paper (which is carefully washed and used again several times over) and serve them up with added goodies. Idlis taste fabulous rolled up with some sliced Goat cheese, or spread with Miso, dips, pestos, salad leaves, pickles, stir fried vegetables, etc. For a pizza type effect, I add Tomato leather and put grated cheese on top that's melted under the grill. These 'Idli Pizzas' are way more healthy and easily digested than normal pizzas.

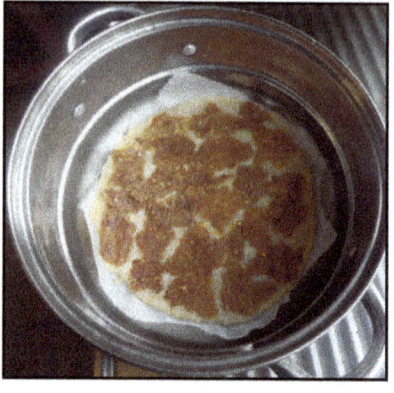

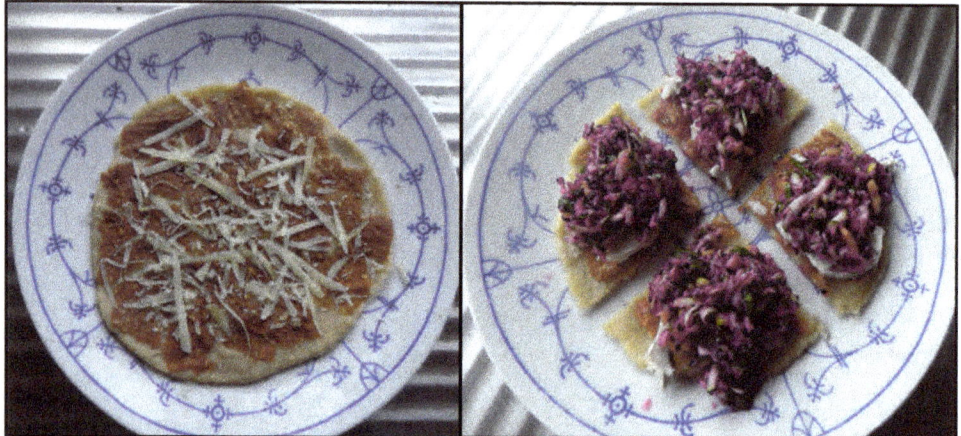

1. New Covent Garden Soup Company's Soup and Beyond, Macmillan, UK, 1999.
2. Fermenting - Recipes and Preparation, Daphne Lambert, Flame Tree Publishing, 2016, UK.

THE BEST YOGHURT

The convenience of buying commercial yogurt is tempered by the necessity to drastically reduce one-off plastic use. I like to re-use plastic containers, but yoghurt tubs were building up at a rate of three or four per week and I could only use a few in my plant nursery. Bagfuls in the garden were waiting to get re-used. I really needed to stop buying yoghurt, which tasted rather fake anyway, and make my own.

In the distant past I did make yoghurt. But after a few batches it would start to go slimey and I'd need a new lot from the shop for a starter culture. Still, it wasn't a satisfying result and I stopped. Years later I bought an electric yoghurt maker and this made results more uniform, although it isn't really necessary. I was able to use organic milk this time, however it came in plastic bottles. So I still ended up with a similar amount of plastic each week. Some old plastic bottles with the bottoms removed were used as frost and Slug protectors, covering small veggie plants at night. But I only needed a few. So I stopped yoghurt making. The plastic yoghurt container mountain started growing again.

Finally, in 2020, I was able to buy lovely glass bottles of raw, unpasteurised, unhomogenised milk from the farmers' market. It's organic, locally produced and the cows are only milked once a day. It makes the best, healthiest yoghurt! Real curds and whey, not like the commercial version thickened with skim milk. When I strain it to make thick yoghurt it can be like cream cheese. The whey is great for Peter's muffin making and for Pig food too. So we get two products from the one bottle. The milk keeps well in a cool room for several days and I can return the bottle back for re-use. Finally, I have a perfect yoghurt making system worked out!

KITCHEN COOKWARE

To eat healthy food is an obvious fundamental to health. But we also need to consider the effects of cooking, as it destroys enzymes and vitamins, as much as it can make some nutrients more available. We need to find a balance, taking plenty of raw foods, as well as cooked. Food quality is also altered by the type of cookware that's used.

Aluminium is a very toxic heavy metal and it can leach into food and us from Aluminium cookware. It only came into home use following the second world war, when bomb factories using Aluminium needed re-purposing, so they started making pots, cans and the like out of it. Bad experiment! Initial symptoms of poisoning include tiredness, stomach upsets and constipation; later on, backache, chest pressure and depression can develop, warns Dr Chiu-Nan Lai, founder of Lapis Lazuli Light, the Taiwan based natural health organisation. [1] Aluminium can affect people differently, attacking the weakest organs and damaging the nervous system, paving the way for Alzheimer's disease, that's epidemic in Western society. Fortunately such heavy metals can be removed with herbal or homeopathic treatments, plus vitamin C to accelerate the elimination process.

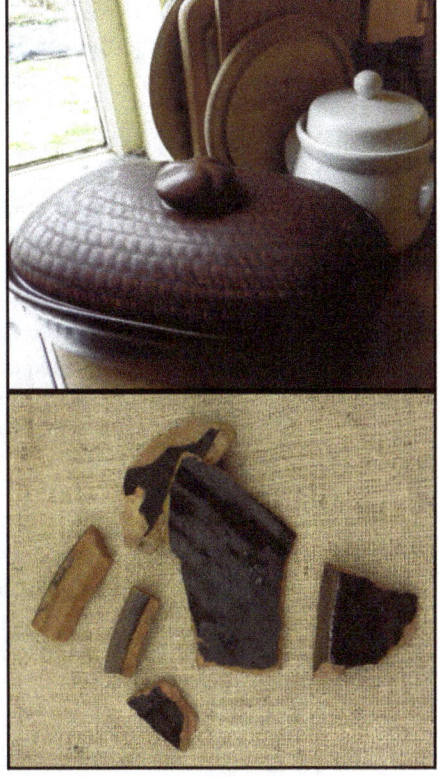

So which cookware to use? This was the subject of studies by German health pioneer Dr Rudolph Hauschka, who boiled water in a variety of pots, then used it to water Wheat seeds, comparing the growth of seedlings after ten days. Unsurprisingly, Aluminium was the worst offender at inhibiting seedling growth.[2] Hauschka found the best (readily available) cookware, producing the healthiest, biggest sprouts, was the clay pot. Ceramic, enamel and glass pots were ok too, but less good. He also found wooden eating utensils to be healthier to use than metal. (I find the traditional Chinese ceramic spoons are also much nicer to use than metal spoons.)

Photo top: My old German clay baking dish and new stoneware Sauerkraut making pot. Below: Ceramic dish pieces found in the garden were probably made in Roscommon about 200 years ago.

Hauschka determined, with the same method of Wheatgrass sprouting, which is the best cooking fuel to use. Compared to control sprouts that received unboiled water, electrically heated water gave the most detrimental result and they grew the least of all with it. Best growth came from water heated by a wood fire, while gas cooking was in between. Dr Lai's own experiment with microwaved water used on Wheat sprouts gave a dramatic result, with only half the growth as that from electrically heated water. (This hands-on science is an easy way for anyone to test for such.)

>1. The Pursuit of Life, Dr Chiu-Nan Lai PhD, Lapis Lazuli Light, USA, 1993.
>2. Nutrition, Dr Rudolph Hauschka, Rudolf Steiner Press, USA, 2002.

PEASANT BATHROOM

Traditionally, Irish peasants didn't have bathrooms. For toilets, there were green fields and animal dung heaps, and nature got to harvest the nutrients this way. Today, the bathroom has standard features that we rarely question. The flush toilet and power shower have been cemented into our psyche as a normal part of life. But they aren't very sustainable and we can do better for the planet if we adapt the bathroom and deal with at least some of our waste ourselves. One can retrofitt with all sorts of water and energy saving gadgets and there are many brands of commercial composting toilet available on the market. (Such toilets are approved by local authorities in Australia and are fairly common there.)

But a penniless eco-peasant can do a lot without the expense of retrofitting. Toilet waste can be dealt with using buckets, for example. In my standard, water guzzling bathroom I've added a lidded Wee Bucket for harvesting nutrient-rich urine, thus reducing water use and potential environmental pollution. There's no need for imported fertiliser in the peasant's world, we produce sufficient with our urine. Relatively pathogen free and sterile to handle, it's a rich source of Nitrogen, Phosphorus and Potassium which, in terms of commercial fertiliser supplies, are diminishing resources or energy intensive to produce and distribute. Yet we produce them every day, then flush them away. We need to harness the power of pee!

In the growing season fresh urine can be applied to plants by sprinkling it from a watering can onto the soil around stems, avoiding the leaves. It's not usually used pure, as it can kill plants, but this can be useful for the killing of weeds, when it's best sprayed on leaves on bright sunny days. For fertilising plants, dilute urine at a rate of one in five with water, or one in ten for seedlings. In the winter, when plants don't need fertilising, urine is great for sprinkling over compost heaps or woodchips to help them break down quicker. If you don't have animal manure for your compost and don't want to handle the urine much, you might just give it to the compost heap all year round.

For harvesting humanure, a different approach is required. I like to compost it the simple way and have lived happily with the bucket system for decades with no problems. In my new Irish garden an outdoor toilet building was erected and a couple of buckets used for collection, one in use and one waiting to be used. The contents are kept fairly dry and various organic materials, such as sawdust, dry lawn clippings and leaves, are added after each deposit, soaking up any odours. A mixture of cover materials is best. When full the contents are added to a dedicated compost heap that's full of earthworms and it's left to moulder for a year or so.

THE POWER OF PEE

Being kind to the planet
I don't feed my plants
With hen poo pellets from a
Torture chamber,
I don't flush my wee
Down to the sewer,
It's a valuable plant fertiliser!

That's right folks
Don't flush that pee,
It's better to have
A chamber potty!

And flushing that water
All clean for drinking
It's just a crazy waste
Is what I'm thinking.
So wee consciously
And moulder your waste
Or make the world
a desert
In a mindless haste!

That's right folks
Don't flush that pee,
It's better to have
A chamber potty!

Grow tasty veggies
See how they power
When the golden drop
Gives them a shower.
Packed with Nitrogen,
Phosphorus, Potassium too,
And pretty much sterile,
compared to poo.
Dilute it down 5 parts to 1
Apply to the roots and
Watch things boom!

Wee is golden
Wee is good
Give it to the plants that
Give you food!

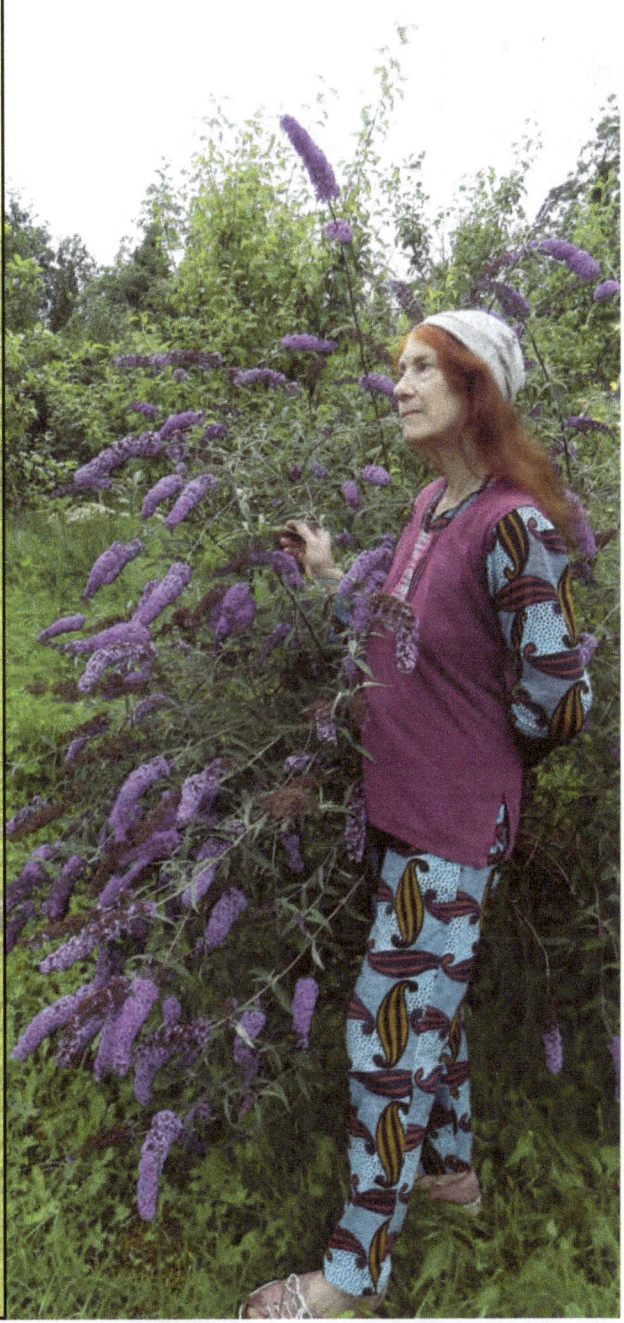

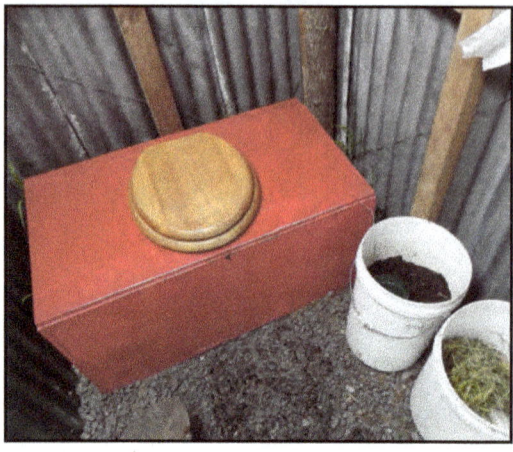

The Koanga Institute in New Zealand, where I visited in late 2019, also has bucket style compost toilets, seen left. Bob Corker, who introduced Permaculture to that country, found that the modern plastic, council-approved compost toilets all break down themselves in the end and are overly-complex. The only dependable (and much more affordable) system uses buckets, he said. As a system that has to fly 'under the radar' I see it as a perfect match with a flush toilet in a house that is council approved. You don't need a license for it and you end up with great compost.

SHOWER VS MANDI

What about Irish peasants and washing? If you were dirty, well, you could jump in a lake I suppose! Today we are so accustomed to having a shower or bath that we couldn't imagine any other way to get clean. But really, the shower is just another icon of the bourgeouisie. Power showers are big electricity and water guzzlers. In the dry continent of Australia, where giant billboards during droughts implore people to take very short showers, they would be frowned upon! Alternative showers can be bought in camping shops - black plastic shower bags that are filled with water, hung in the sun for a few hours, then the tap opened for water to shower down on you from the tiny showerhead. They don't really satisfy. But looking further afield, there are more sustainable ways to get clean.

India is the home of Buddhism, Yoga and the mandi. An Indian mandi is as simple as it gets for getting clean. Billions of Indians can't be wrong! You don't even need plumbing, if you have an outdoor mandi. Washing by mandi is easy and can be as fast or slow and relaxing as you like. You heat up a bucket or so of water to your preferred temperature. Then you lather up your body, or whatever a soap-free version entails, either standing or sitting to do this. Using a dipper, you then rinse yourself off with the bucket water. If you have a garden mandi, the water running off can be channelled to moisten the Mint patch or other thirsty plants nearby. It's a summertime thing, unless you have an undercover facility. A Fire Bath House is ideal, because you can take a quick mandi in the bath in any weather.

TRADITIONAL BATH HOUSE

The Bath House is a great tradition for the eco-peasant today, with a long history of use. An important part of life in northern Russia, Bath Houses were perfect for the forest based culture in a cold climate and they're still popular there today. Looking like a miniature timber house with pitched roof and small chimney, the building was separate from the home to prevent fires and often located at the bottom of the veggie garden. The iron stove inside it heats a cauldron of water set into it. There's an inner chamber where stones or bricks heat up. By opening this chamber and splashing boiling water onto the rocks, steam is created for a sauna effect. One lies on benches to steam, with buckets of warm and cold water close at hand for rinsing. Sometimes herbs or essential oils are added to the steam via the hot rocks.

More than just a place for the weekly, Saturday night high temperature steam bath, they achieved mythic status. Fire, water, heat and steam made them powerful and potentially dangerous places, presided over by a capricious spirit, the Bannick, that had to be carefully navigated. Places of pre-Christian ritual and magic, they were the preferred location for divination and initiation rites that were traditionally carried out at midnight. Ritual flirting games were played there with youths lurking in steamy corners. Wedding eve rituals of brides took place there and babies would be born in them too. Even the Tsaritsa would give birth in the Bath House, as would the serfs. [1]

        1. Russian Magic - living folk traditions of an enchanted landscape, Cherry Gilchrist, Quest Books, USA, 2009.

THE MODERN FIRE BATH

Ireland's Atlantic climate is mild and steam cleaning not so necessary here. But fire and water plus a cast Iron bath tub makes for an equivalent experience. For the simplest Fire Bath, a hole is dug in the ground beneath the tub and here the fire is made to heat the water directly. (Other versions heat it nearby and pipe the hot water in.) The bottom of the tub gets hot of course, so a piece of smooth wood or a raft of small bamboo sticks can be sat on, to prevent burning, while a bucket of cold water is kept nearby, in case it gets too hot. It worked a treat where I lived in Australia, in a dry Mediterranean climate. To soak in a hot Fire Bath on a clear starry night, marvelling at the Milky Way above, is one of the unforgettable joys of eco-living!

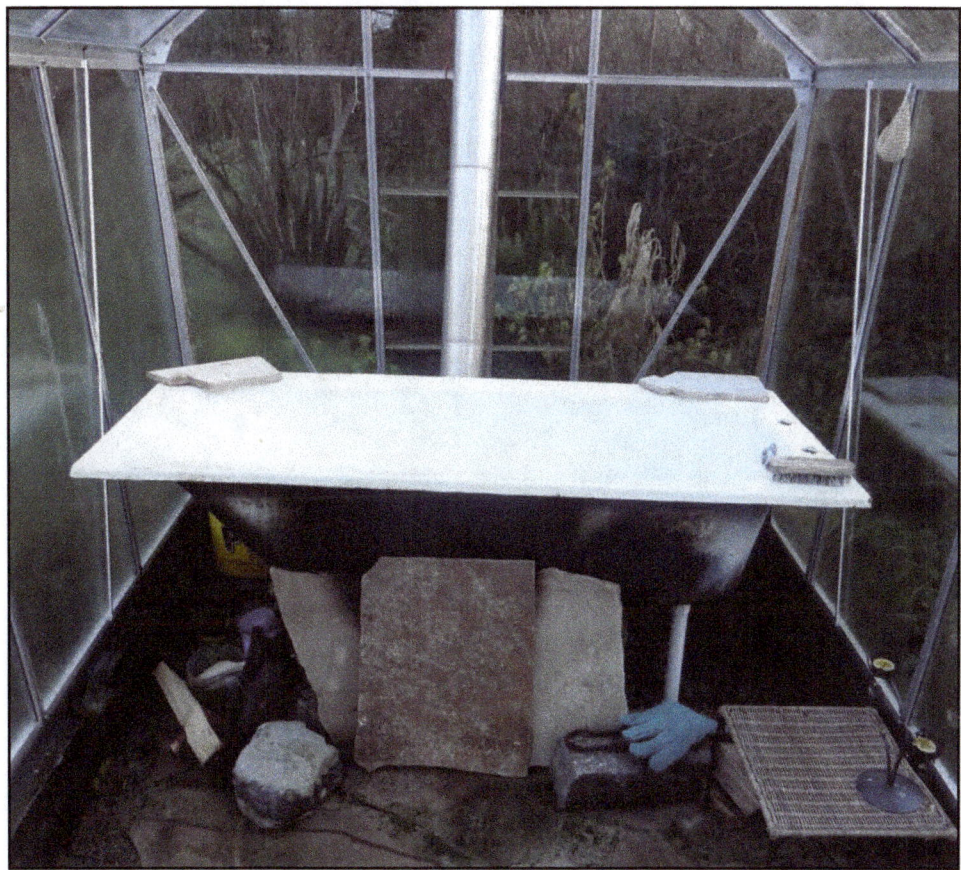

Ireland's damper climate requires an under cover Fire Bath. Mine is inside a small, tempered glass hot house from a garden centre. The bath went in before the walls were finished, as it's a tight fit. I used stones and clay to make a big fireplace, onto which the bath was set. A stainless steel flue takes smoke away from the fire chamber and pokes out through the top of the end wall, where I removed some glass. A drain under the bath outlet takes water away to a pond. (No toxic chemicals, such as sun screen, are ever used, to keep the Frogs alive.)

One can also add substances for relaxation or healing to the bath water. A handful of Epsom Salts thrown in is soothing and especially good for electro-sensitives, helping to boost Calcium levels. Seaweeds, aromatic herbs such as Eau de Cologne Mint and the like are also lovely to use. An odd sock or cloth bag is stuffed with herbs, or a handful of Oats, and steeped in the water as it heats, which usually takes an hour or two to get to the right temperature. The well soaked Oats in the sock feel wonderful when rubbed on the skin. No need for soaps!

All-weather outdoor bathing is just wonderful! Muscles are well soothed and any aches and pains from wear and tear usually dissolve away quickly. Fitting two people comfortably for a one to two hour long soak, we totally chill out, watch the sun setting or the twinkling stars, sometimes surrounded by twining Nasturtium vines with colourful flowers. Unusual sounds have been heard at such times - the cry of Curlews, the shriek of Barking Owls, the soft pelting of hail and snow on the glass roof.

The Fire Bath hot house is also ideal for washing large items, for clothes drying on portable racks, for drying freshly dug root veggies, beans and peas before they go into storage, and for plants drying for seed collection. There could be other uses too, such as a bain marie for keeping food hot for a party, or for herbal remedy making. When the sun is shining, but a cold wind blows, the Bath House is a great place to relax and enjoy the garden views. Folding chairs and table transform it into a Tea House and Writing Room.

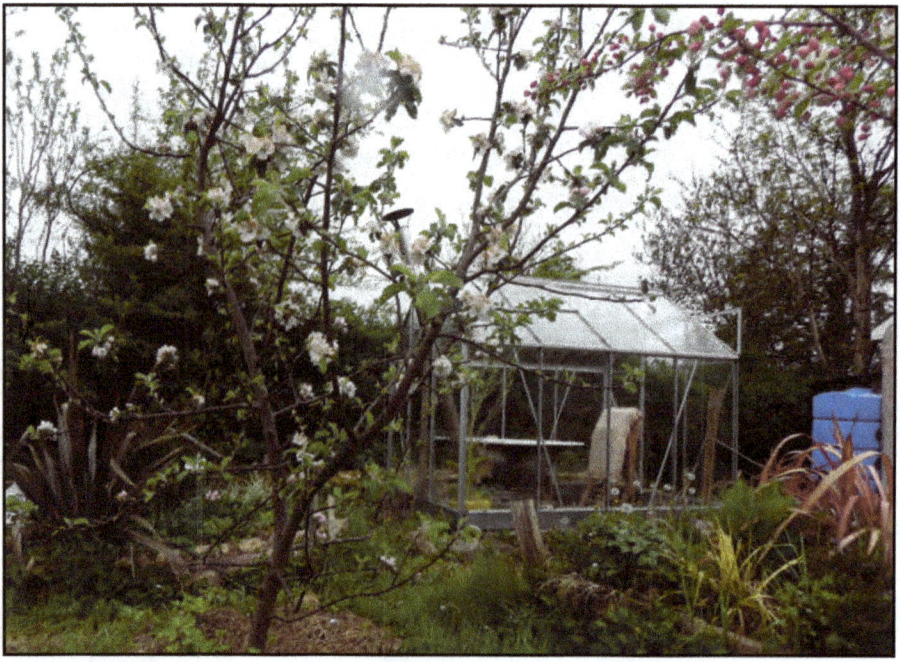

PEASANT CLOTHING

" Fashion is what one wears oneself " **Oscar Wilde.**

An active eco-peasant life requires clothes that are suited to the person, the life and the planet. These are rarely found in fashion shops. One has to create them oneself. If they are beautiful and well made, they can even become family heirlooms. A good example is the classic linen smock of English farmers that were once handed down from father to son, with some surviving examples displayed in museums.

Today, the opposite is usually the case. Cheap clothes are treated as throwaway items. Currently some 57% of new clothes end up going to landfill, 25% are incinerated, while only 10% are recycled and 8% re-used. The disposable fast fashion industry is also the second largest user of water globally, according to the United Nations Economic Commission for Europe. Some 7,000 litres of water is needed to produce just one pair of jeans, for example.[1]

Peasant clothing is characterised as being practical, durable and eco-safe, with natural fabrics such as Cotton, Wool, Ramie, Linen, Bamboo and Hemp etc. Such natural fabrics give our bodies the ability to 'breathe' and act as our second skin for gas exchange, unlike non-breathing synthetic materials. They keep us feeling comfortable and are the healthier choice. Woollen and quilted clothing can be very warm, so there's no need to buy fluffy synthetic clothing that cannot breathe, while it sheds nano-particles of plastic when washed.

1. Sustainable Fashion Matterz, online.

PEASANT CHIC

Peasant clothing can be chic as well! Author of a 1977 American book on the subject, Esther Holderness ran a peasant inspired clothing boutique in California. She wrote that:

"Peasant clothes are always in fashion because their timeless chic doesn't depend on current fads. They contain all the elements of good design - sturdy construction, comfort, classically simple lines, and handcrafted details that make each article unique." [1]

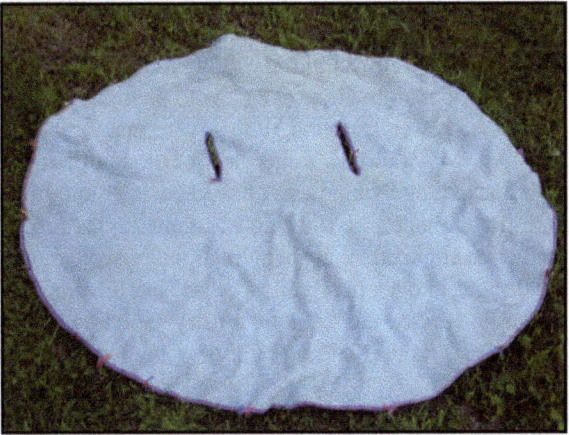

I'm inspired to use the patterns in her book and get creative. Just the job for long winter evenings. I found an old unused blanket and converted it into a Gypsy Cape, as on the right. This can be worn in four different ways and one way is seen in the next photo. The cotton bedspread I never use could become a Monks Robe with a hood and if I can find enough interesting scraps suitable for a patchwork Heirloom Mosaic Skirt, that would be fun to make too.

The modern peasant may find it hard to acquire suitable materials at an affordable price. Certainly there's plenty of new natural and organic fabrics available, such as lovely Hemp-Cotton and Hemp-Silk mixes. But the frugal approach sees me looking for second-hand serendipity. Charity shops can be a treasure trove of interesting pre-loved fabrics and clothes. You can be lucky and find garments that fit or can be adjusted, or use them to make into something completely different. As long as the clothes you get get a good washing or sunning, they should feel great to wear. But don't overdo it. For every item you add to your wardrobe, remove one or two others. Too much stuff can clutter the mind, as well as your home.

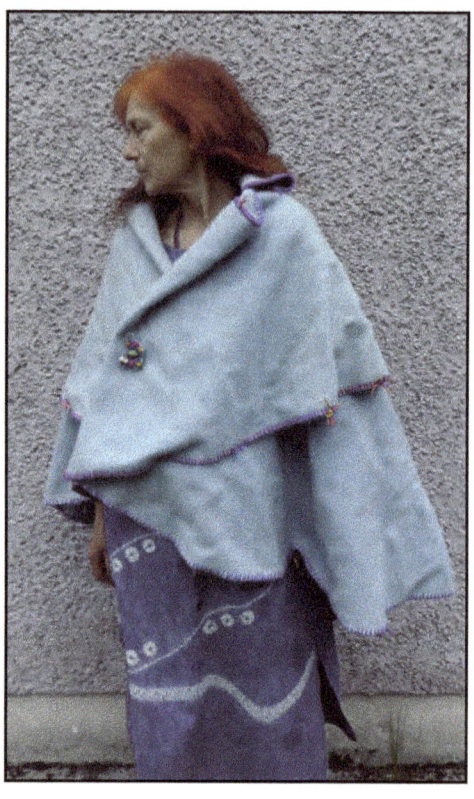

The creative potential is big! I always look in the curtain, fabrics and bedspread section, from where I've made curtains from a lovely piece of thick cotton material. A dress of wonderful African fabric, picked up for just a few euros, was converted by a dressmaker neighbour into an unique pair of trousers and a top. She copied the style of some favourite trousers that were nearly worn out, bought decades ago in an Australian opportunity shop (or just 'op shop'), as we call them there. It's hard to find such groovy material and when I searched online for more African prints, they were hard to find and expensive. (See the outfit on page 37.)

These days most second hand clothing is unfortunately made of synthetic fabrics. One touch and I'm usually repelled. They might also have been mass produced in a sweat shop, plus the styles are generally boring. As for colour, the ubiquitous black, no! I must have vibrant colours! This makes finding something with enough appeal an even more exciting event.

In Ireland charity stores only started to appear in our county town following the Global Financial Crash of 2008. Now there are several of them and they're always full of happy shoppers. Sydney was full of them when I was a youth and it still is. Trawling through them for interesting 'retro' clothing was great fun. It lead to my first schoolgirl business venture and I re-sold them at the first second hand clothing stall in the now famous Paddington Markets. Fabulous dresses from the 1950's were memorable acquisitions. Some ended up in a local museum. My stall was a mecca for colourful people too, like the drag queen performers Cynthia and the Synthetics. A few years later and living in London, I continued op-shopping and also remade old clothing into new styles too. It must have been chic, as my friend Katherine Hamnett, now an internationally acclaimed fashion designer, would sketch some of the designs into her notebook! I heard her on British radio recently, railing against the amount of plastic used by the fashion industry. Good on her! Micro-plastics released by the washing of synthetic clothes end up polluting the oceans in a big way. Another important reason to avoid them.

1. Peasant Chic, Esther R. Holderness, Hawthorn Books, New York, 1977.

COTTON BLUES

So, why not just buy new Cotton material and make clothing from that? It's natural, you would think. But having seen Cotton fields in Australia, no thanks! The cotton growing regions in north western New South Wales are vast toxic monocultures, scary and unreal industrial landscapes, with poisons thick in the air from aerial pesticide spraying. Huge irrigation dams suck water from dying dryland rivers. Everything about Cotton production is unsustainable! Growing Cotton organically wouldn't be a lot different, I imagine, if only the sprays are removed.

Sometimes natural fibres are spoiled by chemical treatments added to the cloth, making them feel synthetic. A good fabric needs to be good to touch. You can't do this online. We have amazing sensitivity in our fingertips; otherwise - read the label. After several washes, chemically treated cloth is improved. This is another reason that second hand fabric can be better than new. (The same goes for cars and homes, with volatile organic compounds and the like emitted by new synthetic materials being literally sickening!)

KHADI - THE REVOLUTION IN HOME MADE CLOTHING

In the fight for India's independence from British rule, Mahatma Gandhi put his central emphasis on encouraging the masses to revert to traditional hand spun and hand woven clothing, known as Khadi. The British had destroyed India's indigenous clothing industry and most people were wearing cheap, imported cloth from foreign mills. Gandhi's freedom movement was egalitarian, everyone wore clothing, so all had the opportunity to participate in the freedom movement. But he realised that switching over to new hand-made Khadi clothes could be unaffordable for the poorest people, so he urged men to proudly wear the simple, traditional loincloth. In 1921 he personally rejected all Western clothing to adopt that of the poorest peasant - the very scanty dhoti and chaddar (loincloth and shawl) - in a powerful act of solidarity. He even took tea with England's King George V dressed this way.

For Gandhi, the spinning wheel was a supreme symbol of self-reliance and self-respect, a declaration of freedom from exploitation and oppression. Gandhi's 'Swadeshi' - to spin and weave as sacred duty and self sacrifice - was a movement taken up by the masses. For many it was done more as a way of boycotting British goods. Still, Khadi became "a powerful visual tool in the creation of an imagined national community, which for the first time incorporated the non-literate majority".[1]

Gandhi advocated for all people to live a needs-based, as opposed to greeds-based life. In his book Clothing for Liberation, Peter Gonsalves says that Gandhi's message was aimed at Indians and British alike. The wearing of Khadi provided a "a symbol of homogeneity, absence of status, simplicity and nakedness or uniform clothing. It was the instrument which made the Swadeshi movement possible, which created the greatest cooperative in the world and which forced the mills in Lancashire to shut down".[2]

To counter India's high rate of unemployment, work opportunities created by the Khadi movement offered a solution and so Khadi became a path to economic liberation for the masses. Today, over six decades later, Khadi is not considered to be an economically viable industry and is no longer a moral imperative, losing some government support. Making up only one per cent of India's textile industry, it still employs some two million people, however. The 'Livery of Freedom' was, and still is today, more than just clothing. In Gandhi's own words, Khadi and Swadeshi carried this important spiritual point -

> "The message of the spinning-wheel is much wider than its circumference.
> Its message is one of simplicity, service of mankind, living so as not to hurt others,
> creating an indissoluble bond between the rich and the poor,
> capital and labour, the prince and the peasant." [2]

1. The Magic of Khadi, Geetika Singh, at
https://www.mkgandhi.org/articles/magic-of-khadi.html

2. Khadi and Gandhiji: looking beyond the fabric, Rajini Nayak
https://www.thehindu.com/opinion/open-page/Khadi-and-Gandhiji-looking-beyond-the-fabric/article15766513.ece

FRUGAL FABRICATION - THE BORO WAY

by Heather Colman

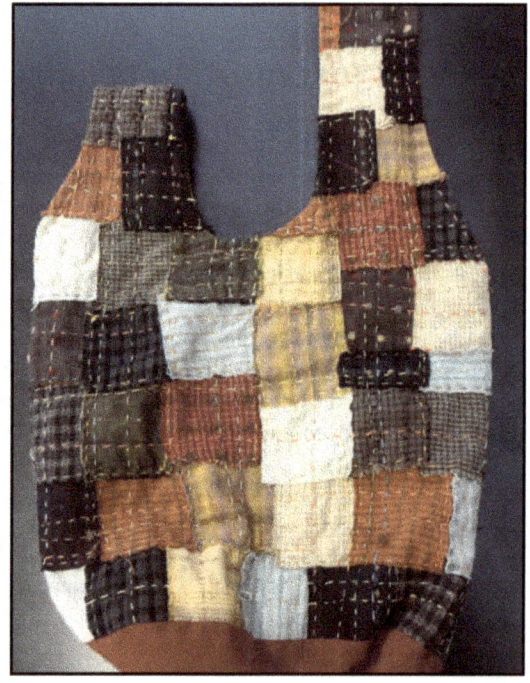

While on a winter camping trip in 2019 some of our clothing couldn't hack the pace and needed running repairs. Luckily our travels coincided with the wonderful Alice Springs Beanie Festival in Central Australia, what a treat! Among the array of offerings was a workshop on Boro, touted as a useful skill for travellers. I went along and was hooked and I've never looked back. The teacher showed us how to make a useful little bag, and she stressed there were no rules. My sort of project.

So, what is Boro? Boro uses a simple running stitch to attach spare or discarded scraps of fabric to mend or enhance clothing to extend its use. Boro started in medieval villages in northern Japan, where the soils were unsuitable to grow Cotton and villagers too poor to afford quality fabric. Thus cloth was precious and every bit was used and never to be wasted.

Before the arrival of a new baby, those who had a special attachment to the coming child would provide pieces of saved cloth to the mother, who would make a wrap to swaddle her baby. And when a loved one died, all those that cared would provide what fabric they could spare to the family to create a burial shroud. The arrival of a new soul or the departure of an old one was wrapped in love through the gift of special fabric and the giver's vibration on it.

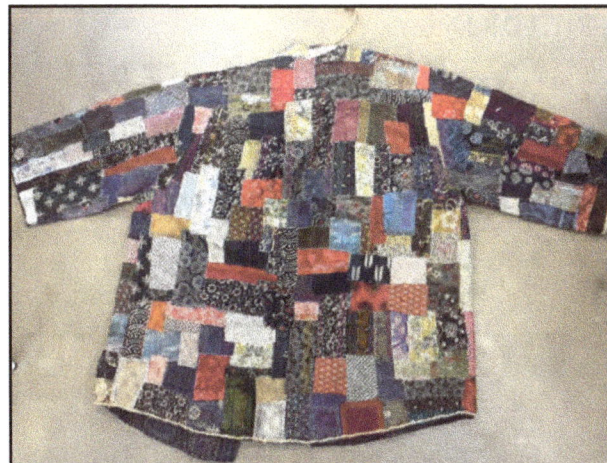

We can do this too!

Boro lives on as a modern art/craft form and can make your favourite clothing and furnishings last longer while, expressing your joy, creativity and resourcefulness. Decorative elements allow creativity and the expression of opinions and ideas not otherwise voiced.

Feel free to embellish your clothing by weaving designs into the fabric, using dyes, painting, patchwork, appliqué, embroidery, or beading. So much can be found in charity shops. If you haven't got the time, a second-hand item may provide the embellishment, such as useful pockets. Braids and trims can be recycled from old items to create new items, there is no limit to what you can make. Anything is possible.

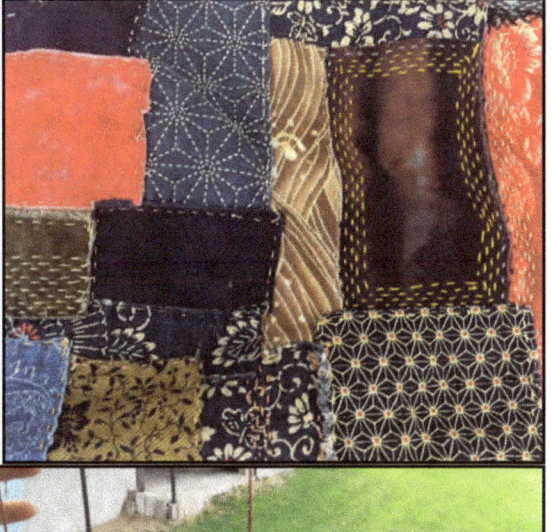

It doesn't have to be in clothing either. I built a puppet from discarded fabrics, as in the photo below. I patched furnishing fabric for two old bentwood chairs by using old tea towels of similar colour that I liked, giving them a long and happy life. You can make shopping bags out of old curtains, embellish over stained table cloths or stained clothing....

The sky's the limit!

Top photo - This coat was originally a discarded shirt, the collar and cuffs were cut off and it was covered over with scraps of fabric. Below - Detail of jacket. Bottom - Heather's puppet.

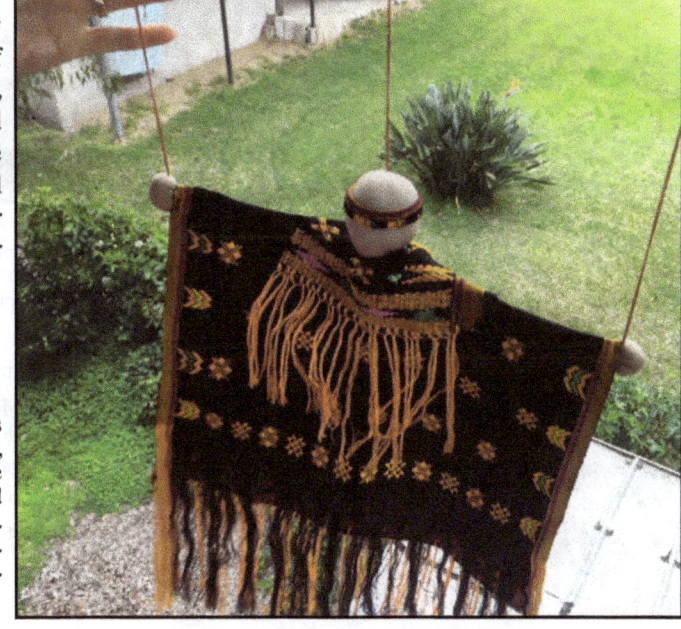

PEASANT TRANSPORT PICTORIAL

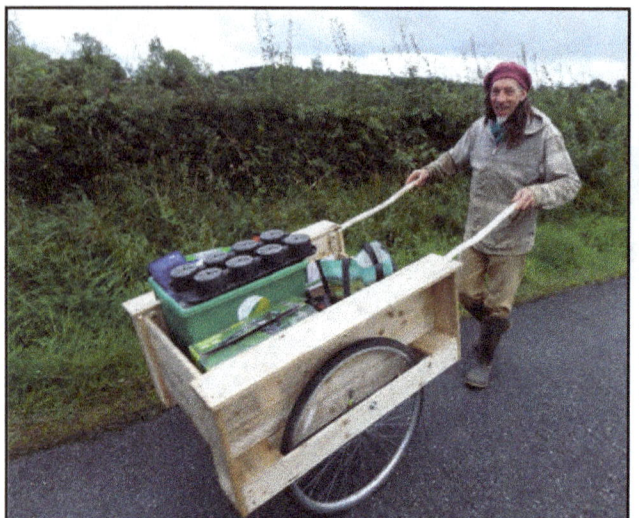

Left and below:
The handcart that Peter built was a design developed by a Peace Corps volunteer in Malawi (Africa) and is based on easily available materials, such as bicycle wheels. The design is available online. It's perfect for commuting between our two homes, along the quiet country lane. It can take surprisingly large and awkward loads.

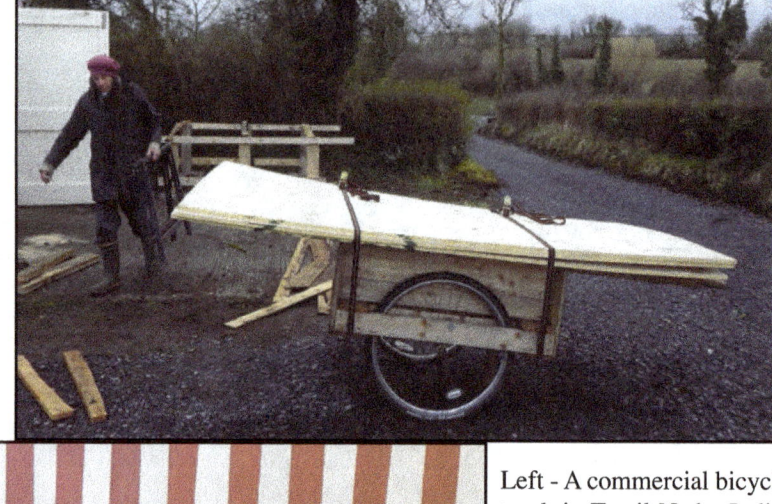

Left - A commercial bicycle truck in Tamil Nadu, India. They also take large loads, and need no registration, insurance or license to operate, however the driver doesn't actually ride the bike, but walks beside, pushing it along in the crazy traffic.

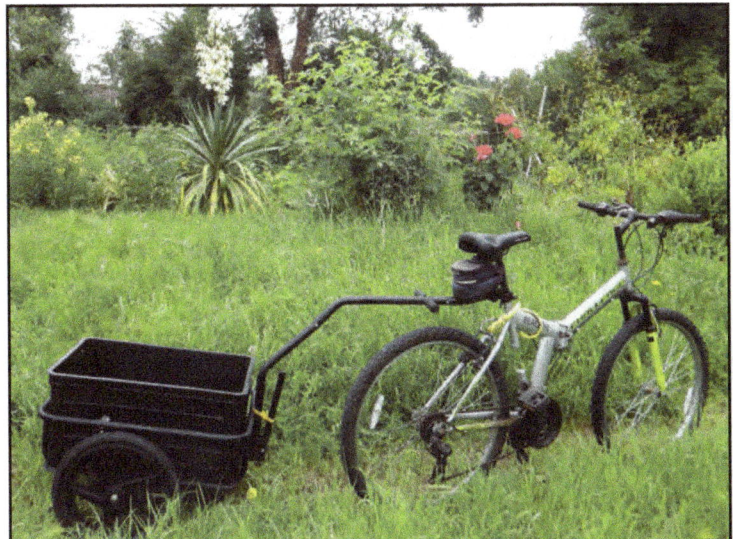

Left - The bicycle is probably the most wonderfully energy efficient device ever invented, as well as providing great exercise. Our folding bicycles can fit into the back of the electric car and they can also tow trailers, making them very versatile.

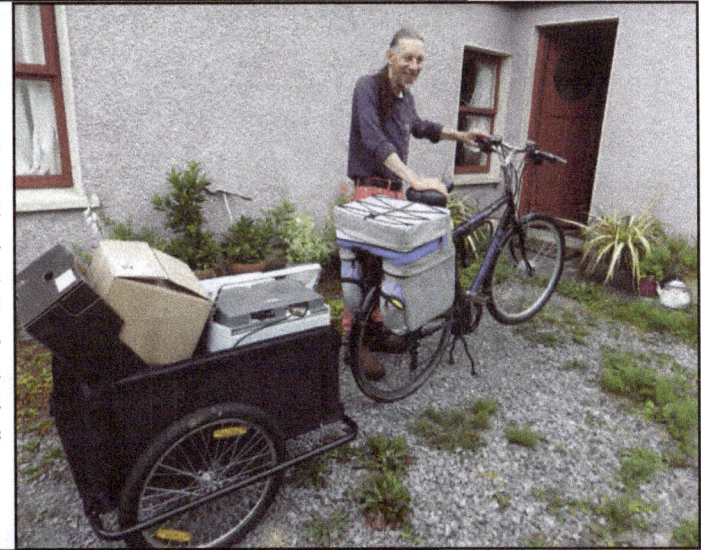

Right - Peter's electric bike and big trailer is really the best transport for now and for an energy depleted future. It would only have a fraction of the Carbon footprint of an electric car. Here, the kitchen is being shifted between households, 'fridge and all, for our weekly house swop-over.

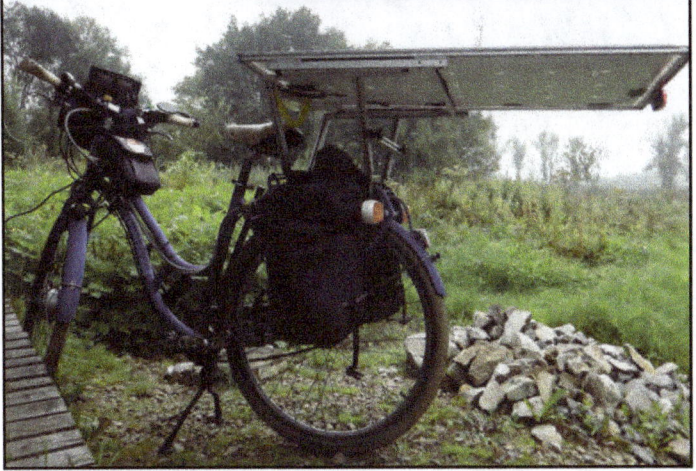

Left - We were impressed recently when Peter Schneider, a solar power expert friend, now retired, came to visit on his solar electric bicycle, after a 80km ride from his home, taking all day at a leisurely pace. He designed and built the clever solar rig himself.

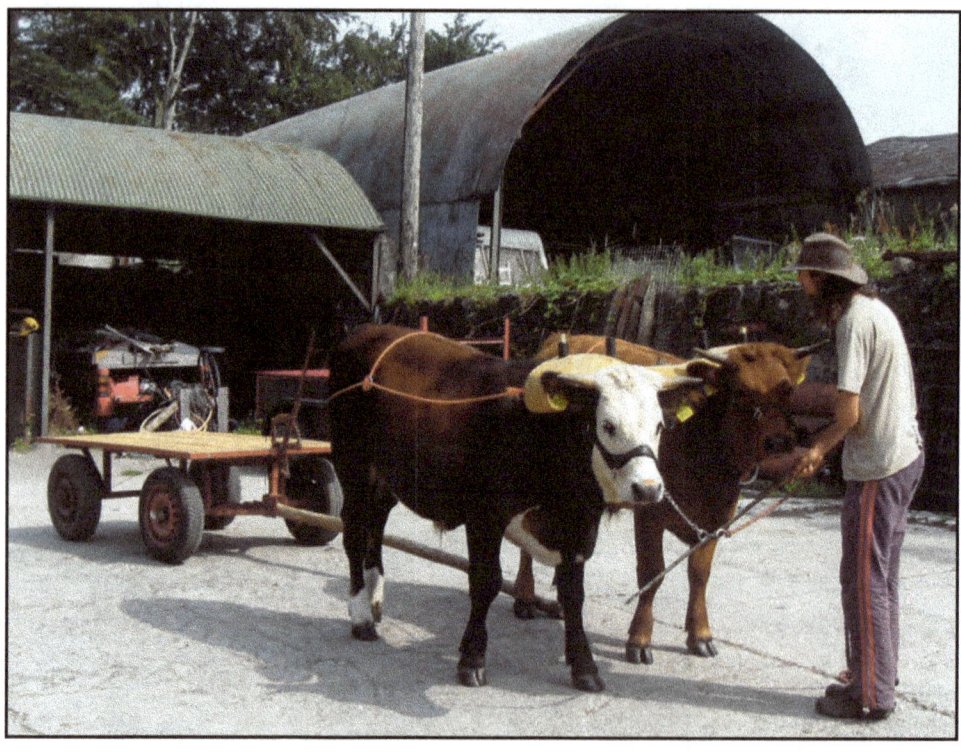

Above - Our friend Noel Higgins and his Bull Cart.
Below - Noel shows a crowd his Tiny Home on wheels.

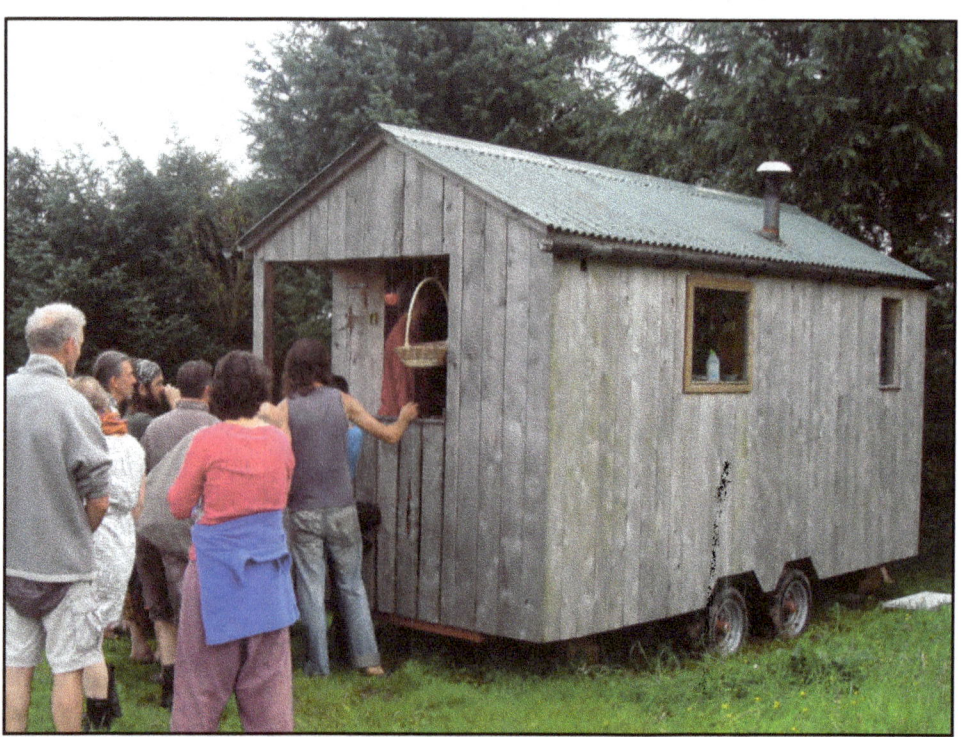

CHAPTER THREE

ECO-GARDENING

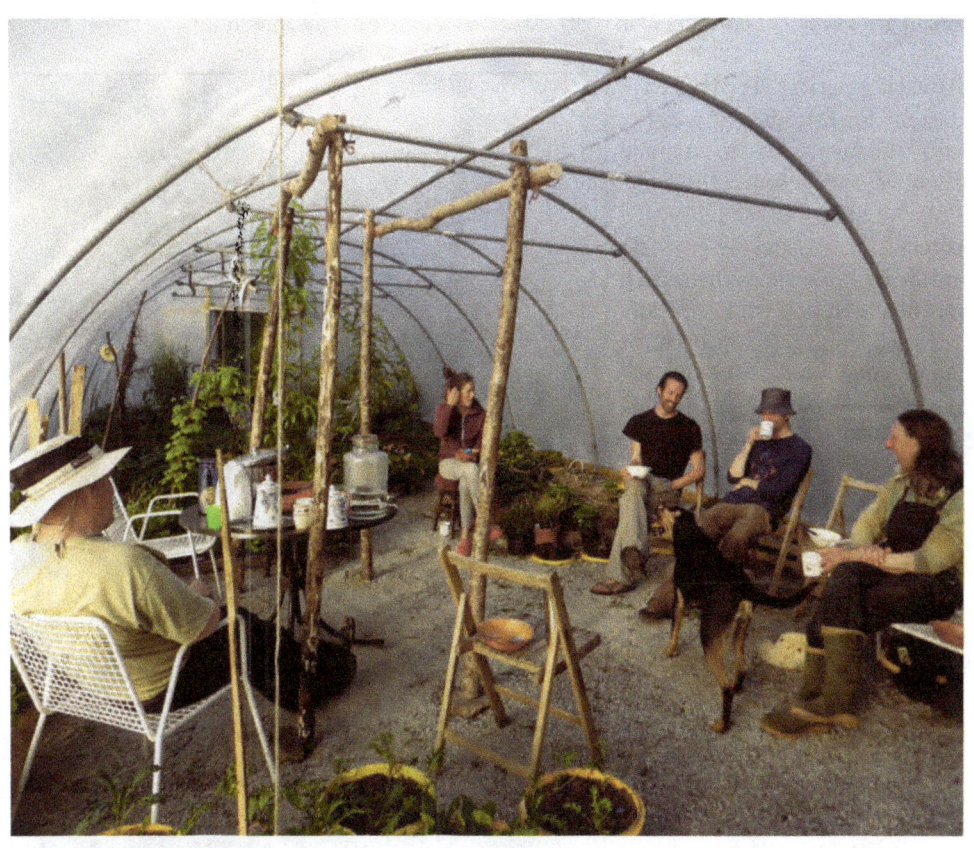

After the garden meitheal, a cup of tea and a laugh in the new polytunnel in 2015.

DESIGN FOR SUSTAINABILITY WITH PERMACULTURE

An abbreviation of 'permanent agriculture' and 'permanent culture', Permaculture is a sustainable design system that was developed from the 1970's by Australians Bill Mollison (deceased) and David Holmgren. Mainly focussing on edible-landscaping, it harks back to global mixed farming and gardening traditions, and aims to optimise the resilience of humans and eco-systems, to create a harmony of plants and animals to sustain us, cycling the nutrients produced between them and not reliant on chemical or fossil fuel inputs.

Permaculture gardens foster high biodiversity and multi-functionality, and follow natural cycles and patterns, such as the forest model. Highly diverse Food Forest gardens in tropical countries were a source of inspiration for Permaculture modelling. These days people in Europe often equate it with Food Forest gardening (more on this subject later), but Permaculture is much more than that. It can apply to society as a whole.

Forests are multi-species communities living in a beautiful symbiosis together. One is humbled to learn of the co-operation and kindness that trees show to each other, as described by German forester Peter Wohllenben and others. The concept of edible forestry, whether backyard Food Forests or broadscale Agro-Forestry, has fired up people's imaginations. Ireland just had it's first Agro-Forestry conference, in early 2021. A leap in the right direction!

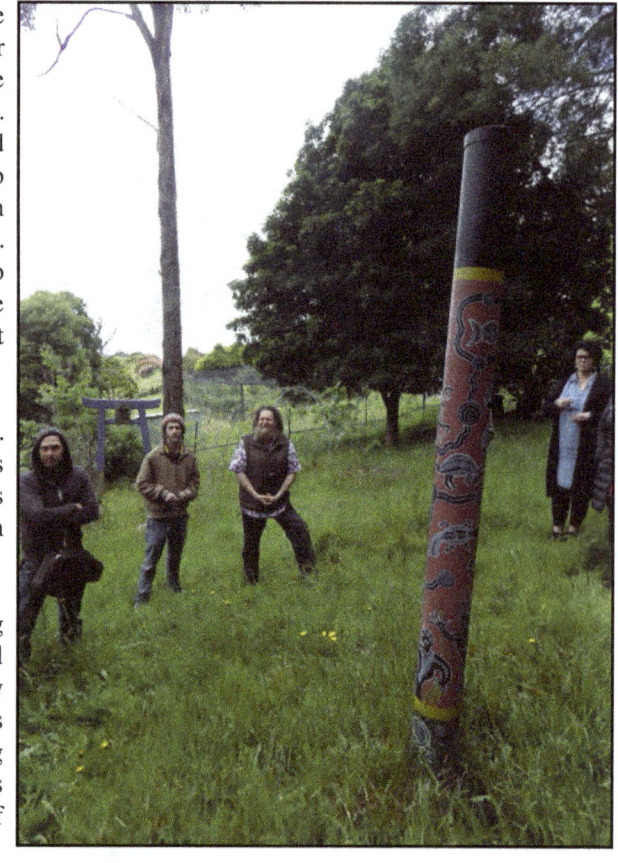

Always practical, Permaculture designs for extremes of weather and climate, using on-site energies and resources wisely. Polycultures of annual and perennial food plants are grown to ensure multiple yields that enrich our diets and nourish nature too. It's the opposite approach to conventional broadscale monoculture food cropping, that sets itself at war with nature.

Permaculture is ethically based. One aims to care for people, as well as the planet, and to share its riches fairly. But still, too much Permaculture might burn you out!

I spent many years working voluntarily for environmental organisations and this led to my own burn out. My spirit was depleted. I had a haunting apocalyptic dream where I was searching across a dark plain of devastation, desparately searching for, but not finding, the Sacred Tree. The sense of loss was intense. I woke up feeling so empty. But it prompted a return to working more with geomancy and spiritual environmental work, and this rebalanced me.

Years later I was encouraged to hear that people at one of the Australian Permaculture conferences discussed the need to add another ethic and this resonated with many there. The fourth ethic of the Permaculture movement, they declared, is to care for spirit.

Renowned Permaculture teacher 'Pete the Permie' (Peter Russell), in the centre of the last photo, has a part of his farm, located in the mountains near Melbourne, that's dedicated to this fourth ethic. The area was once a gathering place for Aboriginal people. We made a Power Tower at this revived sacred space and the energy there now is fabulous!

WINDBREAKS

I studied Organic Agriculture at a technical college (TAFE) in Australia in the early 1990s. The first job to do for cropping land, we were told, is to establish windbreaks. And so I considered the prevailing winds, existing trees and shelter at my Irish homestead. More than just a blank slate, the three grassy fields were bordered by wild, overgrown hedgerows with some tall trees in them. The majority of big trees are in the south west corner. Predominant winds from the Atlantic Ocean blow in from that direction, but are well screened by the row of mature Alder trees beside the stream. Some days I'd hardly know there's a wind blowing, until I come out onto the road and get blasted by it.

Atlantic gales are more prevalent and powerful in recent years of Climate Change. So I reinforced the hedgerow windbreak with another row of closely planted Alders (around 60 cm apart) running parallel to it. These are annually pruned to the height I want them and to reduce shading on veggie beds. The Alder is the perfect candidate for the job, growing like a rocket in the heavy clay, fixing Nitrogen from the atmosphere and so improving the soil while drying it out. Indeed, my neighbour calls these vigorous pioneers 'weeds'.

GETTING HELP TO START WITH

At the onset, transforming land into fabulous Permaculture gardens seems a daunting task. You need help. Luckily for me, friendly locals and neighbours were keen to assist and generous with their attentions. They'd drop by regularly to see if we were ok, if we might need some turf or whatever. Over time the visits tapered off, as we became established under the community's watchful eye. Other newcomers were needing their attention. In a county that has suffered centuries of migration and depopulation, locals are keen for the lights to go back on in the many empty homes here.

I needed all sorts of help at the beginning, so when the old custom of the meitheal was revived in my area and several work parties convened at different people's places, I was well pleased. In the past, peasants would organise a meitheal to harvest corn or bring in hay, especially when the need was urgent, such as if rain was looming. A neighbourly meitheal could bring it in fast. Sometimes when a couple were married, a meitheal was called to do a house raising, making a little thatched mud hut for them. Good relations with neighbours was vitally important and meitheals strengthened community spirit.

Keen to make my meitheals go smoothly, I did much preparation in advance. I selected the most suitable jobs for the size of the group, the weather, etc. Afterwards, everyone enjoyed a bowl of home grown veggie soup and fresh garden salad, or a coffee and perhaps a song. Later we went to other people's places for meitheals and reciprocated the help.

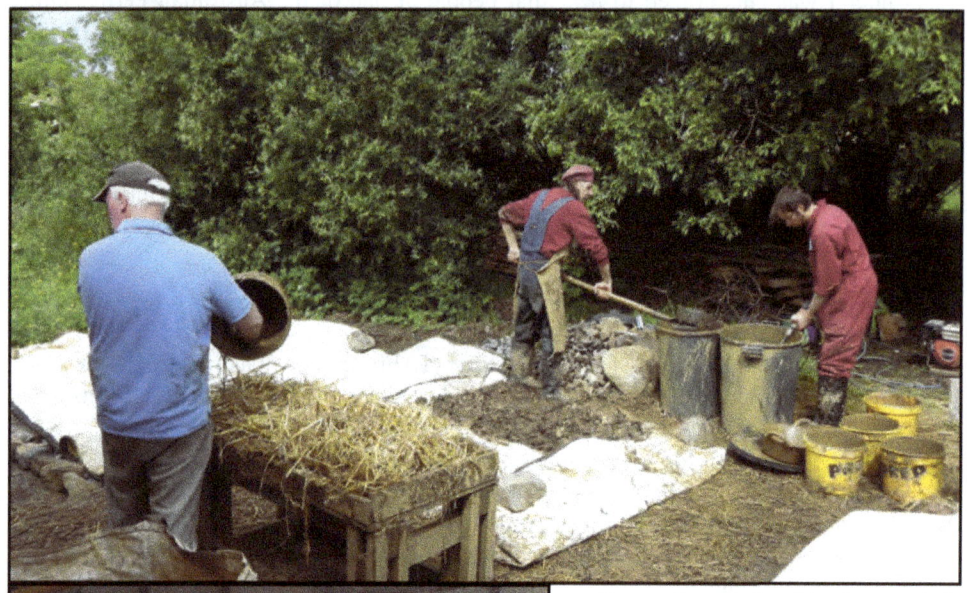

Above - Peter had meitheals to get help with building his clay-straw studio. He often made a delicious paella for the gang afterwards (left).

I've also had helpers from further afield, via the global Willing Workers on Organic Farms (WWOOF) movement that began in the 1970s. WWOOF facilitates people who want to learn about organic farming and gardening, by linking them to hosts who have them work several hours each day in exchange for food, lodging and tuition.

For over twenty years in Australia WWOOF supplied me with mainly young visitors from far and wide. We learnt about other countries and cultures, while lots of projects were done. (However, it must be said that it was generally me doing the bulk of the work!) So in 2015 I joined Ireland's WWOOF and a small trickle of WWOOFers came to stay and work for a week or two. A couple of charming WWOOFers are seen overleaf. By 2018 this trickle had dried up, due to a global drop in WWOOFer numbers, it turned out. All very mysterious. It was just as well my gardens only needed me to maintain them. No need to grow extra food to feed hungry

WWOOFers either. When 2020 came and international travel ground to a halt, once again I was pleased that I didn't rely on WWOOFers coming from distant lands. Plus, I do enjoy my solitude!

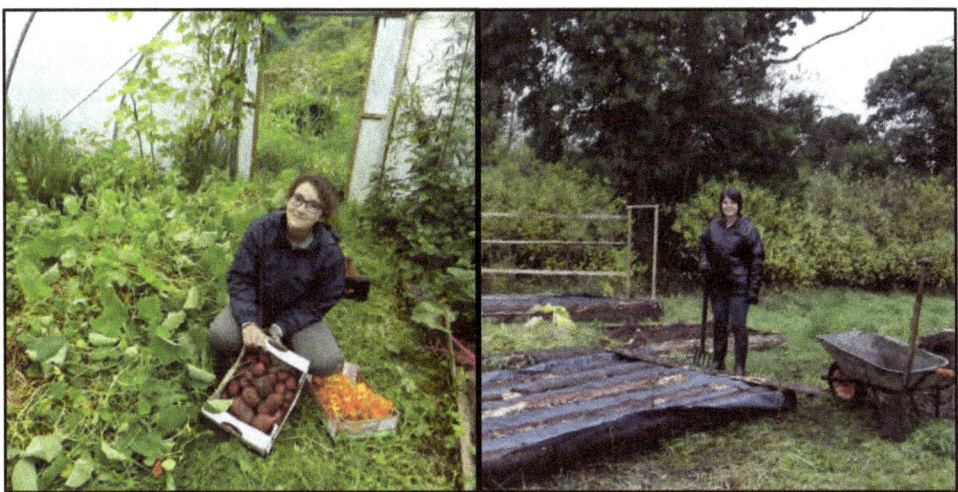

I haven't had a meitheal for a while now either. People get so busy and are hard to muster. Anyway, I don't need so much help these days, as the gardens are maturing. And if I did need constant help, it couldn't really be sustainable, could it?

MAKING SOIL IN LEITRIM

Refugees streamed into Leitrim from western Ulster in the decades following the Battle of the Diamond in Armagh in 1795. They were driven from their homes by the activities of the 'Peep o' Day Boys', protestants 'planted' by the British, the teenage terrorists of their times who were emboldened by the setting up of the Orange Order. Fleeing persecution, the indigenes searched for new homes in the undesirable areas of the less fertile province of Connaught. When passing through County Leitrim many found places to settle on hillsides and bogs, in uninhabited places, remote and inhospitable. There was no suitable soil for food growing. But they were safe from harassment there, so they just had to create soil themselves!

They did this by gathering sand from watercourses in the valleys and hauling it up in creels on their backs to their mountain homes that they built from mud and stones, and thatched with the Heather that grew there. They burned the Heather for its ash and mixed it with the sand and acid peaty soil, along with dunghill compost. They found Limestone rocks in rivers, carried them up mountainsides, heated and ground them to make Lime, to sweeten the soil.

The mind boggles at the effort required to do all this and the amazing resilience of those people! Because they did survive in their new, hard won homesteads. Evident by a plethora of Ulster family names here (Guckian, McLoughlin, McGirl etc), their descendants still live here and also scattered across the globe. [1] They do say that people are 'Leitrim's best export'.

1. Sliabh an Iarainn Slopes - history of the town and parish of Ballinamore, Co. Leitrim, Fr Dan Gallogly, 1991, Ireland.

SOIL DREAMING

Around the world, large scale monoculture farmlands are failing after decades of soil abuse. Drenched in nature killing chemicals, these man-made wastelands function a bit like hydroponics. With no inherent fertility remaining and relying on a barrage of chemical inputs to grow anything, the soil is just a holding medium for plants. Scientists analyse and bemoan the loss of precious farm topsoil globally - from acidification, poisoning, salinity, compaction, erosion and the like.

But hello! We can't sit around crying for the dead soil under our feet. We have to make good the legacy and work to revive worn out, abused soils; to create the ideal soil to match the needs of the crops we grow. In the past, farmers would look for new lands when their's failed. Today there are no more new frontiers to exploit, except for our own backyards and lawn acreages!

The perfect dream soil for food garden beds is a moderately free-draining loam, with a good balance of sand, silt and clay, and a minimum of 3% organic matter. The darker coloured the better, as this indicates good organic matter. Few people start off with such a perfect soil. Luckily there are a host of natural methods to draw upon and Organic and Biodynamic organisations are keen to share their techniques and encourage you. Unsuitable, abused and even poisoned soils can be transformed with the aid of compost, 'green 'manures', microbes, mineral supplements etc. It's a great challenge to take on and it makes you feel good all over when you stand back and see the product of your soil building work as a colourful Permaculture paradise bursting forth from Mother Earth.

Sandy soil is free draining, but usually low in nutrients, while a clay soil is relatively rich but easily waterlogged. Fine particles of clay have only tiny spaces between them for soil to breathe, making it hard for air, water and plant roots to move through it. My local clay soil ('daub') has never been considered good for growing anything other than pasture, and very rough pasture at that. When it rains heavily, water can't percolate down and it stays in sheets and ponds on the surface for hours or days even. Cows can get bogged in it. On the plus side, clay soils are a boon in dry spells. In 2018, when Ireland had no rain for two months over summer, my clay soil proved a winner, retaining enough moisture for plants to thrive, while commercial growers on sandy soils dealt with extreme water stress.

The much-maligned daub was once used for building the traditional mud walled cottages of the peasantry. Peter has used it himself, mixing clay slurry with straw to fill the walls of his studio. Sometimes called Light Earth, it provides excellent insulation at minimal cost, but requires much labour. A meitheal is just the thing, as seen on page 52.

The problems of too much sand or clay in soil, making it 'too light', or 'too heavy', are both helped by increasing the amount of humus (organic matter) in it. This makes the soil a good Carbon bank, so it's climate saving too! You can do this on the small scale by digging ripe compost into the soil surface, or by spreading organic mulch over soil and allowing it to compost down (known as Sheet Mulching), or by planting Cover Crops (also called Green Manures) and digging them in. An increased humus content bolsters the nutrients available for healthy plant growth and earthworm activity.

Sand can also be added to a dense clay soil to lighten it up (and a sandy soil is improved if clay is added), but lots of digging is needed to mix them in, unless you use a cultivator or rotavator type of thing; another way is to just pour sand down any big cracks in heavy clay ground. You might also add finely ground Gypsum (Calcium sulphate), that's recommended as a clay breaking chemical. However Gypsum only improves the structure of sodic clay soil, which is saline.

To improve drainage in wet clay soil areas, a network of small drains is just the thing. These can be open spoon drains, or narrow drains with slotted drainage pipe bedded in gravel, the gravel strip making a dry walking path. I had several such drains (locals call them 'shores') made by a digger in my wet, rushy meadow and now it's transformed into a lovely orchard of heritage fruit trees.

MAKING COMPOST

Compost is an imperative for good gardening, to put back what one has taken out. In the process you transform waste materials into valuable soil and plant food, in a natural alchemy. The art of good compost making can be sublime. And the more you make, the better it gets.

I was trained up in the art of composting in the mid 1990's, when the local council in Lismore, New South Wales, decided to train a team to teach people how to be successful at composting their organic waste and thus prevent it from going into landfill. We were on a mission!

A compost heap is usually a pile of alternating layers of diverse materials of things organic. Anything that was once alive can be composted. Crushed rock can go in too, as well as living micro-organisms and worms. Layers need to be moistened if very dry, because the ideal is to have 60% moisture in the heap. If you squeeze it, a few drops of water should come out.

Nitrogen rich layers, such as manure, kitchen scraps and garden greens, should be much thinner than Carbon rich layers - e.g. dry grass, straw, shredded paper etc. One aims for about thirty parts Carbon to one part Nitrogen, which is a bit hard to ascertain. Be guided by colour - green materials are usually higher in Nitrogen, while brown coloured stuff is more Carbon rich. Grass clippings are great too, but only when used in thin layers, or they'll quickly rot into a slimy mess. (One might call grass clippings - 'vegan manure'.)

SEEDY STUFF

Gardeners often ask me about composting weeds that have seeds. Isn't a no-no? Well, it depends on whether you plan to turn the compost and bury any unwanted seedlings. Turning compost can be physically demanding, so unless you want to build up your muscles, you may wish to let worms do the turning for you. However if you keep adding layers of mulch and compost on top regularly, you'll probably find that weed seeds tend to rot away and don't sprout.

Seedy weeds can also be put in the centre of a large Hot Compost heap for fast break down. Or pre-compost them in a Rough Compost heap. If you add seedy plants to Sheet Compost, make sure they are well covered over with other layers, then seeds should rot down, the damp Irish climate being ideal for mouldering.

WHICH SYSTEM TO USE?

There are several types of composting systems to consider using. Indoors, in the kitchen, you might put all your chopped up scraps into a sealed Bokashi bin to ferment; or into a Worm Farm for vermi-composting. In the garden, a simple pile of organic matter is the easiest type of compost heap. You might box it in with something like pallets, but this isn't essential. In the photo below, a modular compost box system developed in New Zealand is used at north Leitrim's Organic Centre. You add more timber as the level of compost rises.

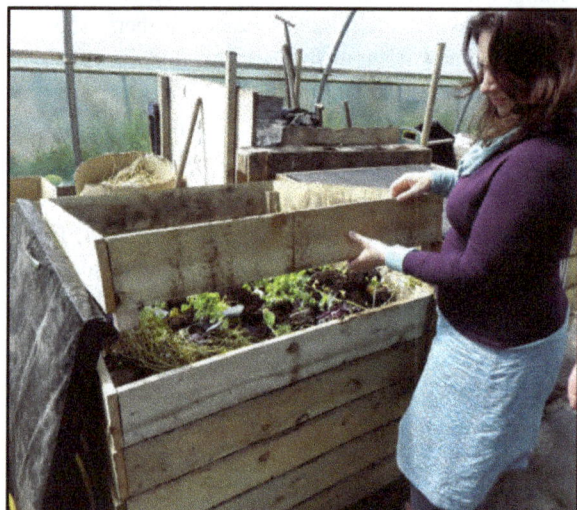

A shady place under a tree can be a good spot to make your compost heap. You might have to turn the pile once or twice, if it is not rotting down evenly. It's good exercise, but you may not need it. Separate out woody material, branches of trees etc, for making wood based Rough Compost and Hugel Mounds. Green waste that isn't seedy and has no invasive roots attached (lawn mower clippings are ideal) can also be spread across garden beds and around fruit trees, Sheet Mulching style. It doesn't need turning.

SEVEN TYPES OF COMPOSTING

HOT COMPOST

A Hot Compost is ideal if loads of manure are available and it's good for seedy weeds too. It's best if you stockpile all the materials in advance and then make the heap in one go. To get it hot enough for a fast breakdown, the heap needs to be a minimum size of one cubic metre. Then heat loving microbes should get it to a high temperature. Earthworms don't like hot compost, but will move in when it cools down. The ready compost is most fertile when it's still a bit warm and isn't fully broken down.

What to make it with: manure, weeds, light garden prunings, leaves and lawn clippings, etc

Over each layer sprinkle a little:
- wood ash, Basalt dust, Lime and/or Dolomite powder
- finished compost, to kick-start the composting process,
- microbial stimulant (such as EM) diluted in water, via a watering can.

WORM COMPOST

This is best for kitchen waste on a small scale. Worms quickly transform it into fabulous vermicompost. It can be made at leisure, adding stuff each day. Veggie scraps are best chopped up into small pieces. Some people even liquidise scraps in a blender, for quicker uptake.

For worm bedding you add torn up wet cardboard or shredded paper. Keep Vermicompost moist, as worms don't like it too dry or too wet, and keep the box in a sheltered spot, not too hot or cold, and covered to exclude light.

BOKASHI COMPOST

Another method for the kitchen, this compost is kept enclosed, so it's smell, bug and mouse free. You need a bucket with an airtight lid to exclude Oxygen as much as possible, to foster a ferment of diverse microorganisms. A tap near the bottom is used for draining off ferment juices. Fruit and veggie scraps are chopped up finely before going in and should be as dry as possible. You buy in the Bokashi EM treated bran and this is sprinkled over each layer as a starter culture. Air is squeezed out as much as possible, via a plate on top, for example, that's pushed down each time after deposits are made. EM microbes thrive on sugars from plant material and rapidly break them down to produce essential foods for plants. The liquid that's drained off is a valuable fertiliser and compost accelerator when it's used diluted 1:100 in water (ideally using rain water, as Chlorine in tap water kills microbes).

HUMANURE COMPOST

Nitrogen rich urine is fairly sterile and harmless, so it's great to use as a plant fertiliser. Research in America found that the average adult Human annually produces enough Nitrogen in their urine alone to sufficiently fertilise around 300m^2 of garden, at a rate of 70kg of N per acre.[1] Diluted with five to ten parts water and applied to soil around plants, it's especially good for Onions, Peppers, Potatoes, Celery and Carrots, but is not well tolerated by Beans and Tomatoes. Urine is a great compost activator too, especially when sprinkled over high Carbon materials such as wood chips, sawdust or straw. A Wee Bucket can also be half filled with such things and these soak up smells and prevent splash backs, the damp contents being an excellent addition to the compost heap.

As for our own Humanure, it is pathogenic so a dedicated compost heap is the go, with plenty of organic materials to cover deposits. Keep it protected from rain and animal interference, apply earthworms and wait a year or so. Worms will transform everything beautifully, given sufficient moisture. If it doesn't work out well, you can turn the heap, mix it up a bit, add moisture and leave it for longer. You may want to only apply the ripe Humanure to fruit trees and shrubs, rather than on annual crops, to be safe.[2]

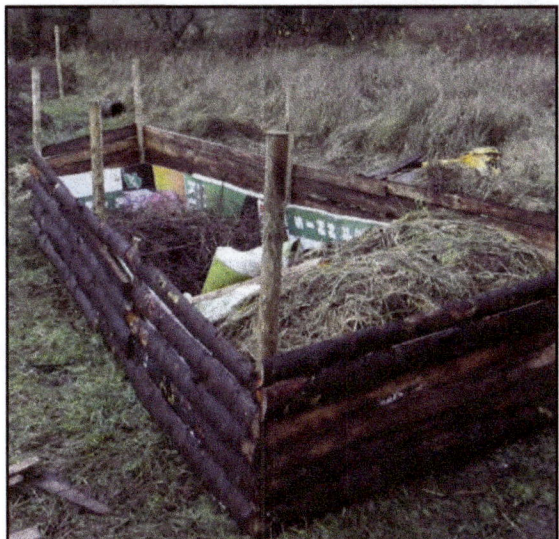

Left - A Humanure compost bed into which berry bushes were later planted. The flitch walls are waste from a local sawmill and the lining is old election boards.

1. Elaine Myers, Permaculture Activist, May 1992.
2. The Humanure Handbook - a guide to composting human manure, Joseph Jenkins, Chelsea Green, USA, 2005.

SHEET COMPOST / MULCHING

> "Mulching is one of the most valuable practises in organic gardening."
> Joy Larkcom[1]

This is the most energy efficient form of composting, because you don't have to turn it or move it when it's ready. Not only a way to transform waste materials into plant food, it's also weed suppressing and a good way to start a garden on barren or weedy ground. When kept covered with organic mulches, soil retains moisture better and becomes more fertile.

Likened to a lasagne, layers of Nitrogen and Carbon rich organic materials are alternated, e.g. manure, straw, grass clippings, hay, spoiled silage, weeds, leaves, twigs and wood chips. A layer of newspaper, six or more sheets thick and well overlapped, or one layer of cardboard, is best laid down first, to exclude light from getting to any weeds below. Beware of using toxic materials, such as old carpets, for mulching. Unless they are antiques, carpets are full of nasty chemicals and have no place in an organic garden.

1. Joy Larkcom, Grow your own Vegetables, Francis Lincoln Ltd, 2002, UK.

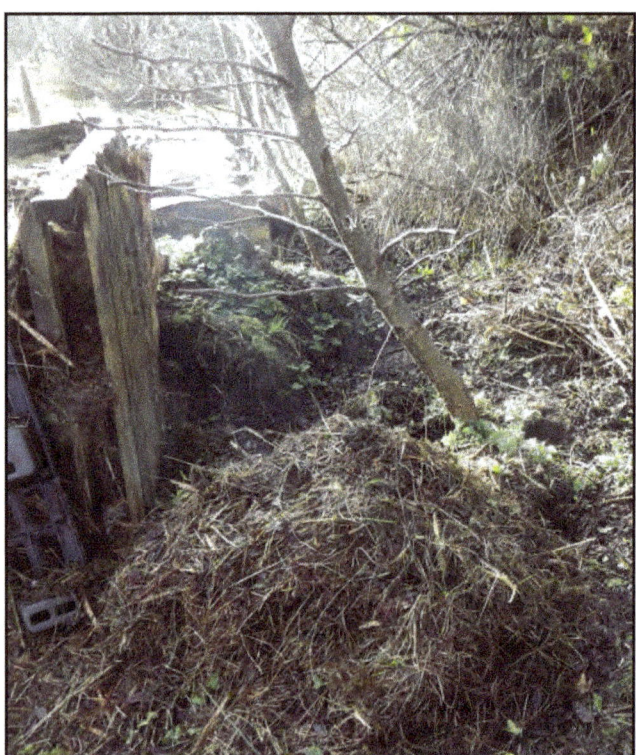

ROUGH COMPOST

This is where tricky items can go, such as seedy weeds, old sticks, prunings and prickly branches. Pile it up in an out-of-the-way corner and let it rot to a less formidable form, for as long as it takes, a year or two. You might want to check it occasionally. Sticks can sprout! Willows and Snowberries are very adept at resurrecting themselves if not left out in the weather long enough to fully die.

Jumping up and down on the pile is a good way to compact it down and speed up the composting process. When semi-rotted, it might be used as layers in other compost heaps, or spread as Sheet Mulch around fruit trees - they love wood based compost. Semi-rotted Rough Compost spread on garden beds can also repel Poultry and Blackbirds from scratching everything up.

HUGEL MOUNDS

Hugel Beds, or Mound Gardening, is an excellent way to deal with woody waste, such as branches, sawdust and wood chips. It developed anciently in China, then more recently in Germany and beyond. After a couple of years in the Rough Compost heap, the woody stuff is piled and compressed into flat topped heaps, mounds or windrows. On top of this, a garden is made, with the addition of upturned grass sods or Sheet Composting material (layers of dead grass, leaves, manure, etc). Into this, pockets of soil or compost are placed for planting into. Americans might call it a Dead Wood Swale and Dan Hemingway in America finds these ideal for Blueberry growing, being so well drained and suitably fertile. [1] Woody compost is generally very beneficial for trees and shrubs.

1. Gaia's Garden -a guide to homescale Permaculture, Toby Hemenway, Chelsea Green, USA, 2000.

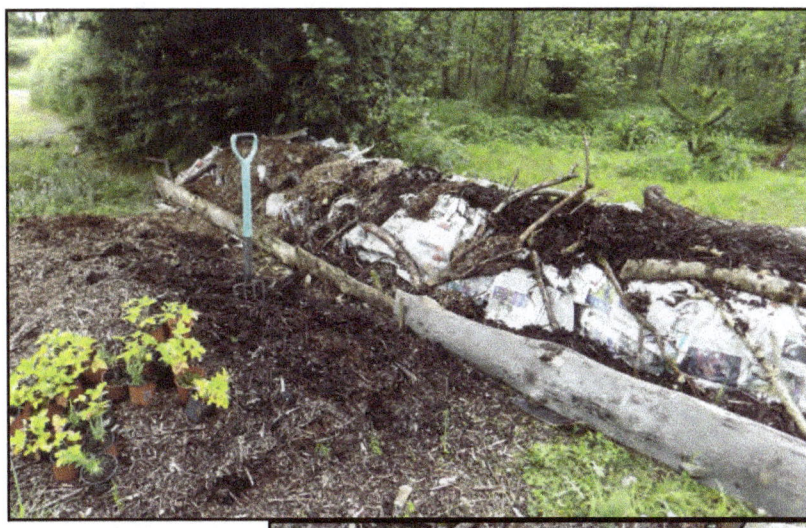

Above and Right - A pile of Willow tree woodchips, gifted to me in autumn, was a mix of twigs, branches and green leaves, that proved perfect for composting. But it needed more Nitrogen to balance all the Carbon. Over winter it was sprinkled regularly, via a watering can, with the 'liquid gold' of urine - a great way to harness the power of pee, especially in the cold months when Nitrogen isn't needed for fertilising plants directly. By summer it looked like black leaf mould and Mushrooms grew over it. In autumn I used it to transform the old boundary wall beside it into a Wall of Food, using flitches, newspaper, Sheet Mulch, compost, branches, etc.

RAISED GARDEN BEDS

Growing crops above ground level prevents water logging in wet spells, while aeration of soil is also improved. Raised vegetable beds are also invaluable for growing food in heavy clay soil, while Rudolph Steiner noted that they receive more cosmic influences than flat beds. Raised beds even got a mention in one of Ireland's oldest books, dating from the Middle Ages, so they aren't new. [1.]

If don't have a pile of soil to make a Raised Bed with, I put plants into mini mounds of soil or compost on top of a new Hugel bed, then fill the spaces inbetween with thick Sheet Mulch, to raise it all up. This is what I did to establish a new Hugel bed for Jerusalem Artichokes, as in the photo. They were sprouting up elsewhere where I didn't want them. I found they transplanted very easily to the new bed and they'll supply future Pig food that will be relished. (Potatoes are also well suited to grow in such a bed.)

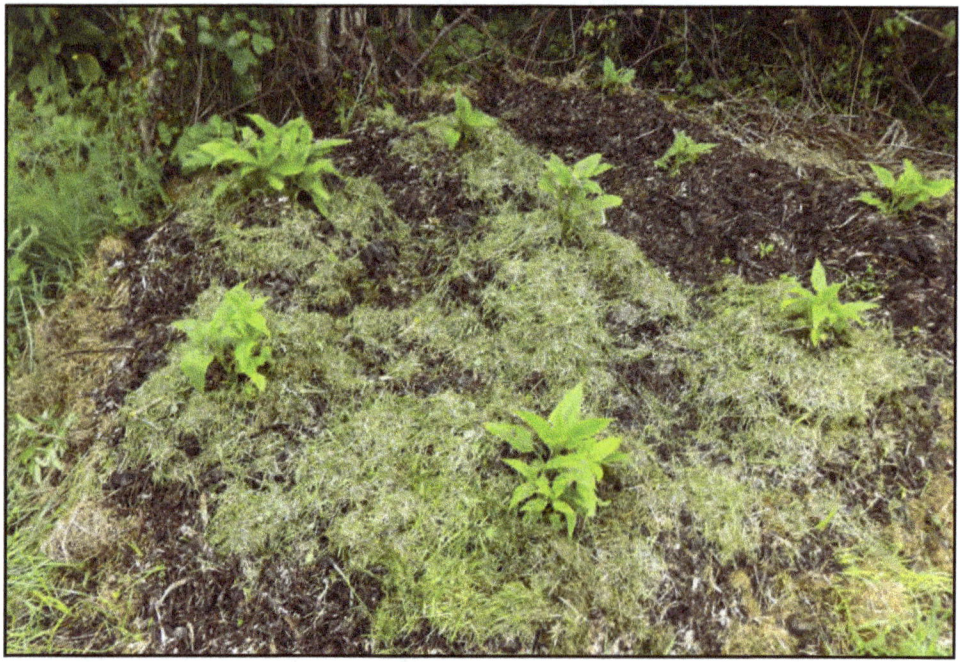

What goes up can also fall down. Sheet Mulch can fall down off the sides, or be pushed off by birds. Weeds can invade from the sides too. So, what to do with the edges? Here are a few suggestions, methods that I've developed.

    1. Taper the slope of the mound's sides so that it only has soft edges that you might easily mow around.

    2. Make a path of black silage plastic, or cardboard etc, around the bed and up the sides, to stop weeds getting in. This is great for an Alpine Strawberry bed, as in the next photo, making fruit easier and cleaner to harvest. The other bed has Blackcurrants just planted.

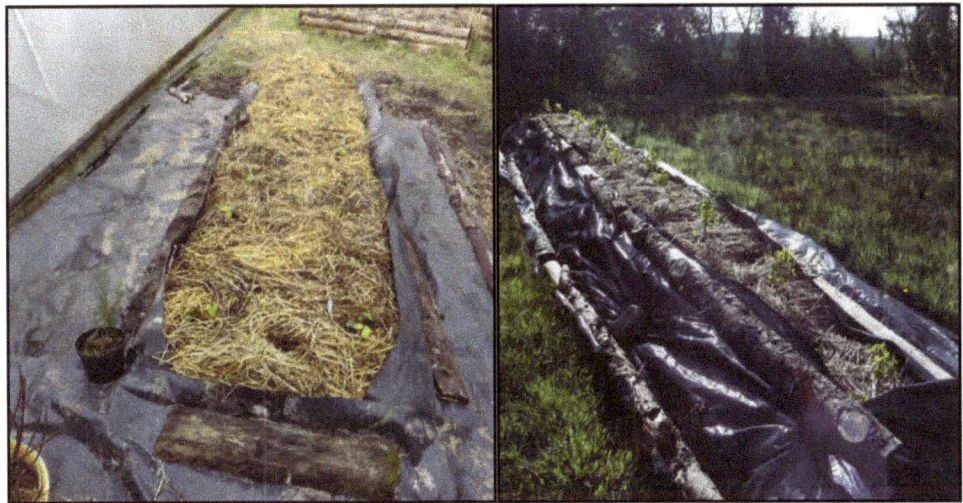

3. Have hard edges to hold in compost, keep out cold wind etc. Flitches (rough timber offcuts, waste from a sawmill) are ideal and 'Flitch Technology' is so simple, using small wooden stakes hammered into the ground, and jamming or tying the boards together rather than nailing or screwing them. The photo below of a new herb garden is an example. I don't use rocks around garden beds, as they become too difficult to weed. Mud walls can also be made, as in the photo on the right.

4. Flitch timber walls can also be laid on the side of the bed without any attachment, as in the top right photo. They hold down stuff by weight alone and thus are moved away easily when it's time for weeding or mulching. This is my preferred method nowadays.

1. Early Irish Farming by Fergus Kelly, Dublin Institute of Advanced Studies, 1997, Ireland.

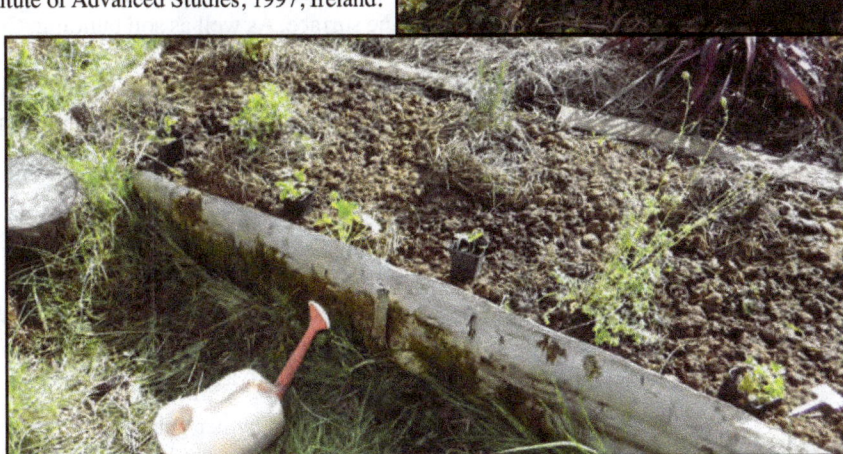

REMINERALISING WITH ROCKDUST

> **"If you can do this in your own garden and orchard and eat fresh, living, mineralised foods, you can give thanks because you are living in Paradise!"   Don Weaver**

Food grown on depleted, mineral deficient soil makes plants and the people who eat them more susceptible to disease. Don Weaver has been promoting the remineralising of farm soils for decades. "Mineral-depleted soil has been directly correlated with increased death rates," he says. "Laboratory studies have shown that trace mineral deficiencies are associated with an increased risk of cancer. Even one trace mineral deficiency carries this risk. Vibrant health depends upon a broad spectrum of all the minerals essential to human health." [1]

How to impart more minerals into garden soils? Crushed rock is the way to go. Ideally the minerals are first digested by microbes, by adding rock powders into compost heaps. A sprinkle of rock dust over each layer does the trick. The minerals feed the microbes, who feed the plants nutrients in more bio-available forms. Basalt, originating from volcanoes, has the highest spectrum of minerals available and I used it extensively in Australia, writing a book on the subject.[2] In Ireland I buy bags of German Basalt dust online, but Basalt is quarried here, so if I had a big farm I would get a truck load.

1. Fruiticulture, David Klein PhD and Don Weaver, 2018, Vibrant Health Publications, Hawaii USA.
2. Stone Age Farming, Alanna Moore, Python Press, Australia, 2001.

COVER CROPS

In broadscale tillage, cultivation with heavy machinery is used to break up and aerate soils to make them workable. But without adding organic matter back regularly, the soil becomes degraded and in the long term it's not sustainable. A better option than cultivation, Green Manure crops can be grown for improving soil, especially heavy clay. Such Cover Crops enrich and aerate soil, protect the surface from erosion by wind and rain, and also control weeds in-between food crops. They're perfect for a No-Dig garden.

The deep roots of Chicory, Daikon Radish, Rapeseed, Alfalfa and Mustard open up heavy, compacted soils and bring extra nutrients to the surface. As well as soil building, Cover Crops foster biodiversity too, with insects flocking to their flowers. By using a mixture of legume and non-legume Cover Crops, a better balance of Nitrogen and Carbon in the humus is achieved too. For improving heavy clay soil, Garden Organic in the UK recommends sowing alternate rows of Broad Beans and Ryegrass in autumn. [1]

Annual Cover Crops are slashed down either a month or so before you want to sow your crop; or just before, or at the start, of flowering. Perennials, such as Clovers, can be cut down after six months growth, to encourage regrowth. In the backyard situation a Cover Crop can be cut with a scythe or sickle - great exercise in the fresh air. There's a wonderful grace and rhythm to scything, when you master the art. Sickling puts more wear and tear on the back muscles, so it's worth doing stretching exercises before and after, to avoid strain and pain.

1. Green Manures - step by step guide, by Garden Organic, UK.

LIVING MULCH

Living Mulches are permanent Cover Crops that food crops are planted into. They protect the soil from erosion, suppress weeds, hold in moisture and benefit insects. Clovers are ideal, as they fix nitrogen too and share it with surrounding plants, especially when regularly trimmed. White Dutch Clover, which only grows to 15-25cm height, is especially good for this. In fact a growing system was devised in Australia around this concept. 'Clever Clover' kits were sent out by government scientists of the CSIRO to encourage people to trial the system. Kits included separate packets of the seeds of Mustard, a couple of Clover varieties and Lucerne.

One day I'll make up my own mix of Cover Crop seeds, when I find out which varieties would suit the soil and region. Actually, Red Clover grows wild here and is beloved by Bumblebees, so that would be an obvious candidate, although it can become over-dominating. My Pigs relish eating it, becoming ecstatic 'Pigs in Clover'.

Natural farmer in Japan Masanobu Fukuoka, who pioneered the No-Dig gardening approach, developed techniques to regenerate desertified land, growing grain without tillage or herbicide, and adapting traditional farming methods into what he called 'Do Nothing Farming'. Instead of machines, he used Cover Crops to open up compacted soils and allow them to breathe. Fukuoka used White Clover as a living mulch in his food growing areas. The lush green Clover sward was simply opened up in little patches to take seedling transplants or crop seeds. He also used Daikon, Comfrey, Alfalfa and trees (Australian Acacias in particular) to open up the hard ground.

WEEDS

A weed is a plant that you don't want. It's an attitude towards plants, because they could be valuable in another situation. Many useful European plants found their way to Australia, became naturalised and are now considered weeds there. St John's Wort, for example. Vast inland plains covered with St John's Wort are a curse for the farmers because it's unhealthy for cows and is classified as a 'noxious weed'. Meanwhile there's a huge demand for St John's Wort products for treating mild depression, such as in Germany where, by 1998, it constituted some 25% of all doctors' prescriptions. Perhaps those 'cow cockies' should become herb farmers? [1]

Some weeds can be considered as a De-Facto Cover Crop, protecting soil from erosion by wind and rain. You can chop and drop them to enrich the soil. Some might also hide a nice crop of berries that goes unnoticed by the birds, so that you get to eat most of them. Only remove them after the harvest is done. Timing is everything!

Persistent, perennial weeds are not so good in the veggie patch. Dig deep to get all their roots out, or chop the tops off and cover the ground with mulch, layers of paper and cardboard, or temporary plastic sheeting (black silage plastic is long lasting). It could take a year to kill them, but it's much less wear and tear on the gardener this way. Who needs to wreck their body when there's easier techniques?

1. The Healing Power of Celtic Healing Plants, Angela Paine, O Books, UK, 2006.

Even Bindweed and Japanese Knotweed, which can be very persistent, can be killed by smothering. Peter covered a large area of Bindweed with silage plastic and used the area on top as a temporary storage place for timber and tree branches. This was handy, because if you stack tree branches on the ground and plants grow up through them it becomes a tangled mess. The silage plastic, treated to resist UV radiation, can be used over and over and you can mend any holes with special tape, to stop light getting in to the weeds below.

SLUG PROBLEMS AND SOLUTIONS

Slugs are a perennial problem for gardeners and especially so in the damp Irish climate. Robert Hart warns that Slugs are a symptom of acidic conditions, that they proliferate in uncomposted manure. So he recommended to repel them by adding a fine layer of sprinkled Lime, wood ash or Dolomite, to sweeten soil and manure.

More solutions for reducing Slug predation -

* Start seedlings in a box, with glass or old window on top, or plastic storage box.

* Seedlings should be well grown before planting out.

* After planting seedlings, protect them with an upturned glass jar or bottle with it's end removed, which also keeps them warm.

* Surround vulnerable plants with a ring of wood ash or Lime/Dolomite, sawdust, partly rotted Oak leaves, Comfrey leaves, a proprietary Copper collar or homemade ring cut from a Tin can, or a mulch of aromatic herbs. (Rain will wash some of these treatments away.)

* Grow the more resistant vegetables - Chicory, Endive, spicy Brassicas such as Mustard, Mizuna, Mitsuba etc. Slugs don't like strong flavours.

* Check plants after dark with torchlight and pick Slugs off. Check their hiding places, look for them underneath plant pots, pieces of wood etc.

* Allow Ducks to harvest Slugs in the garden daily, with brief foraging visits. Or collect the Slugs yourself and feed them to the Ducks.

* Slugs can be put in a sealed jar with water to kill them. The resulting Slug Soup can be sprayed on plants as a repellant. (This might repel you also!)

* Saucers of beer will trap them.

* The Biodynamic approach is to burn dead Slugs at particular times (found in the BD calendars) and also to spray leafy plants and soil with Horn Silica on days that are best for leaf growth, early in the morning. [1]

1. Maria Thun Biodynamic Calendar 2021, Matthias Thun, Floris Books, 2020.

MIRACLES OF MULCHING
- TRANSFORMING LAWN INTO A POTATO PATCH

Sheet Mulching and No-Dig growing is a revolutionary and transformative act when you use it to convert lawns to food gardens. Because lawns are typically high maintenance energy and chemical guzzlers, every bit of lawn that is converted is a great win for nature in the war against wasting the planet. It's especially satisfying if you get to have a feed from what had essentially been a wasteland. A crop of Potatoes is particularly suitable for helping to break in such new ground. When the most suitable spot has been discerned, with good solar aspect, some protection from wind or frost etc, and you have decided what style of bed to make, follow this simple process.

1. Cut grass short, ideally with a lawn mower, as clippings will be useful. Make sure there are no lurking roots of brambles or other pernicious perennials, these can be dug out.

2. For the first layer it's good to have aeration, with woody material such as half rotted sticks and branches or tree bark spread over the plot. But it's ok if you don't have any of such, just plaster wet newspaper or cardboard over the ground, well overlapped, then go to step three.

3. Cover the base with layers of -
    Weeds, plant prunings and waste
    Grass clippings, spread thinly
    Sods of earth turned upside down
    Animal manure
    Straw, dry grass, spoiled silage
    Sawdust, wood chips
    Tree leaves
    Kitchen scraps
    Seaweed, Nettles, Comfrey
    Urine and water to moisten it all.

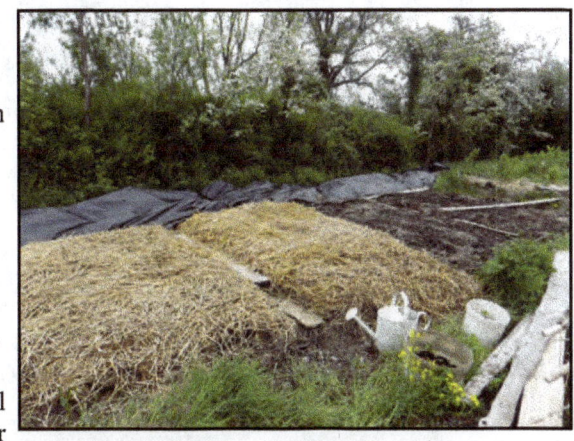

4. Cover the bed all over with a well overlapped layer of cardboard, or several layers of newspaper. Water well to keep them from blowing off in a wind.

5. Make holes through these papers and put a pocket of compost or soil there to plant your sprouting seed Potatoes into. Cover each Potato with some compost or rotted manure.

6. Now spread straw, dry grass or hay over the whole bed.

8. When Potato plants have grown to 30cm high it's time for them to be 'earthed up'. With the No-Dig approach you simply spread compost, grass clippings, straw or hay (or all these) around each plant, without covering the leaves. Do this at least twice as they grow.

8. If there's any danger of frost, cover Potato plants over with a layer of straw (or proprietary 'fleece', real sheep fleece, bubblewrap etc) overnight to keep them warm.

9. Harvest is easy and Potatoes will come out fairly clean.

MAKING AN OCA BED

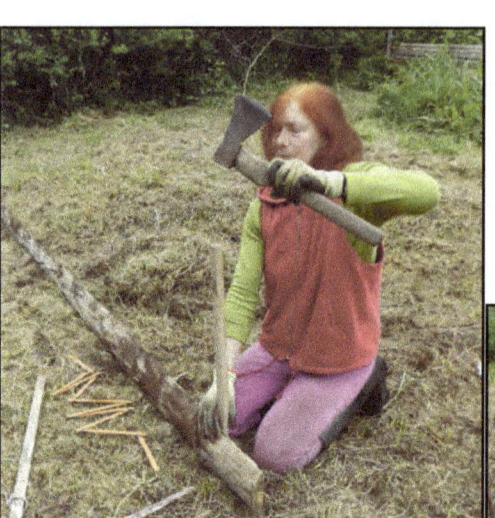

The same technique as just described was used here to make a bed for Ocas, the South American root crop. Starting with the flitch walls, left, then filling the bed with bark, below, and then with Sheet Mulch and planting Ocas into pockets of soil.

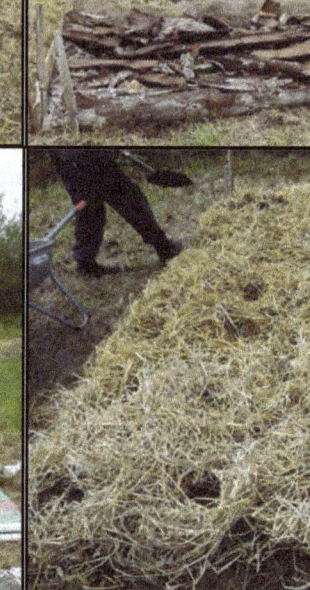

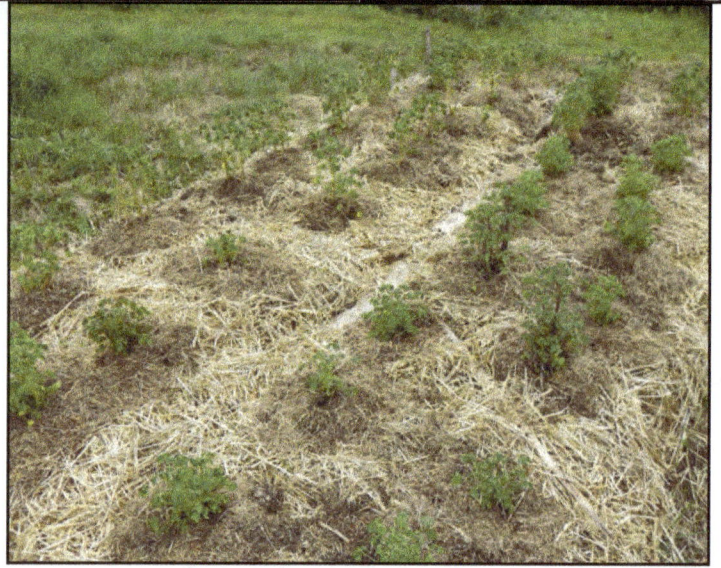

MICROBE POWER

Magnificent living soil in our gardens is what we aspire to. The best fertile soils have a rich microbiota, teeming with zillions of microbes that provide essential food and services to plant life, in a finely honed ecological symbiosis. As long as microbes are provided with minerals and organic matter for their own nourishment, they in turn nourish plants in ways that are only just beginning to be appreciated by scientists.

In times past people discovered how to culture beneficial microbes for adding to soil and enhancing the growth of crops. Rudolph Steiner observed traditional methods and went on to devise a way to culture microbes under ideal conditions. He suggested that Cow manure could be stuffed into Cow horns and buried underground over winter to ferment. The result, known as '500', is a bacterially charged elixir for the land when sprayed over it in highly diluted form on a 'soft' (damp) day.

Scientists of Steiner's day were dubious of the merits of such elixirs as 500. They knew nothing about microbes. The emerging Biodynamic farming movement however was able to enlist people who could see the benefits of this system in plain sight. They quietly got on with adopting and developing the techniques of Biodynamic farming, which is able to consistently produce the best quality food in the market.

Meanwhile, in the more material world, microbes have had a bad press generally. From around the 1950s people were bombarded with advertising that demonised 'germs' and extolled the virtues of 'germ' killing products such that it became instilled into our general thinking about health and hygiene. But it was just propaganda for profit.

The reality is that microbes are essential to life. Our own bodies contain several kilos of microbes and these are essential to health and wellbeing, especially the two kilos of them in our guts. When people take antibiotics it's a genocide on our gutbiota and can lead to serious health consequences if they are not replaced.

Aerobic bacteria, thriving in an Oxygen rich environment are typically considered the 'good guys' of the microbe world. Anaerobic, sour smelling ones from a low Oxygen environment, are all 'bad guys', so we were led to believe. When I was trained to be a teacher of composting we were told it was a no-no to have anaerobic conditions in a compost heap. However life is never so simple.

BOKASHI MICROBES

Along came Japanese agricultural scientist Dr Teruo Higa, creator of 'Effective Microrganisms' (EM). His new and vital observation was that there are aerobic and anaerobic microbes which can work together beneficially for many applications. He developed EM as an unique, balanced blend of eighty different microbes from nature, in five families that work synergetically together and are pathogen and disease suppressing. These five families are the photosynthetic and lactic acid bacteria, fungi, yeasts, and actinomycetes. It turned out to be ideal for composting kitchen waste and even worked a treat on municipal waste on a large scale. Added to my own compost heaps, I've seen it speed up the maturing process dramatically. The process of culturing Bokashi compost is actually more akin to fermenting, the pickling of vegetables, than your average composting process.

EM has many uses, including -

* Producing higher quality food
* Purification of soil and water
* Odour reduction for livestock
* House cleaning products
* Improved animal health
* Repelling insects
* Medical and cosmetic uses
* In clothing, building materials, paints.
(There is even an EM hotel in Japan!)

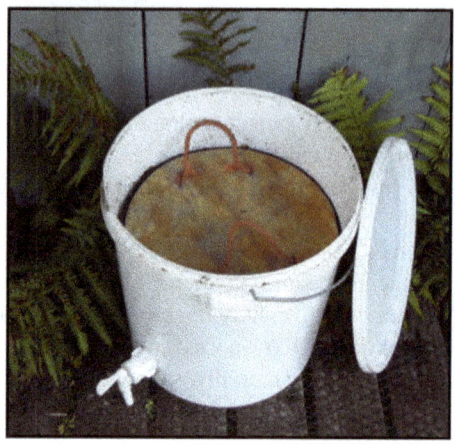

INDIGENOUS MICROORGANISMS IN KOREA

Meanwhile in Korea, Natural Farmers culture their own indigenous microorganisms on cooked Rice, in a do-it-yourself version of EM that's based on centuries old practises in Asia. The techniques hinge on indigenous biology and local inputs. Founder Cho Han-kyu was concerned about the lack of new farmers in South Korea and, as a student, he rejected the hype of so-called Green Revolution technologies as irrelevant for Asia. So, from the mid 1960's he took it upon himself to study the best forms of natural, traditional Asian agriculture and compiled them into the system he called Korean Natural Farming.

The KNF system relies solely on local inputs as much as possible, making it low cost, thus environmentally as well as economically sustainable. It proved superior to Green Revolution strategies, upsetting the powers that be and even landing Cho in gaol several times.

The key ingredient in the system is Indigenous Microorganism #1, IMO1, which is cultured in a natural forested area plus a range of other environments, being mixed together for a good diversity of microorganisms. IMO1 is cultured up to the equivalent of EM's Bokashi, and then again into a super compost that's directly applied to the planting area.

A range of other KNF fermented soil additives are described in a South Asia Rural Reconstruction Association publication[1], along with the way to make them from easily acquired ingredients. This is freely available online. The main training place is Dr Cho's centre at Janong, the Global Natural Farming Living School and Reseach Institute, South Korea.

**Dr. Cho has been reverently referred to as belonging to
"the pantheon of post-modern Krishi Rishis
[saints or sages of post-modern agriculture]
and he is ranked with Masanobu Fukuoka,
Rudolf Steiner and Bill Mollison".**

1. Dr. Cho's Global Natural Farming, Rohini Reddy, South Asia Rural Reconstruction Association, Karnataka, India, 2011, a free pdf download online.

GARBAGE ENZYMES

While I'm happy to use EM in my garden, one needs to buy in the starter culture of EM bran for making the Bokashi. It's not so easy to make your own microbe starter and proprietary secrecy of other commercial versions may prevail. Not so the exponents of 'Garbage Enzymes', as I discovered in Malaysia, where my friends make this type of ferment at home. Garbage Enzyme was developed in Thailand by scientist Dr Rosukon, who was involved in enzyme research and promotion of its benefits for home and planet for over thirty years. It's another way of dealing with kitchen scraps, ideally just fruit (citrus is perfect) and vegetables.

Waste fruit and veggies are packed into an airtight container and left to ferment for three to six months in water with added sugar. Dark, never white, sugar is used in a ratio of ten parts to one, e.g. 10 lt water to 1 kg sugar, into this mix you add three parts of kitchen scraps. The container needs to be 'burped' (gases released) daily for the first month, or you might use the lid taps from home brewing suppliers.

The product of this fermentation process has a multitude of handy uses around the home and garden, due to it's anti-bacterial, anti-viral and deodorising effects - from house cleaning, adding to bath, shampoo and washing water, for air and water purification, cleaning drain pipes, and as a plant fertiliser (diluted 1000 to 1 in water) and pest repellant.[1] But it hasn't caught on in the West, perhaps due to names such as 'Garbage Enzyme Shampoo' being not so appealing?

Dead, barren ground can be brought back to life, its proponents say, when land is constantly watered with Garbage Enzyme solution for three months. (This may take longer in a cooler climate.) There have been some controversial claims, such as the ability to clean up ex-mining land polluted with heavy metals, via improved plant growth.[2] Try it yourself and see.

1. Garbage Enzymes, Pertubuhan Sudarshan Kriya Pulau Pinang, blog at http://enzymesos.blogspot.com
2. Effects of Garbage Enzyme on the Heavy Metal Contents and the Growth of Castor under Mine Tailings, Guangxu Zhu et al 2020 IOP Conf. Ser.: Earth Environ. Sci. 474 022010

FOOD GROWING AND CLIMATE CHANGE

Food growing at home is a great way to reduce one's Carbon/energy footprint and help protect the climate globally. Meanwhile, chaotic climate events have become the new norm and are worsening. We have to adapt to an already changed world, as we anticipate more weather that's 'promised bad'.

Australia has one of the most erratic of climates, with swinging extremes of drought and wildfires followed by floods being typical. I always planned for the worst conditions for growing. This meant investing in shade cloth and trellising, to shelter tender plants from fierce summer sunlight with no ozone to filter it. With the high evaporation rates of summer, I learned ways to keep plants well hydrated without having to water them constantly. Some of those techniques I later found useful in Ireland, where I grow many food crops under large plastic tunnels (called 'polytunnels' here) that extend the growing season with increased warmth.

Climates are never static and we are lucky to live in an Inter-Glacial period. Climate Change has been a cyclic occurrence and in Ireland over the past few millennia it resulted in huge population shifts and adaptations. In the mid Bronze Age, the fertile Ceidie Fields of north Mayo, farmed since Neolithic times, started to get massive amounts of rain. The fields were abandoned and over a long wet period peat bogs developed that completely covered them over. Some 3m of peat, representing 3,000 years of bog growing, lay on top of stone field walls and the foundations of buildings. These came to light again when turf cutters uncovered them, as in the photo below. Previously, a Pine forest grew there and the turf cutters found well preserved Bog Pines under the ground there too, as seen in the museum at the Ceidie Fields.

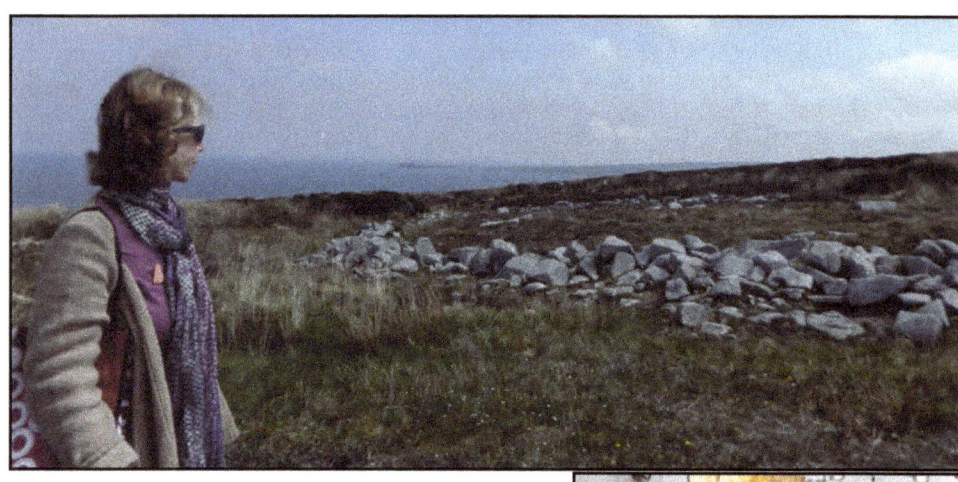

Climate Change scenarios predict more powerful storms in Ireland, indeed, Atlantic hurricanes have been coming ever further north in the last few years, battering the western seaboard. Heavy rain events and droughts have become more common too. Otherwise Ireland is said to be relatively well placed. Then there's also another Ice Age on it's way, while in 2019 NASA warned of an approaching Grand Solar Minimum period, starting 2020, which will be the weakest solar cycle in two hundred years. The last time this happened, Earth experienced the forty year 'Dalton Minimum', with dangerously cold weather, disastrous crop losses, starvation and volcanic eruptions.

Certainly there has been much global volcanic activity since then. Fallout from volcanoes can be very toxic. The same with nuclear fall-out, such as what blanketed Europe after the Chernobyl nuclear power plant meltdown. Some gardens have to contend with polluted, acid rain as a constant threat too. So, protected cropping is the way to go in these times.

POLYTUNNEL FOOD FOREST

A polytunnel (or equivalent) is a great pleasure to work in, a warm sheltered environment amidst the beauty of lush vegetation. I'm often singing or writing in there, escaped from the four walls and artificial lighting of home. I love my polytunnel and my plants grow well in it. It's a tunnel that grows with love!

After having a single large polytunnel for a couple of years I decided I needed another one. My new, second hand, tunnel (below) is for serious annual vegetable growing and and maximum production. The original one is now more of a place to relax, with a table and chair under the shady canopy of warmth loving fruit trees and flowers all around me to delight the senses.

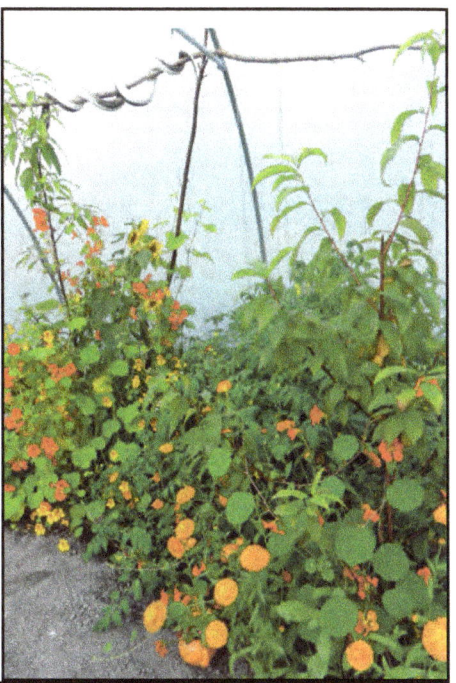

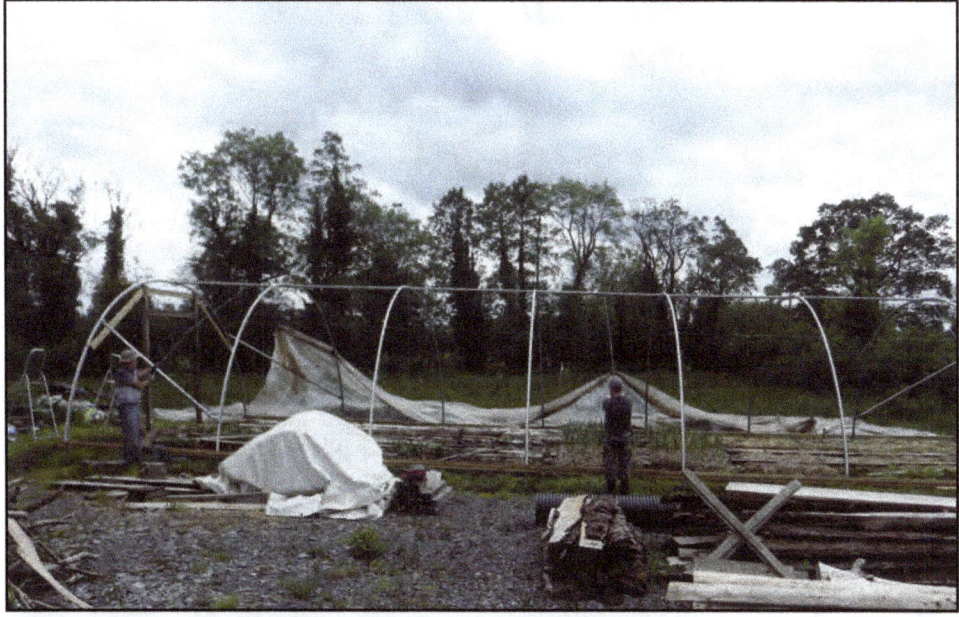

Creating a Polytunnel Food Forest in the first tunnel is a truly delightful project. I'm replacing annual plants with more fruit trees, ones that are a bit frost tender and grow on dwarfing rootstocks. I'm also sourcing perennial edible ground cover plants that can handle some shade. With the addition of my neighbour's horse poo to fertilise, it has quickly become an edible jungle! Grapes and Squash vines twine around the tops of fruit trees and tangle through them. Early salad crops beneath the trees thrive before being shaded by leaves in late spring. It's my own little Garden of Eden, where it never rains and never a cold wind.

FRUIT FOR THE POLYTUNNEL FOOD FOREST

Apricot
Blueberry
Cherry
Chilli
Fig
Gojiberry
Goldenberry
Grapes
Mulberry
Nectarine
Peach
Strawberry

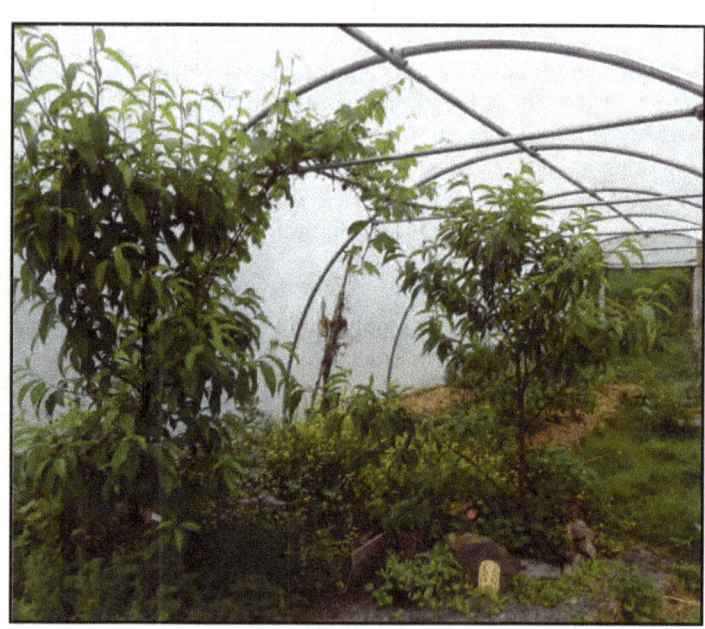

ANNUALS FOR THE POLYTUNNEL

Asian greens
Broad Beans
Chicory
Corn Salad
Cucumber
Endive
French Beans
Garlic
Leaf Celery
Lettuce
Kale
Melons
Mizuna
Onions
Parsley
Peas
Peppers
Quinoa
Spinach
Squash
Tomato
Winter Purslane
Watercress

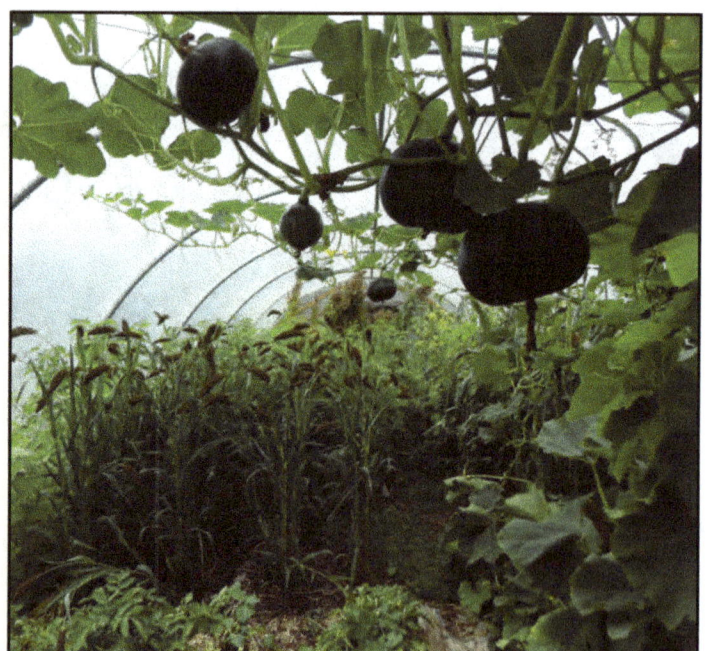

Above - Young Peach trees and Grape vines.
Below - Foxtail Millet on left and above it Hokkaido Squash grows prolifically throughout the polytunnel.

PERENNIALS FOR THE POLYTUNNEL

Good King Henry
Hyssop
Ice plant
Lavender
Mashua
Mitsuba
Rosemary
Sage
Stridolo
Sorrel
Tetragonia
Winter Savoury

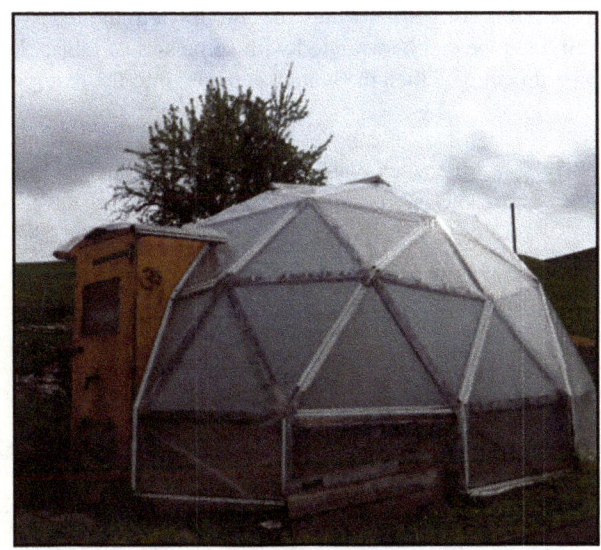

Above - If you don't like the straight lines of a polytunnel, there's always the geodesic version, such as this one in Switzerland.

WICKING BEDS AND BUCKET GARDENING

For many people, the obstacles to veggie growing seem too great to warrant an attempt. Many have limited outdoor space, or are in temporary accommodation, and can only dream of growing fresh herbs and veggies. Not everyone wants to be a slave to a garden, doing daily watering when summer weekends or holidays away are beckoning. Witnessing marauding Slugs destroying crops could also make you give up. So a resilient growing system is a must, if you want a stress-free food growing system.

There is a solution. Retired Australian water scientist Colin Austin invented the Wicking Bed system. His motivation was to find a way of conserving water on a dry continent, where evaporation from intense heat quickly dries up the moisture from any precipitation or watering. In the mild Irish climate it would seem unnecessary. But we have had droughts that saw most of summer without rain, such as in 2018. And the very dry conditions of polytunnels and other covered areas means that this solution has universal merit. Wicking Beds may only need to be watered once a week, they can also have automated watering systems incorporated. Certainly the plants grow lushly this way and though it sounds unnatural, they do love it!

The usual method is to lay a sheet plastic liner in a hole in the ground before backfilling it with soil, creating a reservoir of water under plants that overflows at some point so they don't become waterlogged. The theory goes that plants prefer to get water from below, rather than being sprinkled from above. (The potential for fungal outbreaks on leaves is reduced too.) Rising from below, water naturally wicks its way upwards through the soil to nourish plants. At first some overhead watering is needed to get them started, but after roots have grown there is much less watering to do.

To enhance water delivery in a large Wicking Bed it's common for a slotted (drainage) pipe to be put it, for getting water straight down to the reservoir. To stop it from clogging up with soil, the pipe can be wrapped with some sort of fabric, like a big sock. So a hose can fill the pipe up quickly, then the water seeps out into the reservoir.

Below - A Wicking Bed experiment made in Dunolly, Australia, it takes grey water from kitchen and bathroom basins into old bath tub beds, planted with Canna Lillies and Mint.

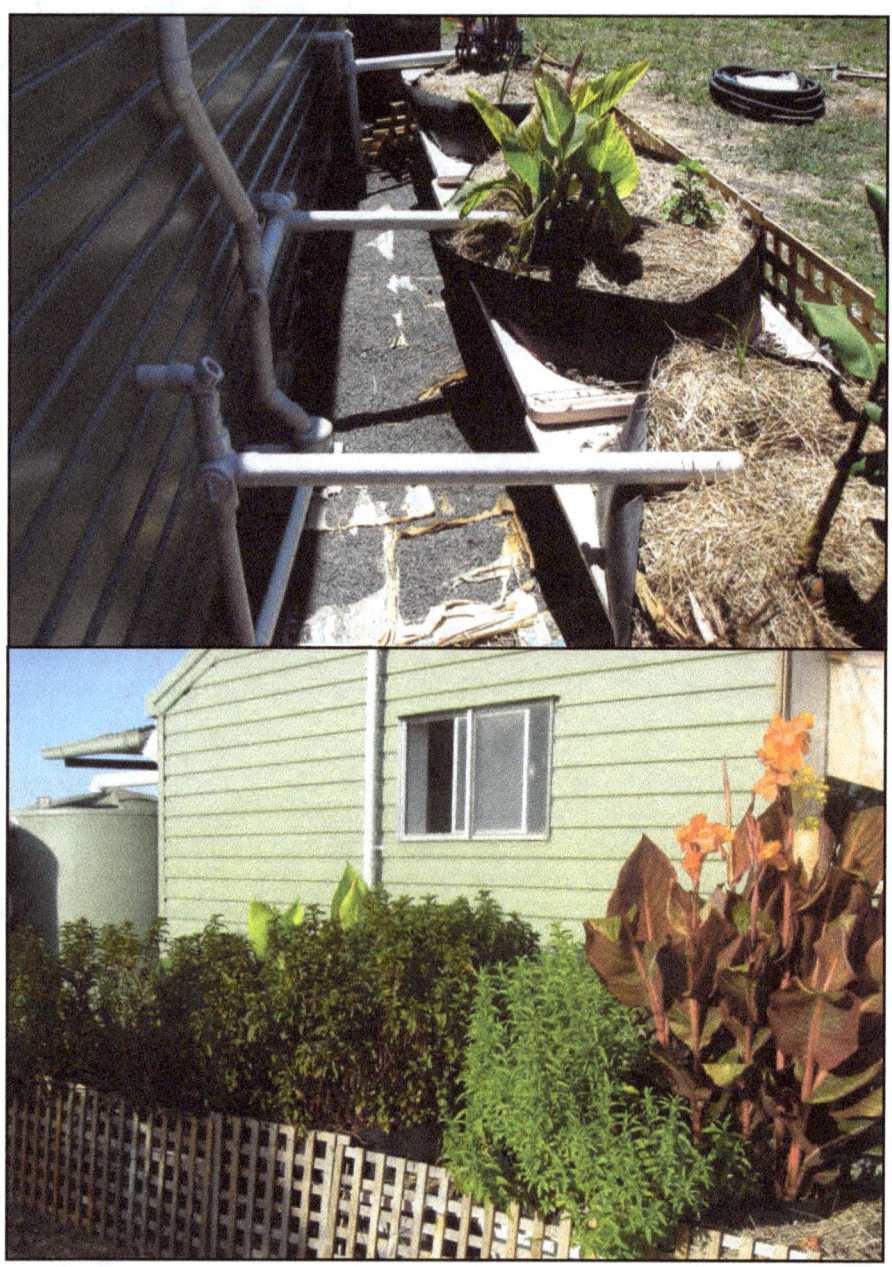

MAKING WATER WICK

You would think this simple growing technology would be fool-proof. But no, somewhere along the way the basic lesson of water wicking in the soil was lost. I have conversed with Colin Austin about this. (Actually, his approach has changed focus onto more larger scale food production and installing electric pumps to stop water stagnation in beds.)

Perhaps people have not taken up Wicking Beds as much as they could have, because of the major mistake of understanding. People were going online and seeing it done incorrectly and copying that. Basically, they were using gravel or small rocks in the water reservoir. Colin had advocated putting straw, dry grass or just soil at the bottom, because this allows water to wick upwards through soil capillaries towards the roots of plants. Rocks have the opposite function - they drain water away. (They are also very heavy!) To make this clear, an experiment was set up. Two Wicking Bed mini gardens were made in two glass aquariums, one with rocks, the other with straw at the bottom. You could see what was happening through the glass. The bed with rocks did not have a wicking effect and the soil dried out. But the bed with the straw did had moisture wicking upwards.

WICKING BUCKET GARDENS

For people who don't have gardens but still want to grow some food, a small portable bed system is the go. A Wicking Bucket garden works on the same principle as the Wicking Bed. I like to re-use food grade buckets sourced from a restaurant, this also reduces waste. Such buckets kick-started my Irish gardening adventure over ten years ago. The outcome was luscious! It worked perfectly for crops of green leaves for salads and stir fries, and Strawberries also thrive in them. It's amazing what can be grown in a 15 litre bucket!

Frost tender plants in Wicking Buckets are moved into warmer places when necessary. Buckets with greens ready to pick are moved closer to the kitchen. Seeds can be sown directly into fine compost and a piece of glass or clear plastic put over the top of the bucket to keep them warm. After harvest, buckets are tipped over, emptied and refreshed with new soil or compost.

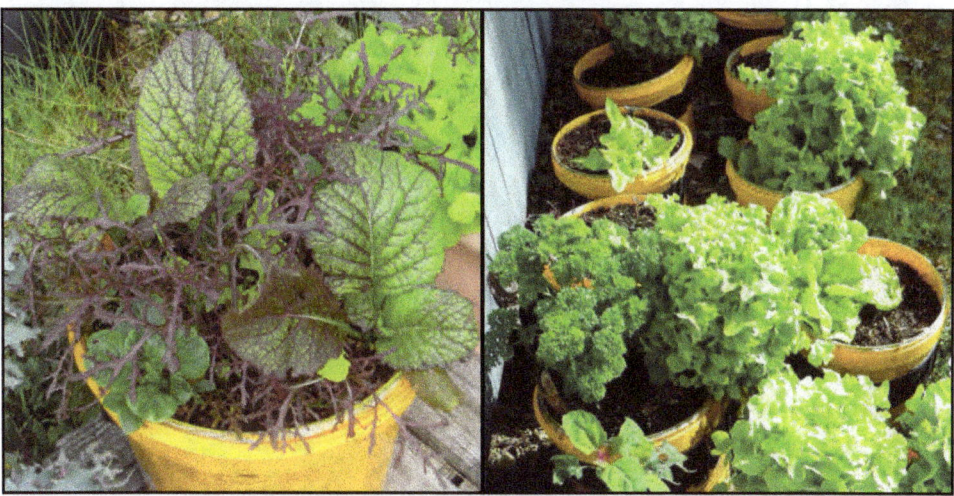

So, here's the simple basics of how I make Wicking Bucket gardens.

1. Drill several small holes into the sides of 15 litre buckets at a level that's about 5-7 cm/2" - 3" from the bottom. Big enough for a nail to poke through, so if they get clogged up you can poke them clear. This allows for overflowing of the water reservoir, so your plants don't drown on a wet day if outdoors. When watering, you'll know the reservoir is full when you see water coming out of the holes.

2. Pack the bottom of the bucket with fresh straw or dry grass to just above the level of the holes, to help stop soil from clogging them up. (Many people use a piece of woven shade cloth or old fabric to separate the straw from the soil. But it isn't necessary and less plastic is the go!)

3. Now you can fill the rest of the bucket with good topsoil or compost. Fill it to the very top then bang the bucket (gently) on the ground a few times to allow the materials to settle down. Be aware that most small veggie plants need only some 15 cm of soil to thrive. If you don't have much soil, put more straw in the bottom.

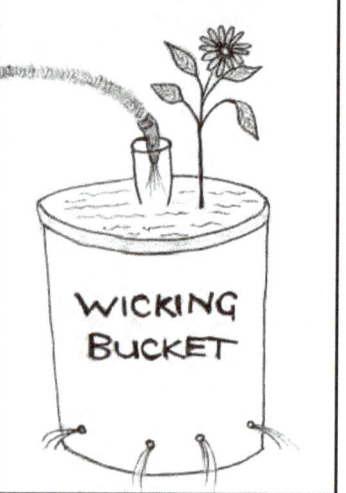

4. Find a good sunny site for the buckets. Ideally on a deck or flat ground. If not a level site, check the level with and adjust. This way your water reservoir will work best.

5. Plant out with a few young veggie plants or sow seed in a fine compost layer on top. Water them frequently for the first week or two. You might want to insert an upturned plastic drink bottle with the end removed into the bucket soil. A hose can be inserted into it to deliver water more directly to the reservoir.

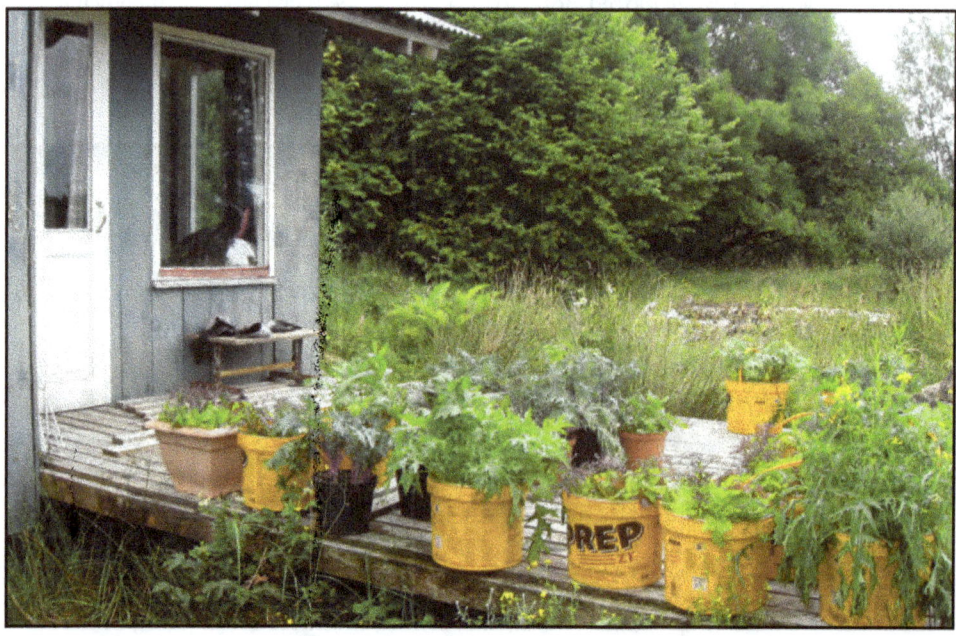

6. Liquid fertilise plants regularly.

7. Repeat with another bucket every two weeks or so, for an ongoing supply of fresh greens.

8. If Slugs do find their way into the bucket plants, find out where they are coming from. Make sure there's no vegetation overhanging that Slugs might slide down onto your greens from. Commercially available anti-Slug Copper tape can be attached around the bucket. Slugs get a nasty shock on contact with it and are deterred. However, it has to be kept clean, as they'll glide obliviously over dirty ones.

STRAWBERRY BUCKETS

Strawberries dangle juicily over the sides of Wicking Buckets, well above Slug level. You will harvest more than ever with this system and they will be clean and easily picked!

Cropping inside the polytunnel over summer, plants are protected from bird predation and damp. When the fruiting season is finished, Strawberry buckets go outside for the rest of the year, until January or February. Returning to the tunnel then they get a makeover, as seen left.

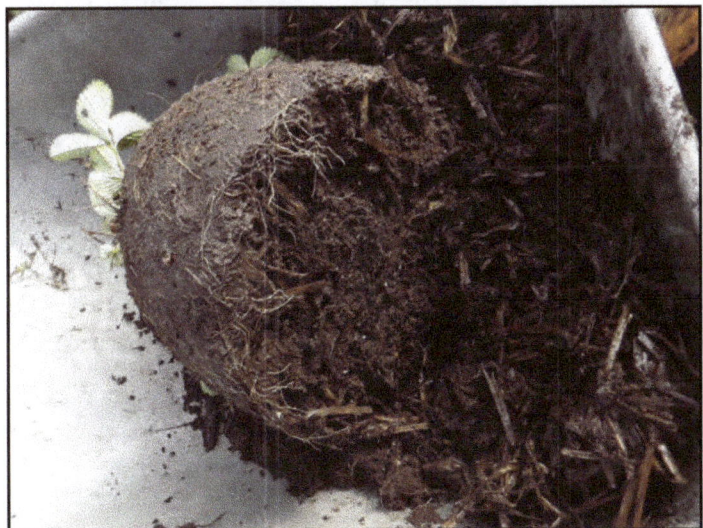

Dead and sick leaves are pruned off, the bottom straw layer is refreshed, the old soil ditched and new soil and compost added. Plants are returned to the buckets and compost is tucked around them.

It's the best way to grow abundant Strawberries that I've ever used!

IMPROVED WICKING GARDENING

Colin Austin grappled with the problem of water stagnation in Wicking Bed reservoirs, deciding that installing electric pumps was the way to deal with it. I suggested he look into EM, because these microbes would thrive in the anaerobic environment. Diluted Bokashi liquid could be added when watering, to keep the system in good health. Others have also thought of this solution. An online search found a practitioner of the art, Brett Prichard, a Permaculturist in tropical Queensland, who wrote in a 2016 blog discussion about his 'Biowicked' beds that he calls 'urban Carbon sinks'.

"I call them Biowicked beds, as opposed to Wicking Beds, as a mix of water plus nutrients plus beneficial bacteria wick up from the saturated anaerobic zone, while only water wicks up from conventional Wicking Beds as you strive to keep this reservoir layer inert to avoid Methane.….This turns what is normally a problem (anaerobic soil going sour) into a solution. I have been trialling these socked-slotted-pipe/soil only/Bokashi Wicking Beds for a year now and the growth rates are better than standard Wicking Beds. They are also a lot quicker and easier to build, and in addition to keeping the bacteria healthy, the Bokashi provides all necessary nutrients for plant growth".

When watering such beds with EM it's important to avoid tap water with Chlorine, designed to kill the microbes. Ideally use rain or spring water.

GARDENING FOR BIODIVERSITY

> "We must restore biodiversity… We must re-wild the world."
>
> **Sir David Attenborough, 2020.**

The Irish government has declared a biodiversity emergency because we are in an era of the 'sixth mass extinction', due to all the environmental degradation, including from conventional farming, which can be deadly to insects. Meanwhile, there are over two million domestic gardens in Ireland, covering some 360,000 acres. Much can be done in one's backyard to redress this problem. Some 70% of our food crops rely on pollinating insects, so choosing pollinator-friendly plants for our gardens is a must. Useful and edible plants such as Lavender, Comfrey, Rosemary, Dandelion and Borage are great for insects. However, many other common garden plants, such as Daffodils, Tulips, Geraniums and Petunias, have virtually no pollen or nectar, so are much less insect-friendly. [1]

Garden plants that birds love to feed on include Evening Primrose, Honeysuckle and Sunflowers. The Ivy that covers so many trees is also high value for birds. Robins, Blackcaps and Thrush love to eat Ivy berries in winter, when little else food is around. Ivy also provides dense cover for nesting birds in spring. I do remove the Ivy that's strangling trees in my gardens, but I only cut Ivy that's growing on the south side of the land, which reduces shading. I leave the Ivy growing on the north side for nature.

1. Juanita Browne, Irish Examiner, https://laois.ie/gardening-for-biodiversity

FLOWER MEADOWS

Lawns have been called a 'totalitarian regime' forced on nature. They are a sterile desert for wildlife. But this can be reversed. Lawns and road verges can be transformed into wildflower meadows. It can be difficult to get wildflowers to establish in a monoculture of grass. But with a regime of mowing the lawn at certain times you can create a flower-rich meadow. Mow the grass first after the middle of April, then at the end of May, the third cut in mid to late July, the fourth cut at the end of August and the last cut after mid-October. This allows various wildflower species to move in and flower and seed naturally, and thus provide food for wildlife. When mowing the flower meadow, it's good to remove all the grass clippings, as wildflowers prefer an infertile soil. Mulch your trees and food plants with the clippings.

You can also start from scratch with wildflower seeds, but they are best sown into a good seedbed, so you might have to first cover the lawn with a sheet of silage plastic for a few months to kill it. Collecting local flower seed is better than buying in seed from elsewhere. Starting with seeds of Yellow Rattle is a good idea, as it acts as a pioneer, reducing grass domination and paving the way for more diverse plants to grow there. No wonder it's nickname is 'Meadow Maker'.

Bug hotels can be placed in sunny, dry places. A number of small ones is better than one big one. A bare section of south or east-facing bank makes an ideal nest site for solitary Mining Bees, if you keep vegetation away from it. In a wild corner of the garden where Nettles can grow undisturbed, these can sustain various butterfly species, providing food for caterpillars. A pile of logs left to moulder in the wild corner is heavenly for bugs too, as is a compost heap.

NATIVE TREES

If you want to feed wild birds naturally, plant native trees and let them feast on Hawthorn and Blackthorn berries, which are also enjoyed by Wood Mice and Foxes. Hazelnuts and Rowan, Guelder Rose, Spindle, Bird and Wild Cherry, Crab Apples, Whitebeam, Yew and Holly berries are also relished by birds. Willow trees are very popular with wildlife and are said to support two hundred and fifty insect species, especially the Goat or Grey Willow that has lots of pollen and nectar when in flower. Oak trees support over two hundred insect species.

A small garden pond is another must. It will invite a wide range of wildlife, including beautiful Damselflies and Dragonflies, Frogs and Newts, which live mostly on the land but need to return to water to breed. Just don't add fish, because they will eat their eggs.

HEDGEROWS

Fly over north western Europe in late summertime and you'll see vast swathes of golden grain crops, huge monocultures of uniformity. Nothing much green breaks the scene. Fly over western Ireland and the contrast couldn't be greater. It's a higgly piggly chequerboard of hedgerows enclosing small to tiny fields, a glorious geometry that often preserves evidence of ancient roads, 'ringfort' homesteads and stone monuments.

Hedgerows, of which there are some 300,000 km existent in Ireland, were developed as living fences to keep livestock enclosed and more protected from wind and rain. People didn't have money to buy fencing materials and timber wasn't available. In the hey day of hedgerows there were no other farmland trees left to offer animals shelter, with forests reduced to only 1% of Ireland's landmass.

Hedgerows were mostly planted in the 18th and 19th centuries, following parliamentary acts pushing for the enclosure of lands by making permanent boundaries. Hedgerows growing along townland boundaries often date from medieval times or earlier and are particularly important from a cultural/historical perspective, says heritage body Teagsc.[1]

1. https://www.irishtimes.com/news/environment/ireland-s-historic-hedgerows-the-essential-corridors-of-nature-1.3471425

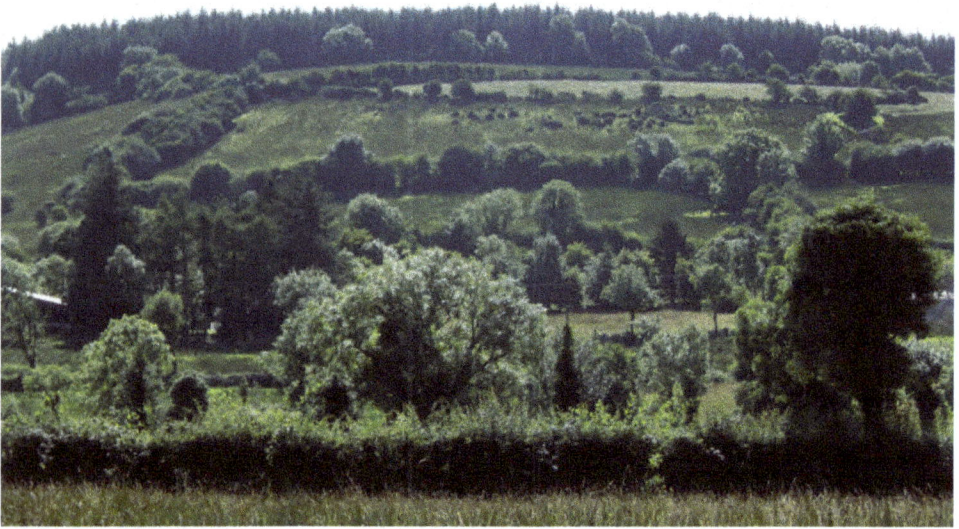

WILDLIFE VALUES

Hedgerows are living fences that provide healthy treats for browsing Cows, Sheep and Goats who, when feeling ill, will naturally seek out healing herbs.[1] Hedgerows are important for wildlife too, as homes, nest sites, larders and thoroughfares. Criss crossing the landscape, they are vital for animal movements, helping to ensure genetic diversity. Preferring not to cross open fields to avoid predators, small birds, bats and butterflies travel along hedgerows; while Barn Owls hunt along them at night, looking for prey, such as Field Mice.

Typically planted with prickly thorn bushes such as Haws and Sloes, they made effective animal barriers, that also produced berries for wildlife. Birds visiting to feast on them deposited various seeds into the hedgerows and so these green ribbons became a biodiverse refuge for nature, in otherwise bare grassy landscapes.

1. Herbal Handbook for Farm and Garden, Juliette de Bairacli-Levy, Farrar, Straus & Giroux, 1991, UK.

WILD FORAGING

Not just an asset for the environment, people went to hedgerows to forage for edible flowers, leaves and berries, craft wood, medicines and other useful wild crops that have been eaten since Neolithic times. In nearby Drumshanbo town there used to be a jam factory for which local people would go out picking the wild Raspberries and Blackberries along the hedgerows, receiving much needed cash for them. Nowadays the berries growing on roadside hedgerows get slashed off by huge tractors well before they ripen, so nothing gets to eat them.

The food foraging potential of hedgerows has been largely forgotten about in our 'age of convenience'. There are laws to protect them and penalties for removing them, but no recognition that hedgerows can be as important to people as well as wildlife, contributing to human food security. Recently a study by John de Montfort looked at the potential economic value of a hedgerow growing on someone's land. The study looked at how products from the hedgerow could be used to replace bought in items, such as vinegar made from wild windfall apples. There can also be financial profit from selling value-added products, with hand made goods being ideal for bartering too.[1]

Montfort calculated a potential annual benefit of over €5000 from 100m of hedgerow! Products that could be sold include berry jams, Hops flowers for beer and decoration, medicinal herb teas and cosmetics, Elderberry cordial and cooking wines, Hazel poles and other coppice woods; plus there are the pollination services provided from hedgerow trees, the shelter and soil improvement that hedgerows might bring to nearby crops, as well as forage for livestock.

Realising more of the true value of hedgerows, we might consider them in Permaculture terms as a sort of linear Food Forest that brings multiple benefits to all beings. And with a revival of the old traditional techniques of hedge laying, rather than the usual awful annual trimming that is more like 'hedge-slaying', hedgerows can be conserved all the better.

1. Hedgerows - Suggested Economic Value of 100 metres, John de Montfort, 2019, Ireland, pers. comm.

FOREST GARDENS

> "The Forest Garden is much more than a system to meet the material needs of humans. It's a way of life; it also nourishes our spiritual needs with its beauty and the vitality of wildlife living in it."   Robert Hart.

People often equate Permaculture gardening with Forest Gardens, that are also called Food Forests. The model of a natural forest provides a pivotal blueprint. A forest is "a society of living beings", as tree planting pioneer Richard St. Barbe Baker put it, that share space co-operatively, with plants and animals occupying specific niches. We honour the forest model and emulate the wisdom of nature when we make a Forest Garden.

Like a natural forest, several layers of vegetation grow in a multi-storey Food Forest. To the untrained eye we see perhaps three layers in a forest - the tall trees, the shrubs beneath and the herb layer beneath them. Robert Hart, the first pioneer of their development in the UK who grew over a hundred different species in his Forest Garden, talks about seven layers.[1]

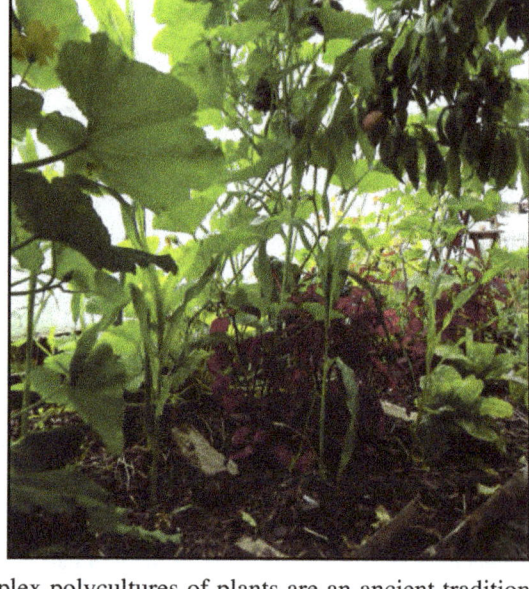

1. Tall fruit and nut trees
2. Smaller fruit and nut trees
3. Shrub layer
4. Herbs and vegetables
5. Ground cover herbs & creepers
6. Root crops in the rhizosphere
7. Vertical layer of climbers

1. Forest Gardening , Robert A de J Hart, Green Earths, UK, 1996.

ORIGINS OF FOOD FORESTRY

Bill Mollison was so inspired by the Forest Gardens he saw in tropical regions that he used the concept in the Permaculture design system. These complex polycultures of plants are an ancient tradition where the verticality of the forest gives a huge increase in diverse harvests. In Java, with its very dense population, rural homes are often surrounded by dense vegetation, looking like the local jungle, but all having been planted for food, medicine and other crops.

Such tropical areas enjoy abundant sun, heat and water. In cooler, temperate regions productive trees are necessarily more spread out, to attain sufficient light and air and reduce the potential for fungal outbreaks. So there are much fewer traditional examples, such as in the south west of Britain, where Plums would be interplanted with Blackcurrants, or the gaps between orchard trees filled with Gooseberry bushes.

DEVELOPING A FOOD FOREST

Usually only perennial plants are selected, unless an annual can sustain itself by self-seeding. Plants with some shade tolerance are ideal, however a fruit crop may be small if it's too shady. With sunshine at a premium in Ireland, it's wise to plant narrow Food Forest belts and Edible Hedgerows, with the tallest trees to the north. This maximises solar exposure, rather than planting a block of trees that will grow to out-shade each other.

The autonomous Forest Garden requires minimal maintenance and the ground is never dug. Falling leaves from the trees provide mineral rich fertiliser, naturally mulching and feeding the top soil. In the formation of a natural forest there is usually a successional factor. Vegetation often evolves into woodland after land has been cleared then allowed to regenerate. Seeds of trees blow in, or are deposited by birds, and pioneer species take hold first. These are short lived, rapid growing tree species, such as Silver Birch and Alders. Fortunately, Ireland has the fastest tree growth rate in Europe.

I planted my woodland in 2016 with mostly Alders (600 of them) plus fifty others of different tree species, into a nearly one acre (3200m^2) field with heavy soil and rushes. Below you see it after six months of growth. It's a perfect habitat for the Alders and they've dried out the wet soil nicely. Having grown rapidly and created a sheltered environment, they are acting as a 'nurse crop', where other plants can get established more easily. The Oak and Monkeypuzzle trees grow much slower, but will get huge eventually and dominate the canopy, at the climax of the succession. When I prune or remove Alders to make room for other trees I can use their wood for fires, while my Pigs love to eat the leaves. Four years after planting, in 2020 I pruned some of the Alders in the sunniest part and started to intensively plant a Food Forest around them, as in the photos overleaf.

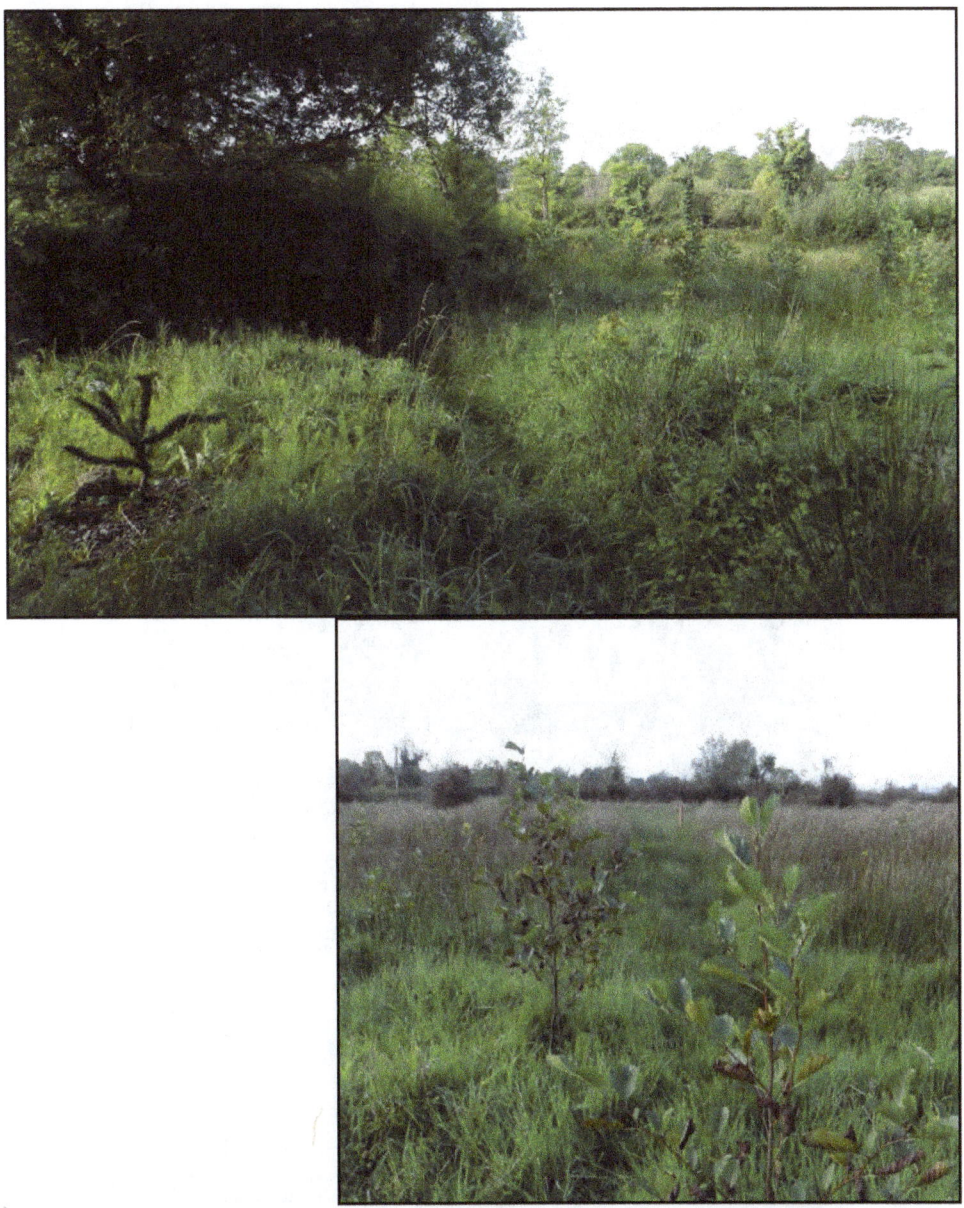

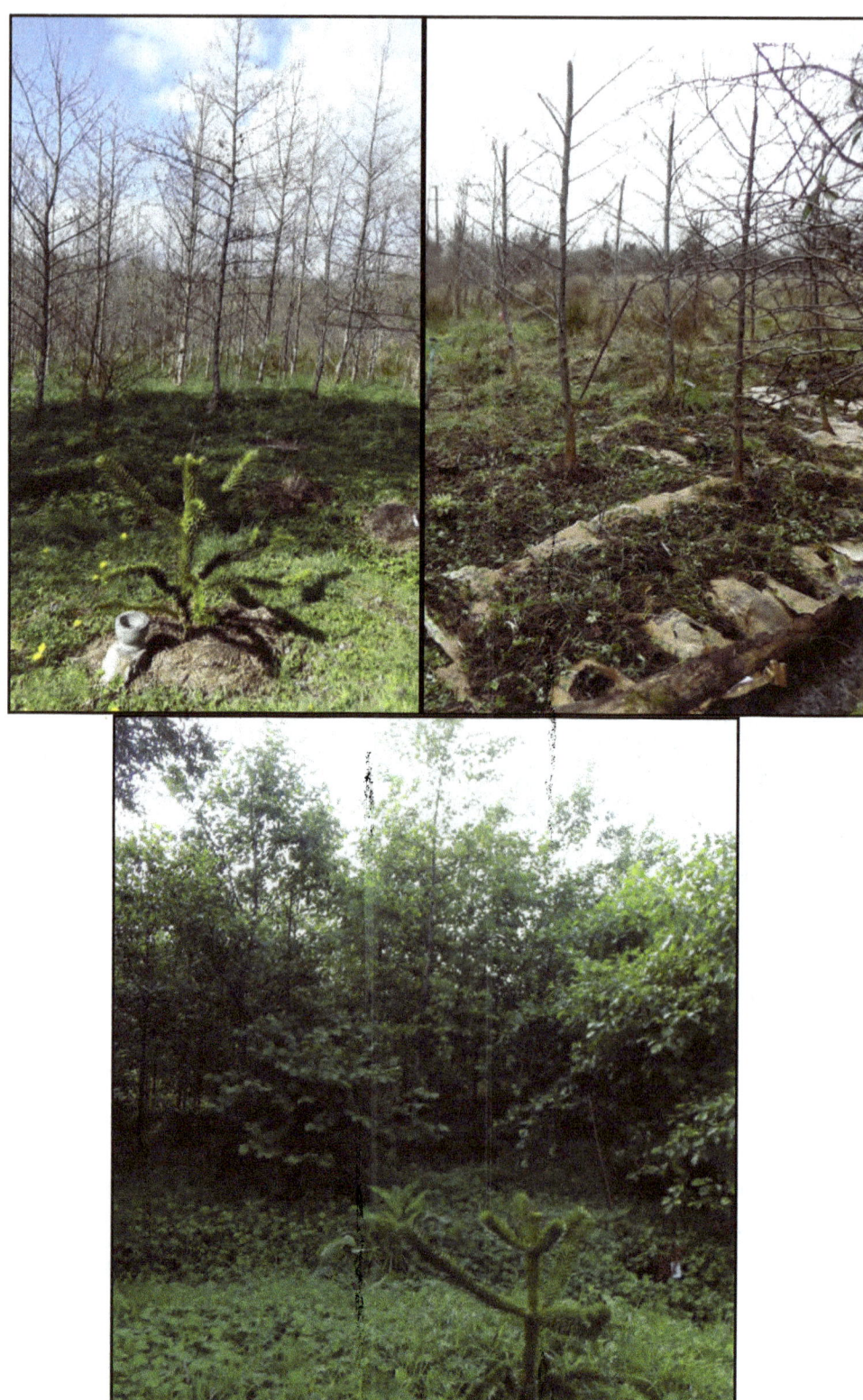

IDEAL TREES AND PLANTS FOR TEMPERATE FOOD FORESTS

1. TALL TREES

These tallest canopy trees can include domesticated varieties of fruit and nuts, those grafted onto the largest rootstocks, Hart suggests; plus seedling trees for genetic variety. However, I would normally grow valuable fruit trees closer to home, rather than in the Food Forest. Being a semi-wild place, I select the tougher, wilder varieties of fruit for planting in my Food Forest.

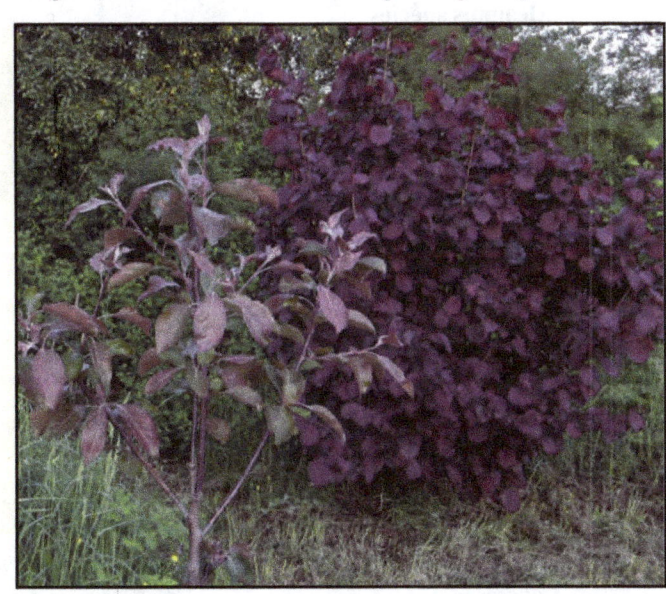

Alder
Apple
Beech
Bullace
Damson
Monkeypuzzle
Oak
Pear
Plum
Serviceberry
Silver Birch
Small Leaved Lime
Spruce

Above - Bakran (Iranian) Apple has red leaves and fruit, Red Hazelnut behind it.
Below - Rowan tree.

2. SMALLER TREES

Fruit and nut trees on dwarfing rootstocks are suggested for this layer. I planted small native trees with edible berries along the edges of paths and clearings of my woodland. Birds will be able to have a good feed and perhaps have less appetite left for my domesticated fruits.

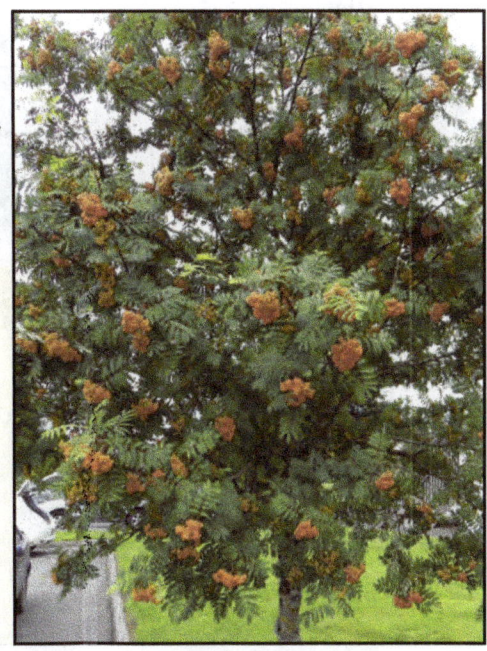

Bamboo
Cherry, Wild & Bird
Cornelian Cherry
Crabapple
Elderberry
Gingko biloba
Hawthorn
Rowan
Strawberry Tree

3. SHRUB LAYER

   Bay
   Berberis species
   Blackberry
   Currants
   Dog Rose (right)
   Eleagnus species
   Gooseberry
   Juneberry
   Juniper
   Mallows
   Raspberry
   Sumac

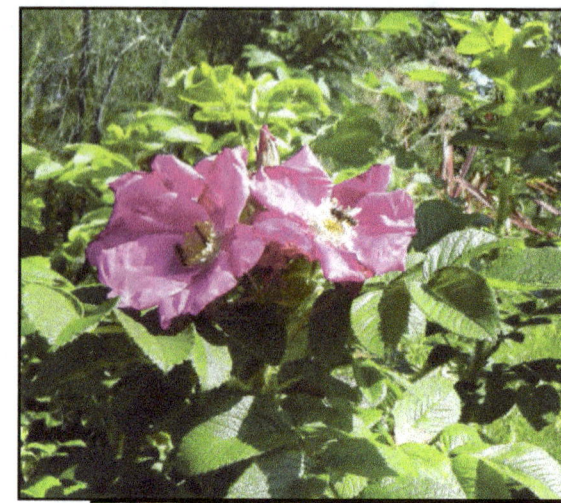

4. PERENNIAL HERBS AND VEGETABLES

   Asparagus
   Chinese Artichoke
   Comfrey
   Day Lilly
   Good King Henry
   Fennel
   Globe Artichoke
   Kale, Daubenton
   Lovage
   Korean Mint
   Marigold
   Mint
   Mitsuba
   Nine Star Broccoli
   Rhubarb
   Sorrel
   Sweet Cicely
   Watercress

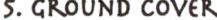

5. GROUND COVER

   Chickweed
   Clover
   Rubus berries
   Sweet Woodruff
   Wild Garlic
   Wild Strawberry

Middle photo - Pineapple Mint
Bottom - Wild Strawberry
groundcover in polytunnel.

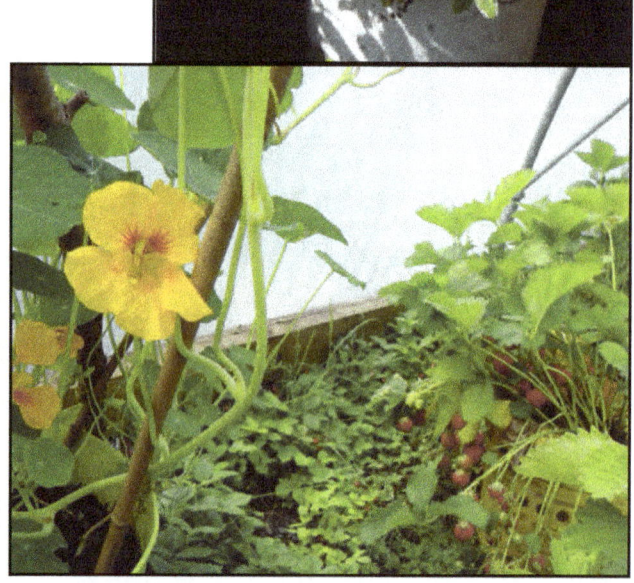

6. RHIZOSPHERE ROOT CROPS

Burdock (right)
Dandelion
Jerusalem Artichoke
Horseradish
Mashua
Maximillian Sunflower
Yacon

7. CLIMBERS

Beans
Honeysuckle
Hops
Nasturtium
Rubus berries
Sweet Woodruff

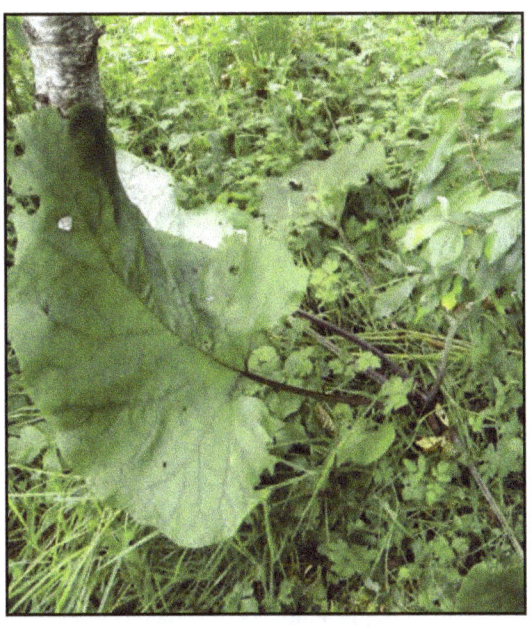

Below - Purple-topped Spinach, right, reaches for the roof of the polytunnel, alongside Celery, Tomatoes, Black Kale, Beans and Corn (top left).

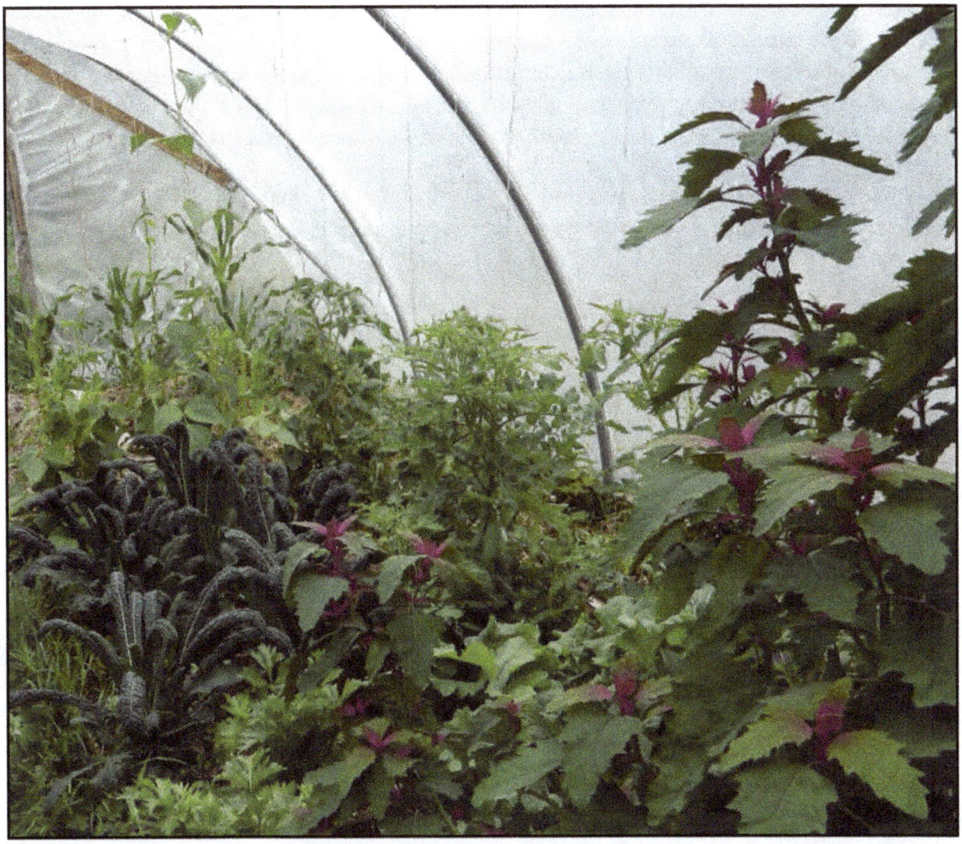

TREES FOR FOOD FORESTS PROFILED

Here's a selection of fabulous trees, mostly Irish or European natives, that are multifunctional, grow well and are easy enough to acquire. Trees that are failing due to diseases, such as Elms, Ash and now some Pine species, are not recommended to be planted, so they don't get much focus, but if you have them, you might as well make good use of them.

ALDER - ALNUS GLUTINOSA
A fast growing, deciduous tree that handles heavy and wet soils. Timber is strong and durable in wet locations (e.g. used for underwater piles of old buildings in Venice), and as firewood it burns with a green tinged flame. Wind resistant, so perfect for a wind break, Alders can be grown as a tall hedge, when planted at 60cm spacing and kept trimmed. Various parts of the tree can be used for dyes, while the bark yields an ink.

Growing to 20m tall and 15m across, Alders are especially vigorous on clay soils. This is one of the best pioneer species to start a woodland with. Mass planted with a scattering of other, slower growing trees around them, Alders nurse a young forest with shelter and leaf mould. They create their own fertility, adding Nitrogen to the soil via bacteria on root nodules that fix Nitrogen from the atmosphere, which is unusual for a non-legume plant.

APPLES, MALUS SPECIES
I rarely see Apple orchards in Irelands, yet they are the easiest fruit trees to grow and tolerate a wider range of soils, climate and aspect than most other fruit trees. Originating from central Asia, there are over 2000 varieties still grown in Britain. So, plenty to select from. In Ireland, heritage fruit trees are available from Danny Gaffey in Co. Leitrim, who says that "Apples are our speciality, and we can offer more than 300 varieties for sale, by far the largest selection of Apple trees for sale in Ireland and perhaps one of the largest in the world".

Below - Winston Apples and Angelica flowers.

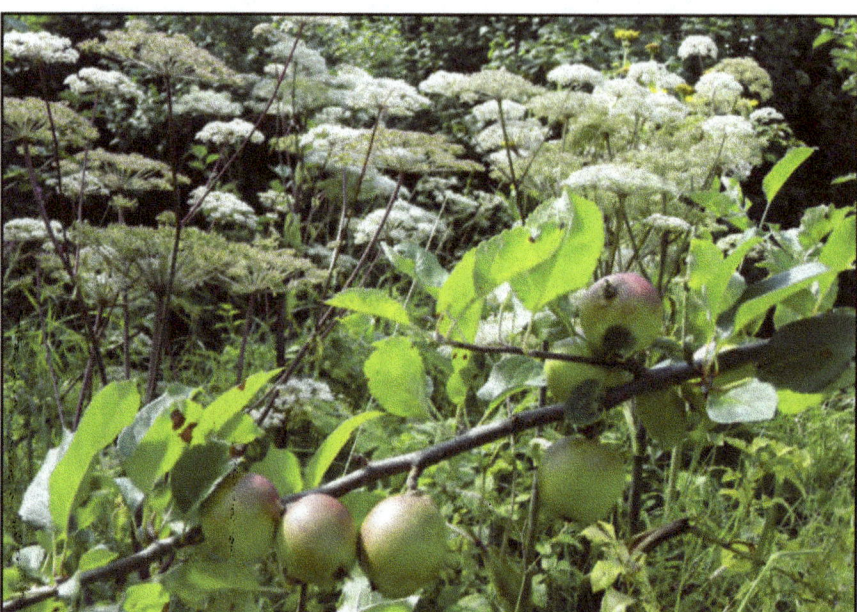

Selecting heritage Apple varieties suited to my area, I go for the hardy ones that thrive in wetter, colder regions and are more resistant to the fungal diseases scab and canker. And with a range of early, mid and late fruiting varieties, the Apple harvest is spread out over several months. (See Danny's tips for fruit tree varieties suited to this region on pages 100-101.) Most Apples are not self-fertile and need pollination partners. This means, for fruit to be produced, at the time of flowering there must be another different variety also flowering. Triploid varieties need two other varieties to be also flowering at the same time.

Apple trees need Bees and other insects for pollination duties as well. If you don't have much space for Apple varieties, consider that your neighbours' trees may partner up, thanks to Bees that travel far and wide, bringing in a range of pollens for cross pollination. Or buy a 'family tree' with compatible varieties grafted onto a single tree. A deep fertile well drained soil is ideal for Apples (and most other fruit trees), but not crucial. If Apples need pruning, it's done when they are dormant, between December and March.

ASH – FRAXINUS EXCELSIOR

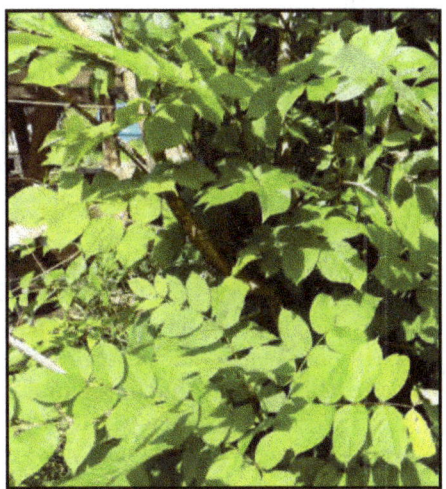

The Ash is a classic tree of Ireland, once the wood of choice for making spear shafts, yokes, furniture and oars by early peoples. Sadly now they are in serious decline in Europe due to disease and are no longer recommended for forestry plantings.

Ash has many uses. Young leaves (seen on the right) can be eaten in salads in early summer. Bark, leaves and seeds have medicinal properties, being diuretic, laxative, helping to loosen uric acid, etc. Seeds strengthen the liver and spleen. The inner bark can be used for bleeding wounds; fresh sap is a disinfectant. People once put Ash leaves inside shoes when their feet were tired.[1]

Ash trees were never allowed to grow near crops, as the hungry roots go far to raid garden fertility.
Around my home they sprout up in hedgerows everywhere but often become smothered in Ivy, which makes them wildlife havens. The dying trees that I've removed make good firewood that burns wet or dry.

BEECH, FAGUS SYLVATICA

A classically beautiful large tree with dense canopy, it can grow to 30m tall and 15m wide, but prefers a freely draining, Limestone or chalky soil. Beech has tasty nuts, which, along with Oak acorns, is traditional Pig fodder ('mast'). However trees only fruit every three or four years. All parts have medicinal use, being mainly used for the astringent, cooling and antiseptic qualities.

Beech leaves, only if very young, are nice to eat in salads and soups. Nuts are protein rich and contain up to 20% oil, which tastes a bit like Olive oil and stores well. The sweet tasting nuts are good in salads or soups, but are small and fiddly to shell. Nuts can be roasted as a coffee substitute drink; or dried, ground and added to flour and cereals. But don't eat too many nuts, as they are toxic if eaten in large amounts).[2]

Leaf tea can be used as a compress for skin problems, while Beech wood ash is used in ointments for sores. Beech Leach is a soapy solution rich in Potassium, good for washing and scrubbing. To make it, soak Beech wood ash overnight in warm water and drain it off for use the next morning.[1] Beech wood is also made into fabrics, I discovered with the purchase of some anti-electro-smog clothing made from 50% Beech wood and 50% Silver.

BLACKTHORN, SEE SLOE

BULLACE, PRUNUS INSTITIA
This thorny shrub with small purple-black, roundish fruits is probably the wild form of the Damson plum. Like the Damson, it handles much worse conditions than other Plums and is relatively trouble free in a soggy, cold climate.

The British Black Bullace has small, acidic, purpley-black fruit and is "virtually a wild fruit" says Ben Pike, who lists it along with varieties Langley and White / Golden.[3] The Black Bullace has heavy crops of acidic fruit in September that are good for jam making. I was able to purchase some Bullace seed by mail order and trees may be available to buy.

CHERRY, PRUNUS DOMESTICA
The Cherry with fruit so sweet and delectable was bred from the much less tasty Wild Cherry (Prunus avium). Sweet varieties, such as Stella, demand drier, brighter and warmer conditions than north west Ireland might provide.

However the sour, cooking varieties, such as Morello, famous for jam making, are much tougher and these were bred from Wild Cherries (Prunus cerasus) in the Black Sea area. Sour Cherries even handle a bit of shade. Old varieties developed in the England's west, such as Mazzards and Tamar Valley Cherries, can handle wet conditions too, but are not so widely available. All have beautiful blossoms.

When a local saw my new Stella Cherry tree and said "That won't do any good!" I hoped to prove him wrong. The tree grew well, but only produced the odd Cherry. Then one day a tour group came that included a man bearing a bag of delicious Cherries grown in a polytunnel. Good idea! I just had to transplant the tree into my own polytunnel while it was dormant. Fortunately, this variety is self-fertile. After being moved in springtime the tree was soon covered with baby fruit. However these were then killed by a series of frosts in May. Better luck next year!

CHERRY, WILD AND **BIRD CHERRY**, PRUNUS AVIUM AND PRUNUS PADUS
The Wild Cherry, often found in Beech woods, grows up to 18m high and 7m wide. A sunny spot with good limey soil is perfect for it. The small Cherry fruits are often a bit bitter, but can be sweet, although the birds may well get to them first.

Bird Cherry, another native, has a similar size to the Wild Cherry. It prefers moister locations but can handle most soils and is ideal for planting on a sunny woodland edge. Fruit is more bitter than P. avium, but is still relished by birds.[4]

CIDER GUM, SEE EUCALPYTUS GUNNI

CORNELIAN CHERRY, CORNUS MAS
A small ornamental tree growing to 5m, it's edible fruit grows to 2cm or more. These days it's mainly valued for the yellow flowers in late winter and early spring. Tolerating most conditions, including wind, it can be kept low by trimming. Seedling trees are slow to produce fruit, but some of the cultivars may be quicker, if you can find some. The fruit can be a bit astringent, especially if not fully ripe, but juicy and Plum-like in flavour. Oil can be extracted from the seeds.

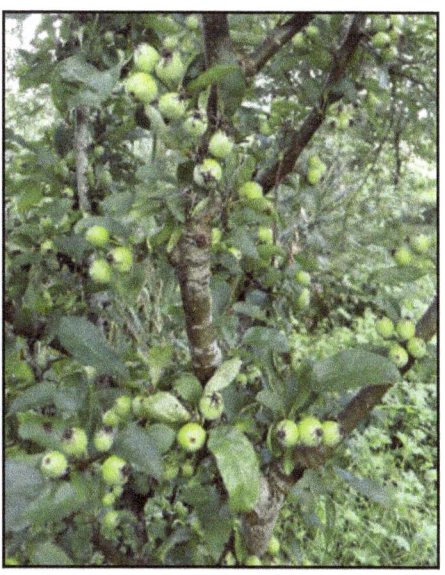

CRAB APPLE - MALUS SYLVESTRIS (seen right)
The native Apple that grows wild on sunny woodland edges and especially in Oak woods, reaching up to 10m in height and 6m across. It can handle most soils, even heavy clays, and is an ancestor of domesticated Apples. The small fruit is edible though rather acid and astringent, however it's great for jams, jellies and juices, and is usually mixed with sweeter fruits. The high pectin content is great for setting jams etc. With many cultivars available, Crabapples are great pollinators in the Apple orchard too, with just one for every twenty Apple trees needed, as they generally flower over a long period. Flowers and fruit can be highly ornamental and are relished by birds.

DAMSON PLUM, PRUNUS INSTITIA
Damsons are closely related to European Plums, but are smaller, tougher and easier to grow. The highly nutritious purpley-blue-black fruit with yellow flesh generally tastes quite sharp with a rich spicy flavour and is usually cooked with added sweetening. Damsons can also be dried to make prunes, other varieties are made into jams, gin, brandy, confectionary and more. Nutritionally, Damsons are rich in Potassium, fibre and vitamins A, C and K, also antioxidants and the amino acid Tryptophan.

Reaching some 3-4m height, Damsons love a sunny aspect and can handle clay soil, though they do prefer good drainage. Self-fertile, they are generally left unpruned, but if you do want to prune them, mid summer is the best time. The most well known varieties, and toughest in exposed locations, are the Merryweather, Shropshire Prune and Farleigh. Merryweather is the commonest and grows large with spreading branches. An early bloomer, its abundant fruit is good to eat raw, unlike most other Damsons. The Shropshire Prune is a more compact tree regarded as the best flavoured of all the Damsons. The Farleigh is also compact, with good tasting, small fruit, but it only crops heavily if cross-pollinated with other varieties.[3]

These 'Plums from Damascus' were probably introduced to the West by the Romans. Succeeding in higher rainfall areas, Damsons were once a big industry in the wetter parts of the UK and are still cultivated commercially on a smaller scale there, but not now in Ireland, though wild ones still persist in old gardens and hedgerows. When cheap sugar became available in Britain (the old slave trade!) Damson jam production became so important that many tenant farmers paid their rent solely with Damsons. Skins also provided an important dye for khaki and blue army and RAF uniforms, hats, gloves, carpets etc. Huge quantities were required and the pulp left over was used for jam making. Synthetic dyes introduced from the mid 18th century ended this. In a few places traditional annual Damson Festivals are still held, such as Damson Day in Cumbria, UK; while in Germany a Damson Queen is annually crowned at the Plum Market in Stromberg, Westphalia. The Italians make traditional Damson and Ricotta Pies, while the Swedes brew Krikonvin, Damson Wine.[5]

ELDERBERRY, SAMBUCUS NIGRA

A short lived, fast growing small tree, Elder flowers and berries have long been used in medicines for respiratory problems, such as winter cordial for coughs, headaches and colds. Both leaves (seen right) and stems are useful but toxic, though this is destroyed by cooking. Leaves bruised and sniffed help clear a blocked nose; if rubbed on skin, they can repel mosquitos, flies etc, and can be made into an infusion (tea) for use as an insecticide.[6] The leaves, with Alum, yield a green dye, the berries with Alum produce a violet colour. Elder flowers are non-toxic, harvested mid-summer (watch out for bugs in them), and they can be dried for a sweet tea with a sedative effect. Don't wash them or the fragrance is lost.[2] Flowers are made into a cold summer drink, medicinal tea and cordial, or an alcoholic 'champagne'.

Berries, which must be cooked before eating, ripen in early autumn and can be turned into jams, jellies, preserves, chutneys, sauces, added to Apple pies and tarts, wine, juice, syrup, and vinegar.[6] Dried fruit taste less bitter than fresh. Berries also supply a good dye. Rich in vitamins A, B and C, Potassium and antioxidants, the berries strengthen the immune system. Daphne Lambert says they are "better than Blueberries" for antioxidant content.[7]

EUCALYPTUS GUNNI / CIDER GUM

I couldn't resist a tree from the Antipodes! A cold climate Gum Tree from Tasmania, it grows well in Ireland and is often seen in gardens and parks. Getting large with roaming roots, it's not suited to grow in small spaces or beside buildings, unless regularly pruned small. Florists use the attractive sprigs of round leaves for

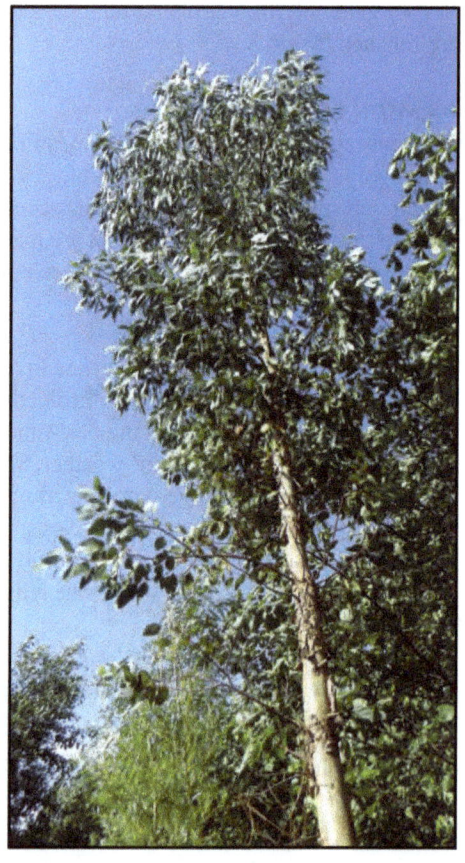

adding to bunches of flowers. Round leaves are only found on juvenile plants in nature, so florists' trees must be kept small by coppicing, then new shoots can be regularly harvested.

The name Cider Gum is a hint at another use of this graceful, evergreen tree. Aboriginals in Australia traditionally used the sap as a source of an alcoholic drink with psychoactive properties. They bored a hole in the trunk and allowed sap to collect in it and naturally ferment; while smouldering Eucalyptus leaves of all species are used for smoking (purification) ceremonies. And don't forget the Eucalyptus oil in the leaves, valuable as steam inhalation for chest and nasal congestion etc.

GUELDER ROSE, VIBURNUM OPULUS

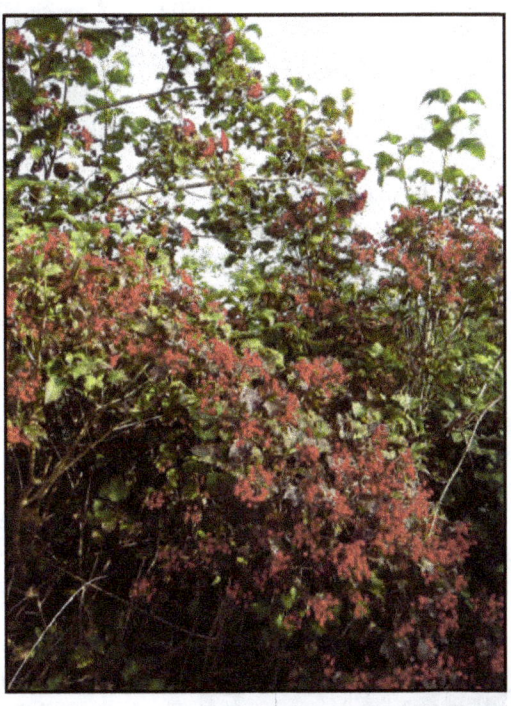

A woody shrub or small tree growing up to 5m and wide, the ornamental variety is found in gardens, with its more showy flowers. However the wild original is the best to grow for culinary and medicinal use. Found in hedgerows, woodlands and in damp areas, they're especially noticeable when the bright red berries are present in autumn. Berries are edible, but too astringent to be enjoyed raw, though popular with birds. But cooked, they are traditionally eaten across eastern Europe and Russia - added to porridge, made into various preserves, jams, jellies, pastes, mousse, pies, vinegars and condiments. Berries can produce red dye and ink; while seeds can be roasted and ground for a stimulating drink. Medicinally, the bark is the best known part, traditionally used for relieving cramps, hence this tree's alternative name of Crampbark.[4]

A special fermented drink (Gilaburu) is made from the berries in Turkey, having valuable probiotic properties and containing strains of lactic acid bacteria that are the subject of scientific investigation.[8]

Good for Forest Gardens, trees can handle a bit of shade, but they don't like acid soils. Cuttings can be made in early summer, but be sure to get them from genuine wild plants.

HAWTHORN / WHITETHORN, CRATAEGUS MONOGYNA

A classic tree once integral to the Neolithic diet, it also has a great reputation as a general heart tonic. The leaves, leaf buds, flowers and berries (young) can be eaten raw, with a pleasant nutty taste that go well on a cheese sandwich. Leaves are best eaten only between April and May.[9] You can make a heart tonic tea from two teaspoons of leaves, flowers or berries by infusing them for ten minutes (berries need to be briefly pre-boiled) and take two cups daily for at least three months.[1] Young shoots are good for salads, flowers can go in fruit salad or flavour syrups, puddings, custards etc [2]. Berries, when dried, can be ground and added to flour for baking. Fresh fruit makes good jam, especially when added to Elderberry and Apple; they're also good in chutney. Haw berries are used to strengthen the heart and balance blood pressure. Dried berry leather can also be made, see the recipe on page 226.

Haw trees are tolerant of many situations and soils, are tough, hardy and easy to grow. To get plenty of fruit, plant them in sunny locations, such as the edge of a woodland. One of the most ornamental of natives trees and sacred to the peoples of the past, specimens are traditionally left in fields to keep the fairies happy.

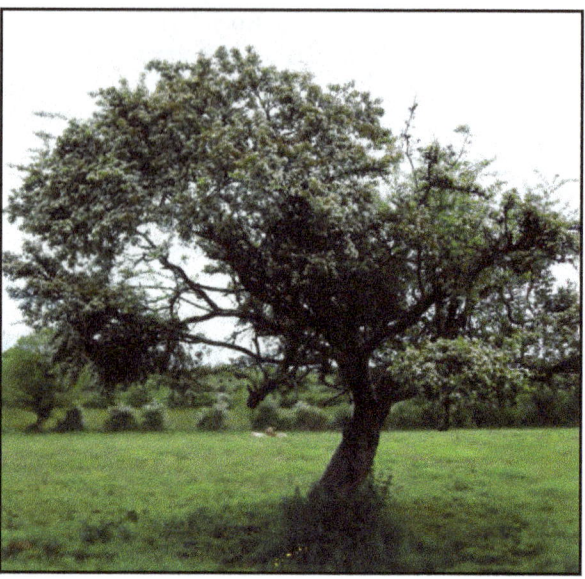

Above - Fairy Haw in a farm field.

Hawthorns can also be used to graft other fruit trees onto. I asked Danny Gaffey of the Heritage Fruit Tree Nursery if he had tried this. Wedge grafting a scion of Pear onto a new branch, it did take, but the tree was very vigorous and kept putting up suckers, so it would need a lot of pruning to get the graft wood established and succeed, he told me.

HAZEL, CORYLUS AVELLANA

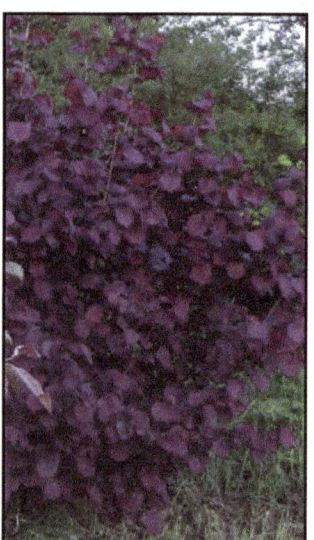

A common tree of hedgerows and woodlands, often dominating the under-storey of Oak and Ash woods, Hazelnuts have long been part of the diet. Timber is small and pliant, and was invaluable for building, furniture, fencing and wickerwork. Trees were coppiced for sticks (called wattles) that were woven into the walls of wattle and daub buildings. The long straight rods were cut to ground level in winter at two to three years age, then every seven to ten years afterwards.[10]

Nuts were an important food in the past. They are harvested when leaves turn to autumn colours. Good for eating raw, they are quite oily and can be roasted to enhance the flavour. Liquidise nuts to make a milk substitute. Oil can be extracted and is good for salad dressings etc. To store nuts for up to one year, keep them in the shell in a dark, dry place. [2]

Trees grow to 6m high and 3m wide. For plenty of nuts, trees needs a sunny spot and free-draining soil of medium fertility, plus shelter from wind. Several varieties of improved Hazelnut cultivars have bigger nuts than the native species e.g. Cobnuts and Filberts. The Red Hazel above is particularly attractive. Self-fertile, you can get nuts with just one tree, however a pollination partner of another variety improves cropping.

HOLLY, ILEX AQUIFOLIUM

A beautiful evergreen native tree with medicinal leaves; its timber is white, hard but easily carved and also burns hot. It's invaluable for wildlife in winter when the bright red berries are relished by birds, but you do need to have both males and females to get them.

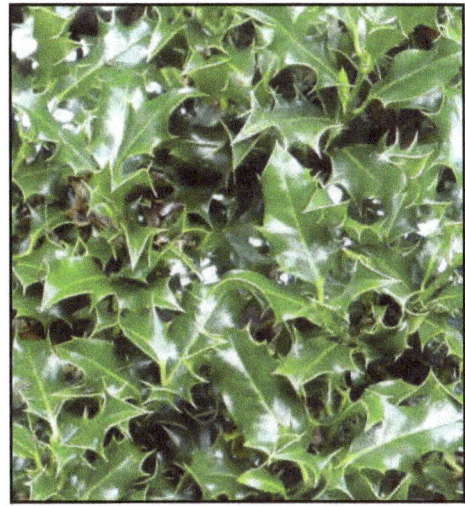

Holly leaves when regularly drunk as a tea are useful for catarrh, coughs, urinary problems, for toxin elimination and preventing kidney stones, says Glennie Kindred. Taken hot they will induce perspiration. Young leaves are eaten by livestock. Berries are mildly poisonous, however. [6]

Trees prefer to grow in well drained soil as a woodland under-storey. Slow growing, they can eventually reach 9m height and 5m spread. Being evergreen, they make a great hedge and tolerate pruning well.

MONKEY PUZZLE, ARACAURIA ARAUCANA

A native of Chile, British gardeners in the Victorian era loved to plant them, so they are fairly common in Ireland. But back in their homeland trees are now so rare because of timber logging that seed has had to be sourced from Ireland! With a striking shape and ancient form, this prickly member of the Pine family has large edible nuts and was once a staple food. Only casting a light shade, it makes a good canopy tree for a Food Forest. Growing slowly up to 30m high with a 15m spread, it needs a deep, well drained soil. After about thirty years of growing, if both males and females are present in the vicinity, it will begin to bear huge seed cones, with around two hundred tasty Almond sized nuts in each.[4] A harvest for one's descendents, perhaps.

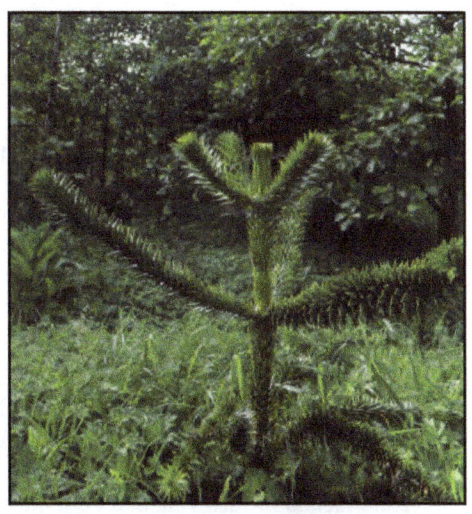

MOUNTAIN ASH, SEE ROWAN

OAK – QUERCUS ROBUR and others

The mighty Oak has long been esteemed as king of the forest. Acorns were important food for people and Pigs, while Oak timber is very strong and valuable. One Oak tree can provide enough acorns to fatten one Pig in a good season, an ancient Irish text states.[11] Bark was used for tanning and as an astringent medicine, while leaves and flower buds are good for a healing tea. Oak bark is also an ingredient of Quick Return Compost Activator, while well rotted Oak leaves are a wonderful, nutrient rich leaf mould great for mulching with, that's repellant to Slugs and grubs. Not to be used fresh, the tannin content of leaves is too high and may stunt plant growth.

Acorns also have high tannin levels, so leaching is necessary to make them edible. But leaching also takes out minerals and vitamins. Ken Fern relates how native Americans in the past would "bury the seeds in boggy ground over the winter and then dig them up in the spring when they were starting to germinate. At this stage they are almost sweet and have retained more vitamins and minerals, so are also more nutritious." [4]

You need a lot of space for an Oak tree, e.g. Quercus robur can reach 35m height and 20m width. Insects love Oaks, with 280 species recorded as frequenting them. Scattered around a new woodland, Oaks will eventually dominate the scene, as a Climax Species.

PEARS, PYRUS COMMUNIS

Pears probably originated in the Caucasus region and prefer warm, sheltered sites, so are not as successful in Ireland. They are classified as either dessert, cookers, or for alcoholic perry drink; they can also be juiced or turned into wine, dried or made into preserves. Pollination partners of other varieties are required. In Ireland the Conference, originating from France, is the most widely grown Pear, says Danny Gaffey, and it has better keeping qualities than other Pears.

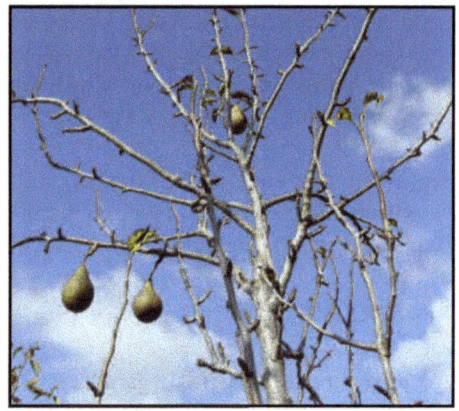

Right - Concorde Pear.

PINE SPECIES

Pine trees, once common in Ireland up until the 9th century, were harvested to extinction for house beams, ship masts and the like.[11] They struggle to grow in the heavy wet clays where I live, but with some drainage will do okay. Not just good for timber, they make excellent evergreen shelterbelts, although not deeply rooted, so unsuited to a windy spot.

Pines are a source of edible seeds, inner bark and resins; they also yield tars, turpentine and dyes, as well as providing medicines. Pine resin was once used for caulking boats and preserving wood too.[11] Pine needle tea is rich in vitamins A, C and K, valuable in spring when other fresh vitamin sources are not available.[16] Even just deeply inhaling the atmosphere around Pine trees, one avails of the therapeutic qualities. As leaves leach out chemicals with rain, however, seed germination of other plants is inhibited in the surrounding area, so they can be anti-social for growing in a Food Forest.

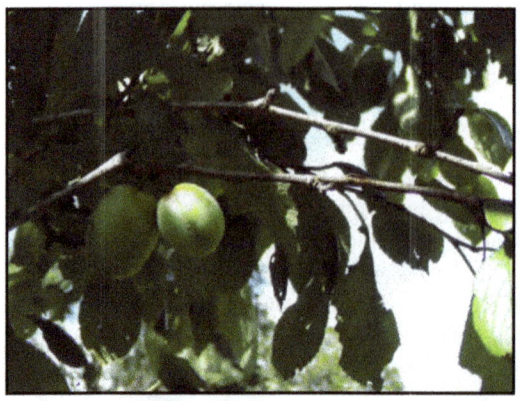

PLUM, PRUNUS SPECIES

The European Plum, Prunus domestica, possibly originated in the Caucasus region, probably from crosses of wild Sloes (Prunus spinosa) and Cherry Plums, Prunus cerasifera. There are now a host of highly bred varieties with bigger and sweeter fruit, such as the Greengages and the popular Victoria Plum (seen left), but these will only fruit and ripen well in the more favourable spots, with rich well drained soils in sunny, sheltered positions. For a Food Forest you are probably better off with the wilder types of Plum. All Plums have a high Oxalic Acid content, so don't eat too many!

As for Cherry Plums, the Mirabelle de Nancy is a fairly common variety, with small, round, sweet, yellow fruit that's used for jam and pies, the juice for wine and Cherry Brandy making. There are other varieties and these all need to have other pollinators, European Plums that flower at the same time will do the job. Mirabelles are wind resistant and can grow to 10m height, they can make good hedges planted at 1-1.5m apart, but they do need a sunny spot for a good crop.[3] Mine grows in the polytunnel.

ROWAN, SORBUS AUCUPARIA

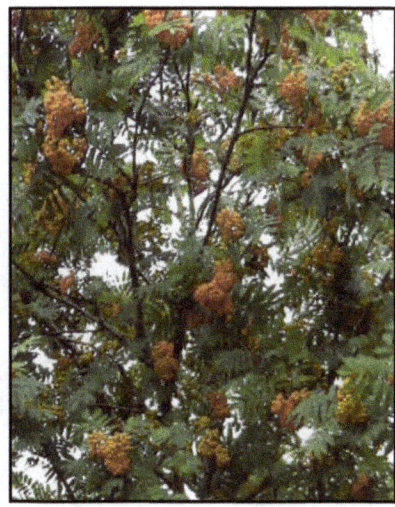

A beautiful small tree with bright red berries, these are edible but rather bitter and best not eaten raw. Berries are very nutritious, with more vitamin C than citrus fruits. Picked in October, they can be made into jelly, with added pectin, such as from Crab Apples. The jelly has a sharp marmalade taste and dark orange colour. They can also be juiced or brewed into an alcoholic drink.[9] Raw and cooked berries are slightly laxative and diuretic, they can cleanse the kidneys, help coughs and sore throat (eat five to eight dried berries or gargle with berry or flower tea).[1] Dried leaves can be drunk as a tea (two teaspoons per cup of tea taken twice daily), while dried berries can be helpful for stomach upsets.

Rowan trees prefer lighter soils, where they may reach 15m height and 7m width. Birds love the fruit, so Rowan berries can distract birds away from your precious fruit trees.

SILVER BIRCH, BETULA PENDULA ALSO B. PUBESCENS

These pioneer species are fast growing and occur across the northern hemisphere. In America, Birch bark was traditionally used for canoes, tepee roofing, buckets, shoes, torches (high tar content), dye and tanning; while sap and leaves have medicinal uses and are a general tonic. Birch twigs are traditionally made into Birch brooms (besoms) in Europe.

The fresh bright green young leaves in spring and early summer can be eaten in salads, made into a tonic tea, or dried for later use. Young leaves and sap stimulate gallbladder, kidneys and bladder, also help arthritis and promote sleep etc. Birch tea is also a scalp tonic, when used as a shampoo (it contains saponins).[1] Leaves for medicine can be steeped in oil for a month before straining off and storing in sterile bottles, and this is good for rubbing on aching muscles and for skin problems.

Sap can be tapped from tree trunks in springtime, by drilling a hole into the trunk before the buds burst and inserting a flexible straw that draws off sap into a container strapped beneath it. After a week's collection you remove it and plug the hole with a twig. Sap can be drunk as is, or boiled down into a syrup[12]. I dont want to try this, as I dont see myself as a sap sucking tree vampire!

SLOE / BLACKTHORN, PRUNUS SPINOS

This small tree is an ancestor of cultivated Plums. The beautiful white blossoms are some of the earliest flowers of spring. Despite tasting tart and acidic, Sloe berries have long been used for food and dying cloth. Archeological excavations at Glastonbury UK produced a barrow load of Sloe stones from a Neolithic lake village.[13]

Sloes are made into jelly, usually mixed with the same quantity of Crab Apples, and are mixed with other fruit for jam, giving a rich red claret colour. Sloe wine and gin can be made; and Sloes can be added to mixed fruit pies. In eastern Europe, Sloes have long been a crop that's wild gathered and sold in markets, for cooking and making into syrup. The berries are used medicinally and have a tonic astringent action. Good for dying also, juice of the berries gives linen a reddish colour that washes out to pale blue.[9] Tannin can be sourced from the bark and also ink made from it. Being in the Prunus family, Blackthorn can also be used to graft cultivated members of the genus onto, being compatible with Plums, Apricots, Almonds, Peaches and Cherries.

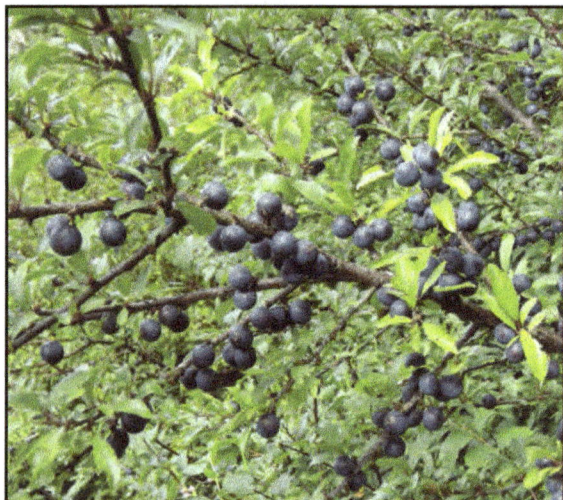

Left - It's best to pick Sloe berries after a frost, when skins become softened and somewhat bletted (half rotted) and they're less astringent. This is something that the birds are aware of also. Went I went to harvest this prolific tree after the first frost, they'd already beaten me to it!

For ripening Sloe berries and making them sweeter, Baracli-Levy describes an old gypsy method of burying them in a straw-lined pit in the ground over several months.[14] Sloe berries can also be preserved by lacto-fermentation. After fermenting them in brine, it's likely that Sloes can provide similar benefits as the famous sour and salty Umemboshi Plum in Japan, adding zest to any dish and also used a medicine, known as 'Japanese Alka Seltzer', for indigestion and stomach upsets, acting on the liver and removing worms. (Umemboshis are sold as whole plums, in liquid form, as tablets and vinegar.)[15] See recipes on page 228. As with all Plums, an excess is best avoided as they are high in oxalic acid.

Blackthorn thrives best in a sunny situation and just about any soil, just not very acid peat. Traditionally grown in boundary hedgerows, as the thorns help keep animals in, these tough trees grow well in woodland edges, reaching 4m height. With their suckering habit, they can develop formidable thickets that are perfect for wildlife refuges. But watch out for those formidable thorns. They can cause some damage if you are pricked. Perhaps because of toxins or bacteria they harbour, pricks from them have caused the skin on my hands to go black and sore for weeks. Fortunately I was recommended the homeopathic remedy Rhus tox and taking a few doses of it quickly gave relief.

SPRUCE, PICEA SPECIES

Spruce plantations are the scourge of many a rural skyline, being gloomy places with little growing beneath them. While I wouldn't plant any, if you already have them, there are many uses other than for timber. The needles of Spruce species, for example, have been traditionally used for respiratory problems. They are taken as a tea, by steeping a few teaspoonfuls of needles in boiling water for five minutes. The tea is high in vitamins, especially A and C, plus chlorophyll and shikimic acid (the base of anti-flu drug Tamilflu). Best nutrient levels are found in needles from three year old trees, sourced from the sunniest side. Heated needles have long been used for fumigation also. The inner bark is edible either raw or dried, then ground and mixed with flour, and this has medicinal applications too. Flower buds can be eaten and the resin is used to make healing skin salves. [16]

STRAWBERRY TREE, ARBUTUS UNEDO

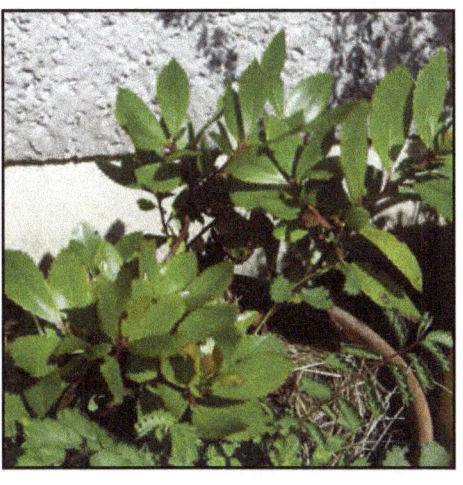

This curious evergreen tree, native to parts of western Ireland as well as Mediterranean countries, grows slowly up to 8m height, but in Ireland it's usually much smaller and often just a large shrub or pot plant. There are magnificent specimens in central Victoria, Australia, where I used to live (as well as many other Mediterranean trees, as well as Oaks, that do well there.) Unusually, the Strawberry tree flowers and fruits at the same time. Fruits are pinkish coloured, juicy and subtle in flavour. It is tolerant of a range of growing conditions, poor soils are ok, but it grows best with good drainage and protected from wind in a warm spot, some shade is tolerated too.

PROFILE REFERENCES

1. The Spirit of Trees, Fred Hageneder, Floris Books, UK, 2000
2. Wild Foods for Free, Jonathan Hilton, Hamlyn, UK, 2007
3. The Fruit Tree Handbook, Ben Pike, Green Books, 2011, UK.
4. Plants for a Future, Ken Fern.
5. A Guide to Damsons, Daiv Sizer, October 2013, online.
6. The Sacred Tree, Glennie Kindred, UK, 2003.
7. Living Food, Daphne Lambert, Unbound, 2016, UK.
8. https://www.researchgate.net/publication/274618752_Diversity_and_probiotic_potentials_of_lactic_acid_bacteria_isolated_from_gilaburu_a_traditional_Turkish_fermented_European_cranberrybush_Viburnum_opulus_L_fruit_drink
9. Food for Free, Richard Mabey, Collins, Ireland, 1972.
10. Irish Trees, Niall Mac Coitir, Collins Press, Ireland, 2003.
11. Early Irish Farming, Fergus Kelly, Dublin Institute of Advanced Studies, 1997, Ireland.
12. Hedgerow Medicine - harvest and make your own herbal remedies
     Julie Bruton-Seal and Matthew Seal, Merlin Unwin, 2008, UK.
13. Prehistoric Cookery, Jane Renfrew, English Heritage, UK, 2005.
14. Herbal Handbook for Farm and Garden, Juliette de Bairacli-Levy,
     Farrar, Straus & Giroux, 1991, UK
15. Healing with Wholefoods, Paul Pritchard, North Atlantic books, USA, 1993.
16. The Healing Trees - the edible and herbal qualities of northeastern woodland trees,
     Robbie Hanna Anderman, Burnstown, ON, Canada, 2017.

FRUIT TREE VARIETIES RECOMMENDED FOR THE WET WEST OF IRELAND

By Danny Gaffey, Heritage Fruit Trees, Co. Leitrim.

These are varieties that I would currently recommend for growing in our part of the world. Even the best varieties can get diseases, but these varieties could well have better disease resistance than most. Some may also have better than average frost and wind resistant flowers, but this would be no substitution for a good site i.e. good soil, full sun, shelter from the wind and away from low lying frost pockets that might be subject to late frosts. Planting on exposed sites and in frost pockets is a risky proposition and could end in repeated disappointment, regardless of varieties chosen and unfortunately you probably won't know until you try.

Plums, Pears and Cherries are more site demanding than Apples, as they flower earlier and would be more likely be subjected to late frost or spring storms at flowering time. I like more vigorous rootstocks on heavier soil and mounding on spots subject to waterlogging. I find dwarf trees do well on mounds also in more sheltered areas. Good pruning and hygiene i.e. raking up leaves, fallen fruit, dead wood and prunings, and removing them from the site can help to reduce disease. If a tree dies and you want to replace it, don't plant it in the same spot. Prune Apples in winter and stone fruit in summer.

I would always recommend going for a good mix of early, mid and late harvesting fruit to extend the harvesting season. In general, late harvesting Apples keep well, mid harvesting Apples might keep for a month or so and early harvesting Apples don't keep at all but some, like Katy can be picked off the tree for a month or so.

EARLY EATING APPLES
Beauty of Bath, Eight Square, Kerry Pippin, Discovery, Katy, Epicure, Tydemans Early Worcester, Devonshire Quarrenden (Blood of the Boyne), and Leitrim variety Golden Royal.

MID SEASON EATING APPLES
Limelight, Greensleeves, Rajka, Ellisons Orange, Prima, Bardsey, Ballinora Pippin, Delcorf, St Edmunds Pippin.

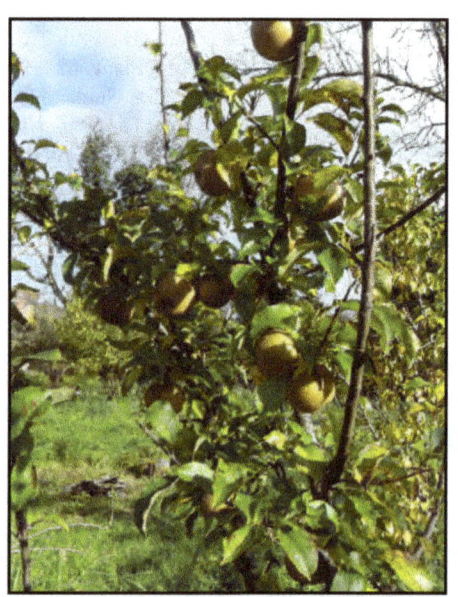

LATE SEASON EATING APPLES
Pinova, Yellow Pitcher, Scarlet Crofton, Red Falstaff, Ecolette, Saturn, Laxtons Superb, Spartan, Sweet Sixteen, Adams Pearmain, Ard Cairn Russet, Egremont Russet (right), Alkmene.

COOKING/DUAL PURPOSE APPLES
King of the Pippins, Lady Henniker, Lord Derby, Keswick Codlin, Golden Noble, Ballyvaughan Seedling, Lanes Prince Albert, Smarts Prince Arthur, Barnack Beauty, King of Tompkins County, Annie Elizabeth, Newton Wonder,

Crawley Beauty, Charles Ross.

PLUMS
Opal, Victoria, Czar, Marjorie's Seedling (seen right), Jubileum, Stanley. (Victoria and Czar have poor enough disease resistance but should still be considered as they are perhaps the most reliable varieties around these parts on a decent site.)

PEARS
Conference, Hessle, Durondeau, Black Worcester (cooking), Invincible Delwinor (with a reputation for reliability in non-traditional Pear growing areas, it can produce a second flush of flowers if the frost gets the first set).

Other Pear and Plum varieties could turn out to be very good but I haven't had them long enough to know for sure. Time will tell.

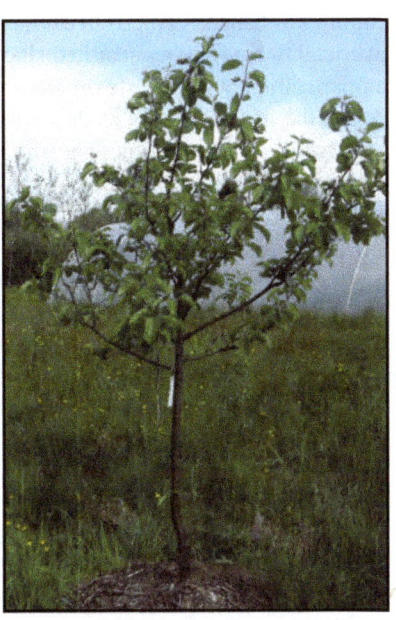

Heritage Fruit Nursery, www.heritagefruitnursery.com

THE VALUE OF WETLANDS AND BOUNTY OF BOGS

Healthy wetlands are a treasure trove of biodiversity that also purify water and reduce flooding, while peatlands (bogs) help the climate too, by storing (sequestering) Carbon in the ground. Peatlands are globally important because they are said to store 20-30% of the world's soil Carbon, three times the amount stored in rainforests![1] A major feature of the Irish landscape, County Leitrim's bogs take up 23.5% of it's area. Nationally, so many bogs have been lost to drainage, cutting and repurposing, that only 15% are left intact. Bogs really need to be better appreciated and conserved.

Millenia in the making, bog plants such as Peat Moss (Sphagnum cymbifolium) established after changes in the climate made it too wet for the original forests. Bogs are highly acidic (or occasionally highly alkaline), low in Oxygen and nutrients. Sphagnum is perfectly adapted and when it dies, it doesn't break down. New Peat Moss grows on top, as the dead stuff is preserved in the anaerobic bog waters, with their anti-bacterial properties. Gradually the bog grows higher and higher above ground level this way.

When dug up and dried out, peat burns well, although it doesn't get very hot. Turf, as the Irish generally call the lumps of peat, was the only fuel available after forests were fully depleted. Essential for heating and cooking, sods of turf were sometimes used for walls and roofing too. Turf was cut with a special spade (the loy), then stacked ('footed') to dry out over summer. People also used bog water for healing, especially for skin problems.

Ancient fallen Oak trees in bogs, lying perfectly preserved, were occasionally discovered by turf cutters, who used them for building timbers that were especially highly valued after tree cutting was banned in the 18th century. Pickled bog bodies have been found across Ireland too, over eighty have been unearthed since 1750. These were people ritually sacrificed and when un-earthed, they were perfectly preserved. No wonder it was a custom to store butter in bogs, where the normal forces of decomposition are prevented by the lack of Oxygen and high acidity. From time to time, ancient butter hoards are found intact after thousands of years immersed in bog water. Some people today store fruit and vegetables in a bed of Peat Moss so that they stay fresh longer. [2]

Since peat became the main fuel and over-stocking of sheep accelerated in the 1980's, the decline of bogs went exponential, such that very little undisturbed bog persists today. Raised Bogs, formed out of lake basins following the last Ice Age, have been reduced by some 93% in Ireland, from the extraction of turf and horticultural 'compost'. Blanket Bogs, the type that hug bare, de-forested hills and western lowlands, are now, ironically, threatened themselves by re-afforestation with commercial conifer forestry. Already some 28% of Blanket Bogs nationally having been drained and put under Sitka Spruce. This releases stored Carbon into the atmosphere and degrades environmental water quality. Blanket bogs on hills are often the location for wind turbines too, wrecking the hydrology and locale with associated earth works; the turbines' spinning blades a deadly hazard for birds of prey and bats; the deep and weighty concrete foundations sometimes even causing 'bog bursts', mud slides that can render farmland unusable, as was the possible cause of a major event in north Leitrim in 2020.

Natural bogs are often carpeted by Heather plants. Ingenious peasants created many uses for this small plant - burning it for fuel and making roof thatch, bedding, floor mats, insulation, fencing, ropes and brushes from it. A few edible berry plants also thrive in the acidic bogs - the Cranberry, Bilberry and Crowberry. Berry picking on hills was once an important feature of the ancient Irish Harvest Festival held in early August, popular with the youth of the day.

As for peat being used as fuel today, I burn locally harvested turf from a nearby farm, where it seems to be a fairly sustainable system. My neighbours have their own turf plots and it's all small scale. Industrial scale peat harvesting in Ireland is not sustainable and is being phased out. If you have some bog land yourself it can be brilliant for growing things. The Heritage Fruit Tree nursery is on the edge of a bog. The rows of fruit trees grow beautifully on long low mounds, enjoying the well drained peaty soil.

PEAT MEDICINES

Sphagnum Moss is super absorbent and able to soak up over twenty times its dry weight in water. This is why it was used in bandages on battlefields in the past, being far better than Cotton wool.[2] Peat products used on open wounds make them heal quickly and reduce infections, partly due to the acidity. There are many other applications, with Peat Moss used over generations both internally and externally for general well being, skin problems, rheumatic complaints, etc. Peat Moss is rich in minerals, humic acids, lipoids, fulvic acids, hyaluronic acid, amino acids, vitamins, trace elements, fatty acids and plant hormones. When used fresh, Peat Moss has female hormones (oestrogens) that is used to correct female disorders and improve fertility. In the early 1940s Dr. Rudolf Hauschka, who started Hauschka body care products in Germany, researched the ancient therapeutic uses of the fluid extract of

Peat and, inspired by Rudolph Steiner's advice about its potential, eventually developed 'Solum uliginosum'. 'Moor extracts' such as Solum uliginosum are produced as an aqueous solution in the separation process when producing peat fibers for textiles.³

In Austria, Neydharting Moor is the most researched Peat Moss region and it attracts 'medical tourists' to bathe in the peat rich waters. As well as bog bathing, people can benefit from the healing potential with cosmetic and skin care products based on Peat Moss that are available commercially.

PEAT MOSS FOR PROTECTION

In 1924 Rudolph Steiner advised, in his famous series of Agricultural lectures at Koberwitz, that Peat Moss would provide protection from unhealthy Earth, electro-magnetic and cosmic radiation, especially so in the future. This has held true. Biodynamic farmers today wrap their containers of sensitive soil remedies with Peat Moss to keep them energetically intact. Geomancers in Holland, I was told, use Peat Moss to line their homes for its protective and insulating properties. Peat Moss isn't a physical barrier against radiation however. To keep out those ubiquitous frequencies from the high-tech world you also need something like a layer of Aluminium building wrap or Carbon based paint. Peat Moss does have unique protective qualities that enhance our wellbeing when living in a 'microwave soup'.

Weaving technology was eventually developed, following Steiner's advice, to create textiles from a common European bog plant, the Sheathed Cotton Sedge, Eriophorum vaginatum (called Bog Cotton in Ireland). The processed fibres are used for insulation, filling duvets, in rugs, mattress covers, furniture textiles and clothes. (In the past Irish peasants would stuff their mattresses and pillows, if they had them, with Bog Cotton.) Peat clothing, often a 50 - 50 mix with wool, is said to confer a great sense of comfort and wellbeing when worn. I found some online that's being produced from 'sustainably harvested' Raised Bogs in Sweden and Finland. I just wish it wasn't so expensive, or I would be ordering some immediately! ⁴

1. Celebrating County Leitrim's Wetland Wealth, Leitrim County Council report 2019.
2. Nature's Way - the Wonder of Peatlands, An Taisce,
The National Trust for Ireland, www.antaisce.org
3. https://drhauschkaaus.wordpress.com/2016/06/24/secrets-of-the-moors/
4. The Current Importance of Peat Textiles, at www.anthromed.org/Article.aspx?artpk=252

WASTE WATER TREATMENT WETLANDS

Treatment wetlands and reed beds are a natural way of treating grey water and effluent from a septic tank or treatment plant. Final cleansing is achieved when these discharge into what are variously called distribution or percolation areas, or drainage fields. These evapo–transpiration seepage systems use soil soakage and plants for the disposal of treated effluent. They typically have perforated pipes laid in shallow trenches that are filled over with gravel, allowing effluent to flow out into the surrounding soil. The area is planted with suitable plants that tolerate wet feet and take up the nutrients for growing, while removing water via the surface of their leaves through the natural process of evapo-transpiration. The cleaner the water is that goes in, the better it is for the system, especially if you want to include some edible plants.

In the past people came up with crazy ways to create pollution. Mixing human waste with water was a disaster for the environment. Separating the water out later in treatment plants requires money, time, space and careful management. Far better for the planet, a dry compost toilet with separate urine collection for garden fertilising is the way to go. Then only the relatively harmless grey water from kitchen and bathroom needs to be cleansed. If you direct that water into a special garden with moisture loving, thickly mulched plants and plenty of earthworms, you may not need any other treatment system. But shhh!, don't tell that to the local authority who might have a different concept. If you live in a house where there is an existing septic tank or sewer connection - perfect! Then you can do whatever you like with your waste and just keep the Water Closet for grandma to use.

If you have a natural wetland already, or need one to satisfy the authorities for a new build waste water system, it can be a beautiful and multi-purpose feature in a garden. If you have heavy clay soil, this can be perfect to seal a constructed treatment wetland and avoid plastic liners. An attractive selection of plants can be used and these host a range of wildlife. Many wetland plants have multi functionality too, so reed beds, wetlands and drainage areas can provide a very useful resource for the eco-peasantry.

USEFUL PLANTS FOR CONSTRUCTED WETLANDS

COMMON REED, PHRAGMITES AUSTRALIS

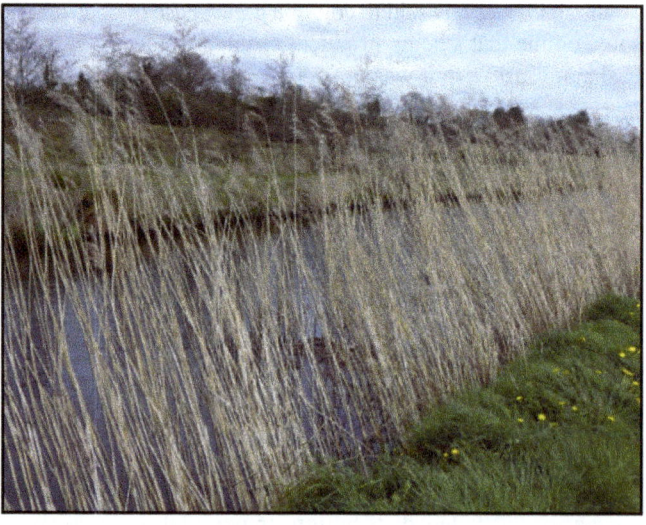

A graceful aquatic reed, ubiquitous in Ireland's wetlands, it grows to some 3.5m tall and has gorgeous plumes of purple flower heads in autumn. This Reed is truly common, being one of the most widely distributed of all flowering plants, with a range from the tropics to far south Tasmania. It's the number one plant for constructed wetlands and reed beds. It grows vigorously, in fact it can become dominant and invasive if you don't harvest it regularly, using the waste to mulch the garden. The cylindrical stems of this reed persist through wintertime (as seen above), allowing oxygen to go down into the underwater roots during the dormant season and thus stay alive - an ability that's called 'snorkelling'. The roots are powerful and can puncture plastic pond liners.[1]

This plant has been used as a food source globally since ancient times. When green and if broken, the stems slowly exude a sugary substance that can be chewed like a sweet and, if put near a fire to melt, tastes like toasted marshmallow. Native Americans would cut Reeds while green and before flowering, they then dried them, ground them and sifted out a sugary 'flour'. Young leaves have been dried, ground into a powder, mixed with other flour and made into dumplings. The young roots can be eaten dried, ground and boiled as porridge. Underground stems are edible too, but are tougher. The newly emerged shoots are also good eating, while seeds are nutritious raw or cooked. [2]

GREATER REED MACE, TYPHA LATIFOLIA

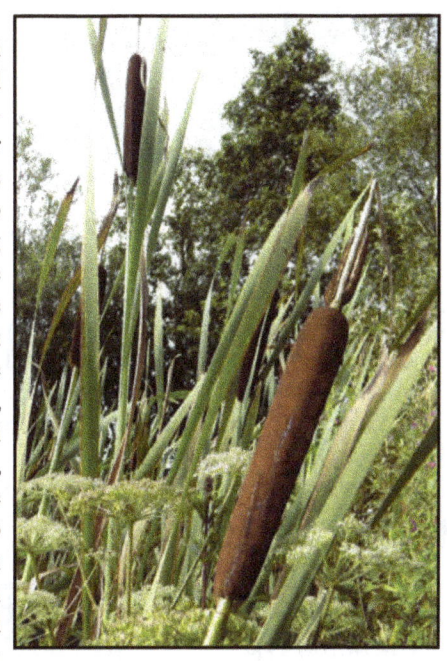

Another vigorous global aquatic reed and food source, it grows in water no deeper than 30cm and gets to 2m tall. Commonly - and incorrectly - called Bulrush, this is another important plant for constructed wetland systems. Like the Reed, it has edible parts and these are available from spring to autumn. Young growing shoots up to 50cm long can be collected in early spring. Tasting like cucumber, they are good raw or cooked as a veggie or added to soups. The flower spikes, when immature, are said to taste like Sweet Corn and are also good in soup. When flowers are mature, turning golden yellow, the protein rich pollen can be added to flour or pancake mixes. The seeds, used raw or roasted and ground to make flour, have a nutty taste but they are probably too tiny to bother. In late autumn the rhizomes, which can grow to 60cm long, can be harvested and are then richest in starch. The central core can be cooked like a Potato, or dried and ground to a flour to mix with other flours, or boiled down to make syrup. [2]

YELLOW FLAG, IRIS PSEUDOCARUS

A beautiful plant of damp meadows, seen left, it has bright yellow flowers over summer and sword-like leaves. It stays green over winter. Dig a few up from the wild, they'll take a few years to establish, slowly spreading in clumps.

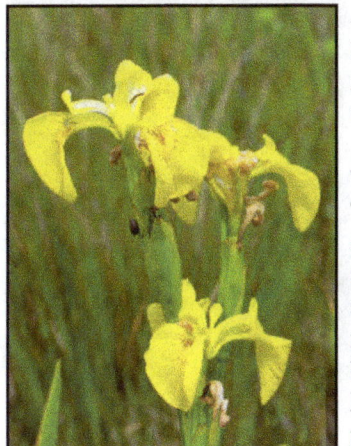

WATER MINT, MENTHA AQUATICA

This wild Mint is surprisingly good made into tea and added to pestos and dips. Its lovely mauve flowers in autumn are beloved by Bees and Butterflies. It's a hardy plant that can become quite rampant.

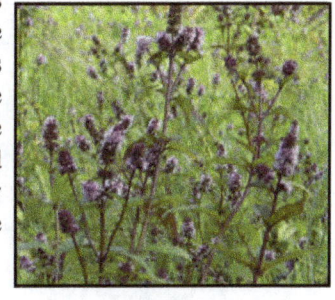

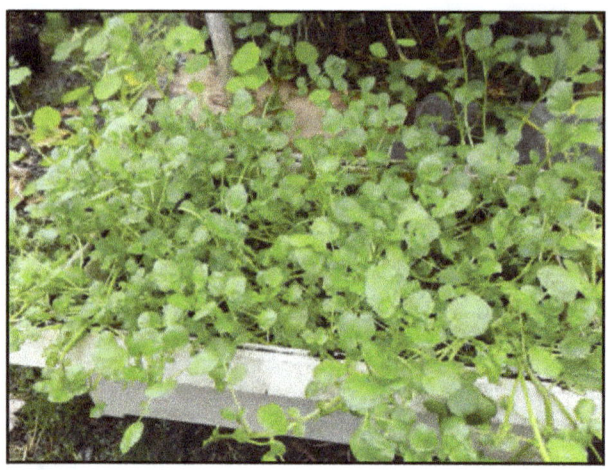

WATERCRESS,
NASTURTIUM AQUATICUM
This thrives in the cooler times of the year. Growing wild across Ireland, like the Mint, it's easy to find some for your wetland. But, if you want to eat it, don't plant it in a sewage treatment reed bed system.

Left - Watercress bed in the polytunnel. It's a variety of Watercress that doesn't have to be in running water.

NON-EUROPEAN WETLAND PLANTS

New Zealand has similar climatic conditions to Ireland, so its native plants often do well here. British garden fashionista in the Victorian era were wowed by certain evergreen plants from there and these were extensively planted and thrived. Two main species, Phormiums and Cordlyines, had multiple uses for Maori people, but this knowledge didn't seem to come over with them. They are sold at Irish garden centres.

Guy Bowden wrote online of the usefulness of such New Zealand plants for wetlands, that "Grasses, Rushes, Flax and Cabbage Trees will perform the task of soaking up and filtering effluent with the greatest efficiency. There are also a number of large trees that will tolerate wet conditions as well." [3]

PHORMIUM TENAX
In Australia we call it New Zealand Flax, the Maori people know it as Harakeke. Now bred into a range of bright colours, it's simply known as Phormium in Ireland.

These large clumping evergreen plants can grow up to 3m high and nearly as wide, with striking flowers and seed pods. Usually green in colour in the wild, they are found growing naturally in swampy places, although they also flourish in a wide range of conditions.

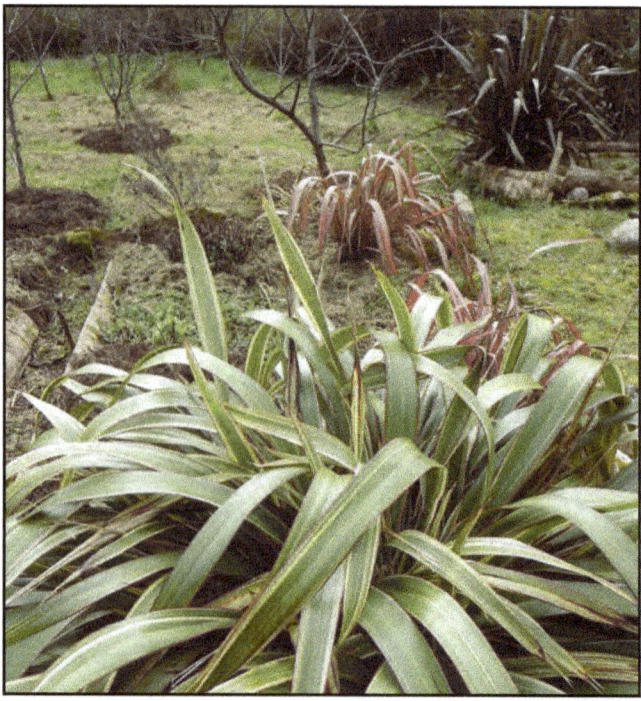

Having no relation to true Flax, Phormiums provided one of the main weaving materials used by Maori people to make a host of essential items, such as warm clothing, baskets and platters, fishing lines, sleeping mats, canoe sails, bird snares and sandals. They also made medicine from the roots, while nectar was obtained from the flowers and face powder from the pollen.

There are two species of Phormiums in New Zealand, with many variations of colour and leaf form. Phormium cookianum, known as Mountain Flax or Wharariki, is smaller with droopier leaves and was not so widely used. This is not the one for grey water systems, according to Bowden.[3]

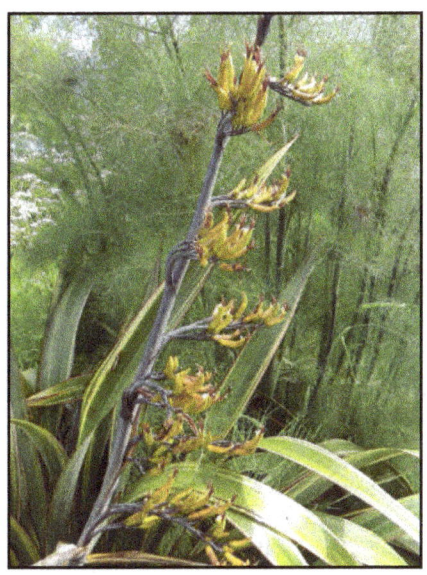

CORDYLINE AUSTRALIS, CABBAGE TREE

This garden plant can grow eventually into a palm-like small tree with a dense mass of long, spiky sword-like leaves up to some 6 – 8m high with a 3m spread. In New Zealand it's known as the Cabbage Tree, because for the Maori it was a food source, though more resorted to as a famine food. The roots were eaten cooked, as were tender young stems. There were medicinal attributes as well. It was also valued as a source of durable fibre, used for textiles, anchor ropes, fishing lines, baskets, waterproof rain capes and cloaks, and even sandals were made from it.[5]

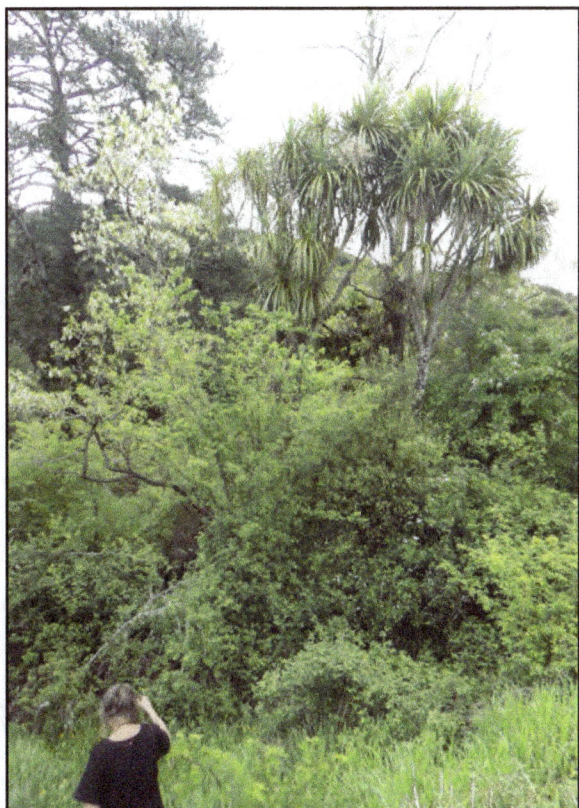

Happy to grow in moist soil and tough in seaside locations, it's useful for giving a wetland planted area character and structure by adding height, while the big bunches of creamy white flowers make it attractive at blossom time.

No wonder the Victorians spread Cordylines throughout the British Isles, where they grew well. They're often seen with large trunks in grand old Irish gardens too and they remain fashionable today.

Left - A flowering Cabbage Tree in the wild is seen top right, at Koanga Gardens, in New Zealand.

PLANTS FOR PERCOLATION AREAS

For these areas Comfrey (see its profile on page 120) and Willow are ideal.

WILLOW

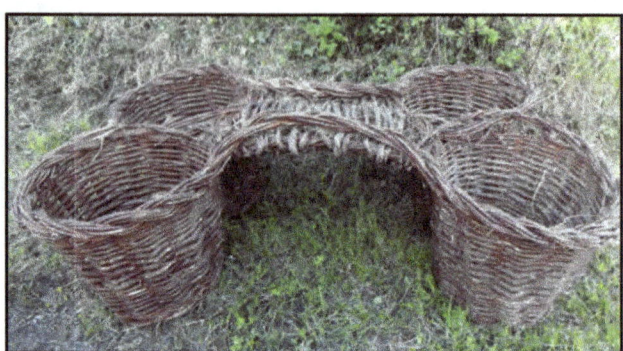

Willow trees have provided essential weaving materials for millennia and plantations of them were called Osier Beds. From baskets, cradles and Donkey panniers (seen right), to coffins, Willow had a vital place in peasant culture, before plastic ruled supreme.

Wet meadows are perfect for Osier Beds, where Willows can grow up to 6 or 8m height in just three years. Willows are generally coppiced (cut to the ground in winter) every three years. The craft varieties have colourful stems that look gorgeous in woven articles. Other hybrid cultivars have been bred to produce huge amounts of biomass for generating heat or electricity.

Willows have a very high evapotranspiration rate, rapidly absorbing nutrients and venting water harmlessly into the atmosphere. This ability has been harnessed in Zero Discharge Willow Beds, developed in the mid 1990's by a Dutch engineer, where the large area beds, sealed with clay or a liner, take treated water, vent it upwards and produce no discharge of water at all.[1]

A downside of Willow trees is that the vigorous root systems can clog up drainage systems and pipes, so they are best grown only in percolation areas or Zero Discharge Willow Beds.

It's easy to establish an Osier Bed. Stem cuttings, some 90cm long, are inserted into the ground to about 30cm depth. Cuttings are ideally kept weed free until they establish. To suppress weeds, cover the ground around them with cardboard and paper (there's really no need to buy plastic weed mat sheeting). A layer of wood chips over the paper will keep it in place and eventually feeds the soil too.

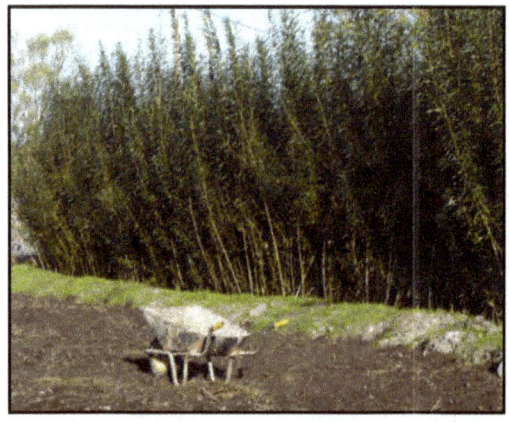

1. Permaculture Guide to Reed Beds - designing, building and planting your treatment wetland system, Féidhlim Harty, Permanent Publications, UK, 2017. See - www.wetlandsystems.ie/shop.html
2. Hilton, Jonathan, Wild Foods for Free, Hamlyn, UK, 2007.
3 http://www.tawapou.co.nz/about-native-plants/planting-for-treatment-of-waste-water
4 Fun with Flax, 50 projects for beginners, Mick Pendergrast, Raupo, New Zealand, 1987.
5. https://maoriplantuse.landcareresearch.co.nz

Left - Two year old Willows.

CHAPTER FOUR

PLANTS AND ANIMALS

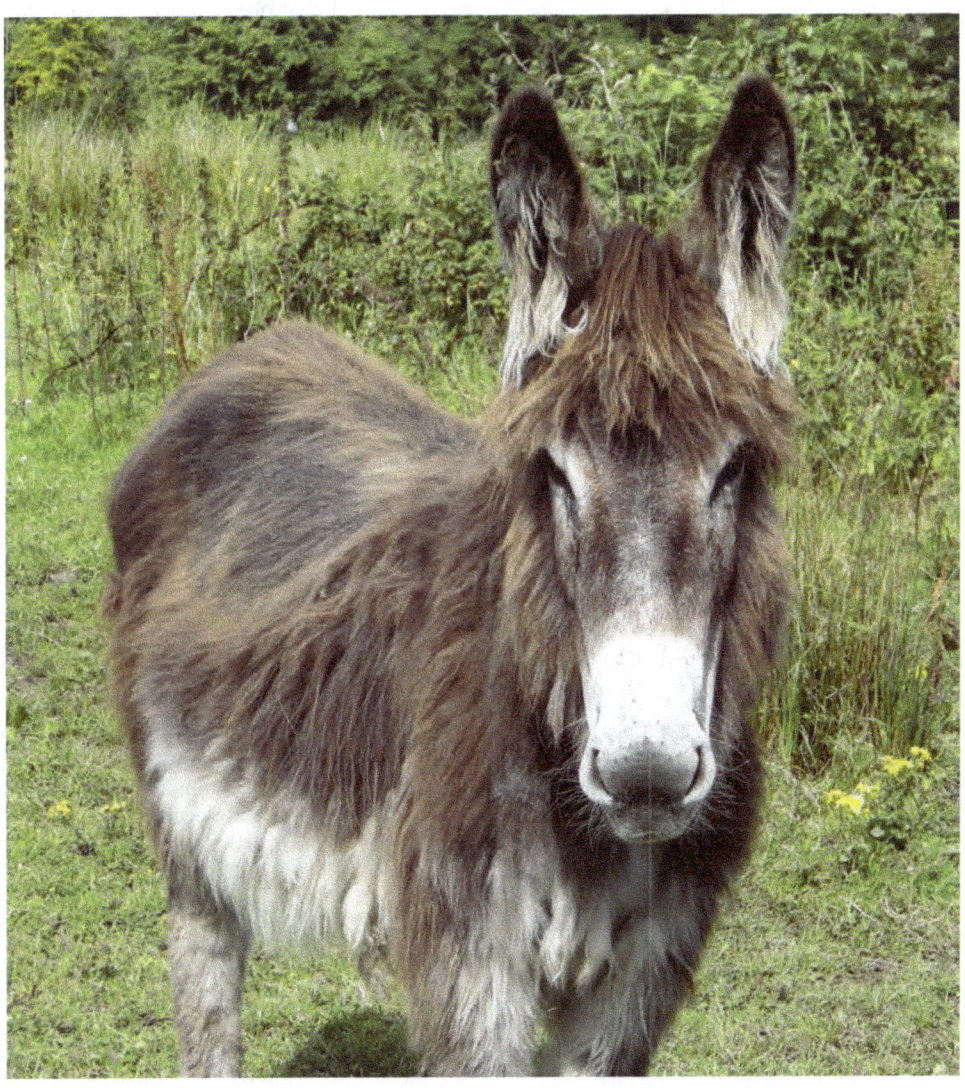

This friendly Donkey lives on the banks of the River Shannon.

STAPLE CROPS

Some crops grow so easily and have superior nutritional qualities, that they are much more worthwhile growing than others. These plants became the dietary staples that fuelled many a mighty civilisation. While I love to grow diverse crops, I also focus on growing plenty of staple vegetables - Potatoes, Beetroot, Celeriac, Broad Beans, Peas, Onions, Garlic, Squash, Kale and Asian greens being favourites. The storage ability of most of these is excellent too, so you can often enjoy eating them up until next year's crops are ready. As for fruits, the best and easiest to grow here in Ireland are Apples, Damsons, Currants, Strawberries and Raspberries. If these were all that one could grow, your diet would be great!

Even if you could only grow Potatoes, Broad Beans, Kale, Onions and Garlic, plus Apples and some plus herbs for flavouring - you would still get enough nutrients to not just survive, but thrive. With added dairy products or eggs, meals can be made more tasty or have a different form. But they aren't essential - our protein requirement has been vastly exaggerated by the meat and dairy industries.

Left - An imagined small backyard Permaculture garden design for the urban peasantry. The tallest, the Apples, go to the north end, to avoid shading other plants. Lower growing berries are in front, with four beds of rotating vegetable crops, then a border of perennial herbs and vegetables in front of them, at the sunny south end.

Now to look at those big five staples from an eco-peasant perspective. Not so much their well known attributes or techniques of production, but focusing on lesser known aspects.

POTATOES

A native of South America, where some 4000 varieties are recorded, this was the food powerhouse that fuelled conquering Inca, Mayan and Aztec tribes, who grew them high in their Andean mountain fortresses. With a 2% plus protein content and providing essential fibre, it's an important source of vitamin C too (especially high in new Potatoes) as well as Foliate, Potassium and Iron. One of the treasures brought back from Peru by Spanish Conquistadores in 1540, but it took some one hundred and fifty to two hundred years for Potatoes to catch on in Europe, spread by the peasantry and eventually replacing other less abundant crops.

Before Potatoes arrived in southern Europe, for example, the main starchy crop staple was Chestnuts. In Spain the nuts were harvested in autumn, peeled and dried for storing over winter, and stewed with beans or made into soups, after being roasted.[1] A lot more work than producing the spud, that's come to be the most important root crop traded in the world.

Potatoes grew well in Ireland and the marginalised, land-poor peasants could live well on them. Potato could also be fed (cooked) to Pigs and Poultry, and distilled into alcohol too. Just one acre of land (4000m2) planted to them could provide enough food for a family, a well as a Pig, for an entire year. Not surprisingly, from around 1750 Ireland's population boomed, trebling from about three to nine million over the following century.[2]

The century of exponential population growth ended abruptly when Blight, a deadly fungal pest (Phytophthera infestans) struck Europe's Potato fields in the 1840s, blackening the leaves and making tubers inedible. It possibly came in accidentally with imported guano fertilisers. Mainland European peasants didn't generally suffer as much as the Irish, who had no money to buy other foods and starved to death or emigrated, while at the same time other crops were being exported. (Those times have been referred to as a type of genocide.)

An over reliance on a single variety of Potato didn't help either, as there were no others to select from for breeding up Blight resistance. These days, several Blight resistant varieties are grown, eliminating the need for anti-Blight sprays that contaminate soil with Copper etc. (Old Potato fields may also have toxic Mercury residues from anti-fungal sprays commonly used in the past.)

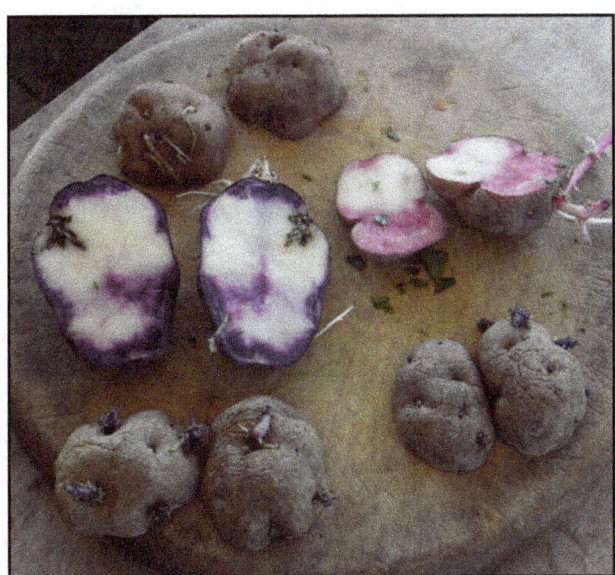

Being 'reduced to Potatoes' became a term for abject poverty. But really, it isn't that bad! We eat them as 'comfort food' and most people love them! A minimum of labour is needed to get a crop and this was the basis of the derogation of the Potato that 'it made the Irish lazy'. What this really meant was that they were made self-sufficient by living off Potatoes, such that they didn't want, or need, to work for the landlord!

Left - Heritage varieties of Maori Potatoes at Koanga Gardens, Wairoa, New Zealand

BROAD BEAN, VICIA FABA

Originating from the Mediterranean and further east, Broad Beans, also called Favas, are eaten in many regions, having been a staple since Neolithic times. The large and tasty Beans are high in protein, dietary fibre and essential vitamins and minerals, the young leaves are edible too.

Nip out the growing tips when plants have grown tall, for a tasty dish of greens.

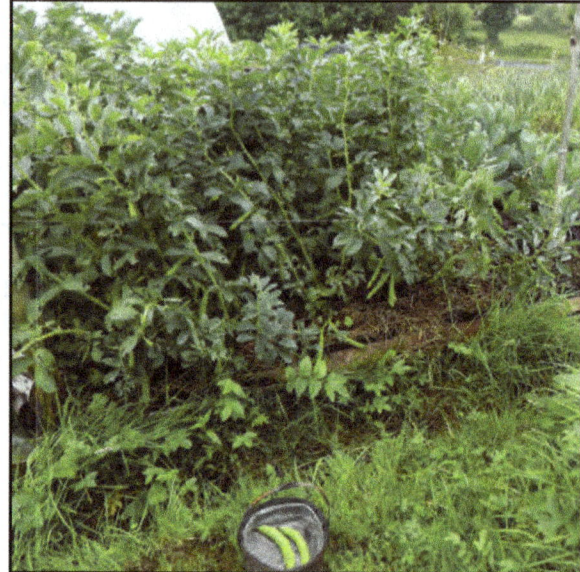

Immature whole pods and shelled larger beans are all used. They are delicious in stews and soups (going nicely with Potatoes), boiled then mashed and made into dips, and also sprouted then cooked. The Japanese marinade them with Shio Koji, a salty fermented product that brings interesting flavours. (As with other beans, when cooking Favas it is better to add salt only after they have become tender and this speeds up cooking time too.)

In springtime you can enjoy fresh young Broad Beans, with the whole pods sliced and steamed, or stir fried, being delicious. Italians savour the young fresh beans that are taken out of the pod and eaten raw with Pecorino cheese. Large fresh beans can be steamed until soft, then skinned and eaten warm, dressed with Lemon juice, salt and Olive Oil. Mature beans also make a wonderful dip when cooked and pureed with Olive Oil, Salt, Garlic and fresh herbs. More recipes later on.

When plants start to die off, leave some mature beans on the plant to naturally dry and be stored. I cut the plants at ground level and lay them in the polytunnel for a few days, then dry them undercover in shade for a week or so before storing longterm. Before cooking, the dried beans are soaked overnight (or half a day in warm water) and the tough outer jacket can be popped off with fingers before eating, or you can liquidise them whole.

I'm always singing the praises of Favas, but is there is downside to them. Curiously, the condition of Favism, a sort of allergic reaction to them, is a problem for many southern Europeans, where they are widely eaten. An Italian friend cannot stand even the smell of them and keeps well away. So, if cooking a meal for people, it's a good idea to check their Fava tolerance beforehand (as I should have!)

Favas are ideally grown in cooler climates and if the weather is too warm they won't flower and set pods, so they're best sown in autumn, to grow over the winter; or make an early spring sowing. Being super cold tolerant, handling down to -8°C, they give the first crop of beans in the summer. They prefer to grow in a well drained, open site with moderately fertile soil.

Removing the tasty top shoots to eat them also helps to prevent Black Fly infestation, while reducing vertical growth and encouraging more bean production. (An old remedy for Black Fly is to make a decoction of old, torn up Rhubarb leaves that are boiled for ten minutes, strained and sprayed over plants a couple of times.[3])

KALE, BRASSICA OLERACEA, ACEPHALA GROUP

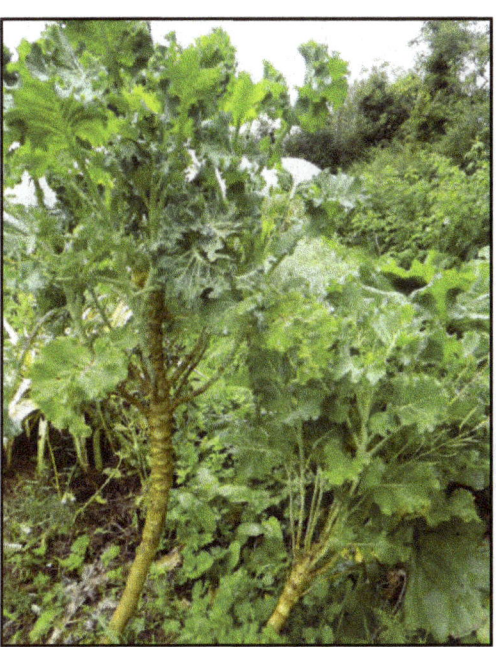

Kale (also called Borecole) is in the Cabbage family, but the central leaves don't form a head as a Cabbage does. Popular in northern Europe, Kale isn't generally appreciated as much elsewhere. I don't think I had ever eaten it until I came to Ireland. It was a revelation and I was so impressed with all the beautiful, colourful varieties, sporting tasty green, red and purple leaves. The young leaves can be good in salads, while the big leaves at the bottom can be steamed and stir-fried briefly to retain goodness. When Kales start producing flowering shoots in spring, these can also be snipped off and eaten like sprouting Broccoli. My favourite Irish variety is John's Kale. Originating from County Cork, where John grew it for 50 years, John's Kale is very tender, with great flavour, being good raw in winter salads, as well as steamed lightly or stir fried with a little oil. Black Kale, with it's dark narrow elegant leaves is a darling of restaurateurs. The photo above shows Daubenton or Portugese Kale, classed as a perennial, that I grew from cuttings.

A powerhouse indeed, Kale is a rich source of dietary fibre, protein, Thiamin, Riboflavin and Folate, and is also high in Vitamins A, C, K and B6, plus Iron, Magnesium, Phosphorus, Calcium, Potassium, Copper and Manganese. Kale is packed with phytochemicals such as Sulphur-containing Glucosinolates and Isothiocyanates that help ward off cancer; plus Carotenoids - powerful antioxidants that also support proper functioning of the immune and reproductive systems, and lowers the risk of cataracts. You can't eat enough deep green leafy veggies - Kale is a perfect candidate for the job.

ONIONS AND GARLIC, ALLIUM FAMILY

In cultivation since earliest times, the bulbs are indispensable for cooking tasty dishes, as well as for eating raw in salads; while young leaves of Garlic and Welsh Onions can be eaten like Chives. The high Sulphur content of all the Alliums has great powers of cleansing and disinfection, both for the body and garden, and they make good medicine. Garlic can be used as an insect repellant and is anti-fungal, often sprayed on crops; or eaten or drunk in water for expelling worms in people and livestock.

Take Garlic regularly, either raw or cooked, or made into juice, decoction, pickle or tincture, for lowering blood sugar levels, as a digestive and respiratory tonic, for coughs and colds, earache and gum infections. It also fosters a healthy heart, reduces high blood pressure, acts as an anti-inflammatory and anti-cancer food, and is a general prophylactic. Some Indian spiritual sects prohibit the eating of Onions and Garlic, due to their ability to 'stimulate the chakras'. So, do they make you more sexy? Indeed, herbalists might prescribe them to 'restore sexual function impaired by illness or stress.' [4] More on Onions and Garlic later on.

APPLES, MALUS DOMESTICA

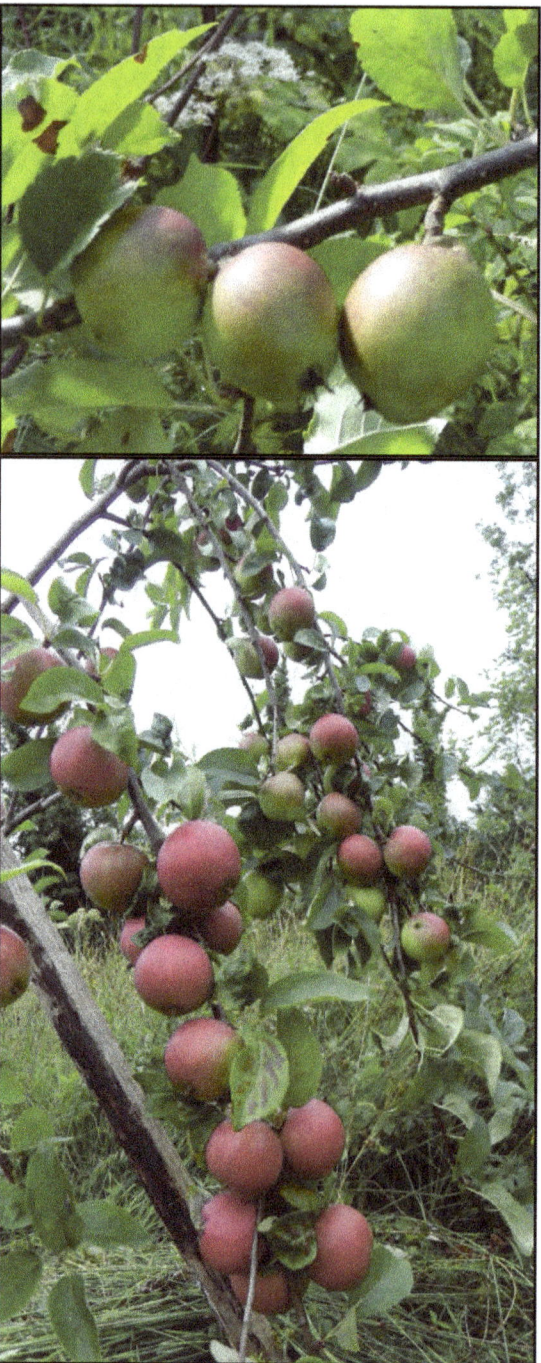

Long a symbol of paradise, the Apple trees that sustained people from earliest times grow perfectly in Ireland's climate and their blossoms in April and May are beautiful. Of ancient mythic status, they have been depicted as symbols of power and wisdom.

Such a versatile fruit, Apples are delicious fresh or cooked, made into sauces and compotes, baked into pies, made into juice (any variety can be, the Bramley Seedling is very good juiced), fermented into vinegar and cider, and dried for mueslis etc. Crab Apples are high in pectin and thus make good jellies and jams that need less sugar to set, while birds love to feast on them in winter.

The other outstanding quality of Apples is that they are very good keepers. Apples will store for many months in a cool, dry, dark place with good air circulation. One method is to wrap each one in a sheet of newspaper and keep them in a drawer or cardboard box in a cool room. Just don't keep them near Potatoes, as the Ethylene gas they exude will make the spuds sprout.

Despite growing well in Ireland, most Apples eaten here are imported.

Left - Late frosts in May 2021 meant that most of my Apple trees had no fruit. But the diversity of having seventeen Apple varieties meant that some did crop well, such as the Winston above, while the Tydeman's Early Worchester had a spectacular first crop, seen left.

PLANTS AND ANIMALS

USEFUL GARDEN PLANTS PROFILED

This list is mainly focussed on perennial plants that grow happily in a moist, temperate climate and can handle heavy soils. The most common vegetables are not all included, as information on growing them is freely available elsewhere.

ANGELICA, ANGELICA ARCHANGELICA

This large biennial herb can reach 2m high and 1m across. It grows wild in the damp, untrodden corners of wet meadows. Dramatically attractive, all parts are subtly aromatic, with medicinal, culinary and cosmetic uses. The striking flower heads are a magnet for bees and hoverflies. A legend goes that an angel revealed the plant's virtues of protection from infection to a monk, revealing a suggestion of much sacredness attached to it in the past. It was once much used as a plague remedy and today is known for its anti-bacterial properties. But it's mostly used for Candied Angelica these days, a deep green decorative confectionary on cakes. This is made from young springtime shoots; when these are stewed together with tart fruits like Rhubarb or Gooseberries, acidity is reduced and less sweetener is needed.

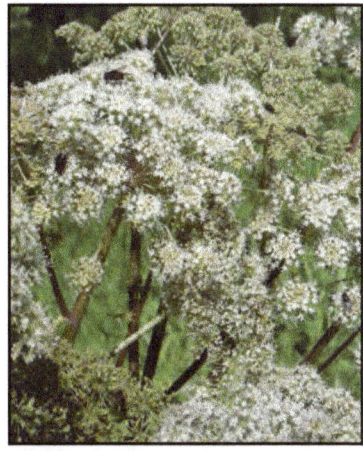

A few young leaves can be added raw to salads, giving a liquorice like flavour. Young leaves are also made into tea for indigestion, tension and headaches and are good for respiratory problems such as colds, as is a decoction of the roots. Large doses are to be avoided, especially by pregnant women and diabetics. Seeds, beloved food of small birds in the wild, are used in biscuits. Both seed and root are used for flavouring.

Easy to grow in damp ground and preferring partial shade, it produces statuesque flowers in the second or third summer and self seeds readily before dying off. Harvest leaves before flowering and dig up roots straight after flowering ends in the second autumn; harvest seeds when they are still green.[5]

ARONIA / CHOKEBERRY, ARONIA MELANOCARPA

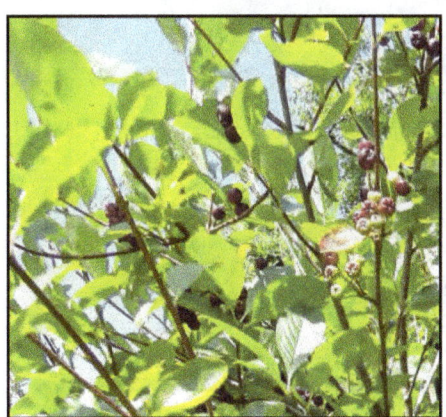

A member of the Rose family, Aronia is a tough North American berry plant, a deciduous shrub growing to a height of 1-4m tall. It grows easily and is widely grown across Europe and Asia, especially in Russia, Denmark and eastern Europe where the fruit is popular for juice and wine production. Little known in Ireland, several varieties are available to buy here. Originating from moist woodlands of the Upper Great Lakes and Appalachian Mountain regions, Aronias are very cold hardy. The pea sized purple-black berries are considered a superfood and the berry juice is valued for making jelly and healthy fruit drinks, containing high levels of Anthocyanins (source of red food colouring), plus Flavonoids, and with higher levels of Antioxidants than Blueberry juice.

For best production Aronias prefer moist but well drained sites, in full sun. They sucker and self-layer, so can be propagated that way and also trained into a hedge. Propagation is also good by seed that has been well cleaned, sown in September and stratified over winter. If the birds leave any for you, that is!

BARBERRY, BERBERIS VULGARIS AND OTHER SPECIES

Barberry species are easily grown shrubs, both evergreen and deciduous, thriving in full sun to heavy shade, that are northern hemisphere natives. Berberis vulgaris, the Common Barberry, grows to some 3m high, has prickly stems and is great for a hedgerow, as a living fence. Its small fruits, loved by the birds, are sharply sour flavoured but ok eaten raw, although they're more often cooked and made into preserves. Berberis berries often taste acidic and lemony, so they are useful as a citrus peel substitute. A forgotten fruit in Europe now, in Persian cuisine Zereshk is still important, used for flavouring Rice pilafs and poultry dishes. Iranian markets sell dried Zereshk, while in Russia it's used in jams with other mixed berries, the extracts popular for flavouring soft drinks and sweets. Ken Fern recommends the evergreen species Berberis darwinii for pleasant and milder tasting fruit, its hybrid cultivars are also good.[6] Berberis roots yield a yellow dye.

BAMBOO SPECIES

Many species of Bamboo are suited to woodland conditions and are not only gracefully beautiful but also produce edible shoots, eaten raw or cooked, plus canes for pea supports, craftwork and construction. There are several genera, Ken Fern recommends the Phyllostachys genus as being more suited to a soggy temperate climate. Luckily the runner species that can become invasive in warm climates don't usually become rampant in colder climates. Fern lists some of the most useful species in this genera as P. auea (Golden), P. nigra (Black), and P. dulcis (Sweetshoot Bamboo, which he says is highly regarded for eating in China).[6] In addition, Bamboo leaves when finely chopped can be fed to poultry, and if added to their dust bath, parasites are repelled by them.

BAY, LAURUS NOBILIS

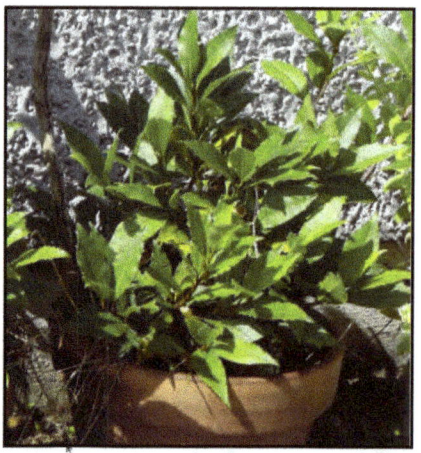

In Ireland the evergreen Bay tree only grows to shrub height, but in a warmer climate it can reach 12m high. Leaves are essential to bouquet garni, adding flavour to many dishes, the fresh ones being stronger than the dried. An essential oil used in soap making can be made from the berries and dried aromatic leaves repel insects, so a few are placed with stored food to protect it.

Bay trees are shallow rooted and, in the first few years, need frost protection of a good thick mulch if it gets very cold. Position them in full sun or semi-shade, protected from wind and given good drainage and rich soil. Root exudates are rather hostile to other plants, so keep them at least 1m away from them, or grow one in a large pot and move it to a sheltered spot over winter.

BEETROOT, BRASSICA VULGARIS

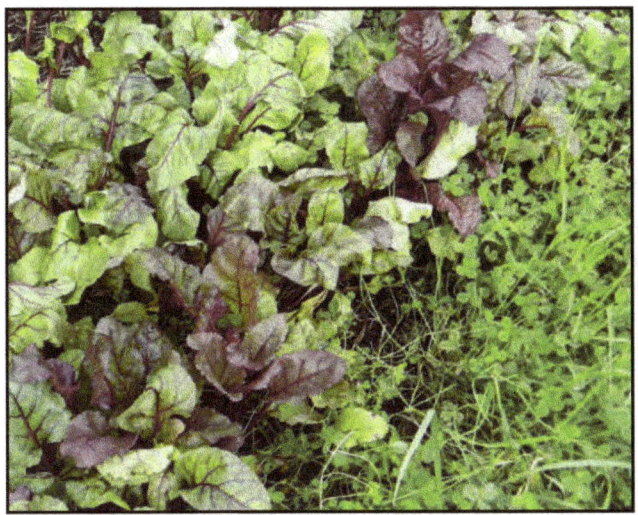

Not only is the root of Beet tasty and wonderfully nutritious superfood, the greens are good too. Young leaves can be eaten raw or steamed, though they are fairly high in Oxalic Acid, so eating them no more than twice weekly is a good idea (like all foods high in this). Beetroots store well in a clamp. And if you leave a few plants in the ground over winter they'll sprout early spring greens for you to enjoy, eaten lighty steamed.

Photo shows Beetroot growing happily with Red Clover.

BERGAMOT / BEEBALM, MONARDA DIDYMA

A small herb plant growing to 1m high and 50cm across, the young leaves are used raw or cooked, while they also make a good potpourri ingredient when dried. An aromatic tea made from leaves is good for digestive problems and, when added to black tea, gives it the classic Earl Grey flavour. The showy fragrant flowers are loved by bees, while the flower petals are good for eating in salads. Bergamot ideally grows in a moist, rich soil, in a semi-shady or sunny spot. Divide the clumps every three years.

BLACKCURRANT, RIBES NIGRUM

One of the easiest of soft fruit to grow, the delicious and nutritious berries can be dried and stored. They were once a key ingredient in Pemmican, the traditional dried food of native north Americans for long journeys and also polar explorers, the dried currants being pounded together with dried meat and the balls coated in fat for long keeping.[7] Delicious jams and syrups are also made from the berries, which have high pectin levels, so they set easily. As with other Currants, flowers are good for salads, but don't eat too many or you'll have no berries.

Young Blackcurrant leaves are aromatic and can flavour black tea when infused for just five minutes (longer brewing brings out excess Tannins). The leaves can be used alone as medicinal tea, also for seasoning dishes, the young ones used fresh on sandwiches and in fruit salads, also made into syrup with a lemony taste. They can be dried for off season use. Berry juice is well known for alleviating respiratory infections, such as sore throat and coughs. The well known drink 'Ribena' was made from them in World War Two. Berries are high in flavonoids, so they strengthen capillaries. Young leaves, twigs and buds are made into tinctures (preserved in alcohol) to treat allergies and joint aches, and were once known as 'Gout Berries'.[8]

The seeds are an important source of GLA (Gami-linolelic acid), a powerful anti-blood clotter and a guardian against arterial disease, also helping with weight loss and acting as a precursor of beneficial hormone-like substance PGEI. Seeds are the commercial source of GLA.[5]

Planting Blackcurrants on heavy clay can reduce their growth size. Mine grow vigorously on raised beds. Harvesting is simplified by cutting off whole branches of fruit and taking them indoors to pluck at leisure. Using a fork to strip branches can reduce berry damage.

BLUEBERRY, VACCINIUM CORYMBOSUM
The plump blue fruits are delicious super food, but plants are very exacting in soil requirements and not easy to grow well. Learning that the famous antioxidant content of fruit is surpassed by that of wild Elderberries and also Blackcurrants, I'm not getting too excited about growing Blueberries. Acid, well drained soil and warmth are essential. You can grow them in acidic potting mix in polytunnels. That's where my unhappy outdoor ones were transferred to in the dormant season. Growth is much improved now and I even got some berries. If you live in an acidic peaty bogland, they could make good sense there.

BURDOCK, ARCTIUM LAPPA
With its prickly burrs and big floppy leaves, this distinctive wild biennial herb grows up to 2m tall and does best on rich moist loose soils in sunny spots. Popular in Japan where it's eaten as a root vegetable, the nutritious roots contain up to 45% inulin. Inulin is a probiotic gut food, a starch that doesn't break down easily and immune stimulating. They're good eating for diabetics and for weight loss, but inulin can cause flatulence. To prepare roots, they can be first peeled (or not), then boiled, sliced, patted dry and sautéed, and served with a lemony dressing. Young leaves and green stems can be steamed and cut up for adding to salads, or boiled and added to soups and stews. Flower stalks, picked before flower buds have developed, can be peeled and the soft white part boiled and eaten with a sauce, or a dash of Lemon juice.[9]

Burdock stems and leaves are also eaten; while the leaf, root and seed are all medicinal, used for internal cleansing, stimulating the liver, gallbladder, spleen, kidneys, bladder and skin, so - great for a de-tox. It's an ingredient of Essiac, an anti-cancer herb mixture based on ancient native American herb lore. The root is mostly used for medicines, harvested from second year plants. Root tea, plus massage oil infusions, leaf compresses and salves for skin problems are also used. The leaf is bitter, a digestive stimulant and diuretic.[10]

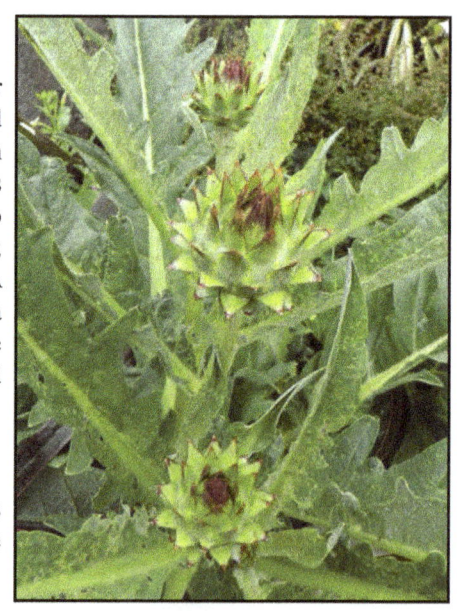

CARDOON, CYNARA CARDUNCULUS
Closely related to the Globe Artichoke, the flower buds are smaller and fiddly to eat. The leaves and stalks are eaten, being rich in Potassium, Calcium and Iron. Bitterness can be removed from stems by blanching them first. Leaf tea is drunk to stimulate the gall bladder and detoxify the liver; while leaves can also yield a yellow dye. A decoction of the leaf (boiled) can be used as a rennet substitute in cheese making. Cardoons are perennial and grow vigorously up to 2m tall and 1m wide.

CELERY LEAF, APIUM GRAVEOLENS
A smaller, hardier and finer form of Celery that's closely related to Wild Celery, all parts of the plant have culinary uses. It provides leaves and

small stems for seasoning stews and soups with a Celery flavour; while the seeds are a component of Celery Salt. Harvest roots in the second year for medicine, for arthritis, gout, asthma and bronchitis in particular.[5]

Originally a plant of marshland, it needs plenty of moisture and a rich, alkaline soil. It's particularly valued over winter, when it survives much better than normal Celery. Red Celery has small red and green stems and is also closely related and useful over winter.[11]

CHICKWEED, STELLARIA MEDIA
A small native herb that's ubiquitous in shady corners, it's nutrient dense and leaves make a healthy tea (fresh or dried), or can be added to mixed salads or made into broth and pesto. If not already wild in your garden, plant Chickweed in moist, fertile soil in semi-shade. It's a good ground cover plant for a Food Forest.

Harvest the green bits with scissors before flowering in early summer. Most valuable in late winter and early spring when greens are few, Chickweed is considered one of the best spring tonics and the most tender eating of the wild greens. When eating it, chop it up small as stalks can be tough. Kress suggests cooking Chickweed by sautéing it in butter for five minutes, then serving with Lemon juice and salt to taste. For a pesto, blend washed Chickweed greens with Olive oil, salt, Garlic and nuts to taste.[10]

Medicinally valuable too, Chickweed can help problems in the respiratory and digestive systems. It can be juiced, added to smoothies and made into cough syrup. Used externally, it is soothing and cooling for itchy skin, burns or bites. Oils and salves are made of it, or you can simply crush the fresh plant into mush and apply it to skin. For a soothing bath, put the fresh plant into a sock or fabric bag with added rolled Oats and hang it under the bath tap as the water runs.[12]

CHICORY, CICHORIUM INTYBUS
A hardy perennial vegetable not often seen in Ireland, Chicory has pretty edible blue flowers and leaves in summer. In winter, the leaves can be forced for salads. Leaves can also be boiled to make a blue dye. The chicon roots are used for salads or are lightly cooked; or roasted, then ground and drunk as a Coffee substitute. Many cultivars exist. Chicory is easily grown but prefers alkaline, light soil. Used medicinally, it has bitter tonic, diuretic and laxative properties.[10] Slugs are not keen on eating it.

CHINESE ARTICHOKE, STACHYS AFFINIS

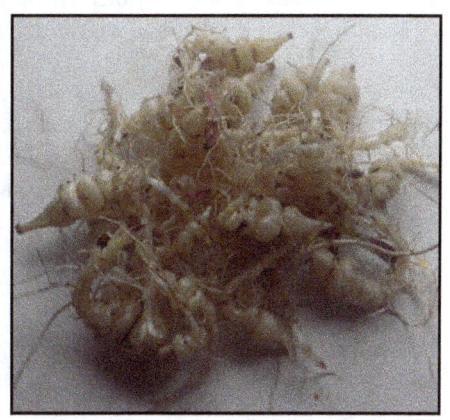

A small plant growing to some 45cm high and related to Mint, the tiny bumpy tubers (seen right) are edible, but small and fiddly to clean. They make a nice crunchy addition to a winter salad and are good lightly steamed also. If small pieces are left in the ground at harvest, it can become rampant. But it's easy enough to weed them out.

To make harvesting easier, I've switched to growing them in buckets, and can move them to a warm spot if frosts are threatening. They get a free draining soil mix and don't take over garden beds this way. As they grow, I mulch around plants with compost or straw, as it's advised to earth them up to encourage more tuber growth.

CHIVES, ALLIUM SCHOENOPRASUM
A perennial vegetable with Onion flavoured leaves that are available for much of the year, these are great for salads or cooked to flavour dishes. Flowers are edible too and attractive to Bees and Butterflies. Plants don't like it too hot nor do the tolerate weeds, but they are pretty much pest free. They grow happily in a polytunnel, where they can be kept drier than outdoors.

Garlic / Chinese Chives, A. tuberosum, are important in Chinese and Asian cuisine, with a mild Garlic flavour, the white part of the leaf stem, below the surface, is particularly appreciated. In Chinese cuisine the leaves are tied in a bundle, dipped in batter then deep fried; the flower stems also are cooked. The lovely flowers are a good cut flower when gathered at the end of the season and if fully dried will keep over winter.[13]

Give plants good drainage and light fertile soil in a lightly shaded, humid environment. Leaves appear early in the spring. Plants may live up to thirty years. Three or four year olds can be divided in spring or autumn to get more plants. Feed regularly with liquid Nitrogen rich fertiliser and keep them weed free.

CHOKEBERRY, ARONIA MELANCARPA, SEE ARONIA.

CLOVER, WHITE AND RED, TRIFOLIUM SPECIES
Lovely ground covering plants, you can eat young leaves and young flowers in salads, or cooked, or make tea of them, with mild medicinal effects. Seeds are great for sprouting as well. Caterpillars of Moths and Butterflies, as well as Bees, love to feed off this plant. Grown in an Apple orchard, Clover is said to help trees produce tastier fruit that also stores longer. But it is not a friend to Gooseberry bushes, as it harbours a mite.[6] Grown as a Green Manure or Living Mulch plant, it fixes atmospheric Nitrogen into soil, sharing it with other plants, especially when regularly mowed. My Piglets adore eating Clover!

COMFREY - SYMPHYTUM OFFICINALE
Comfrey is essential in an organic garden. This native, medicinal species is a rich source of Allantoin and ideal for treating skin problems and for broken bone healing, hence it's alternative name 'Knitbone'. Despite millennia of human use, Comfrey is only used externally these days, for a couple of reasons. The root is the part mostly used for medicine. Leaves and stalks also yield a yellow dye, with added Alum.

Comfrey has been an important food since ancient times, but, as with any medicinal foodstuff, care should be taken. Leaves can be used (sparingly) in mixed salads or infused as tea, cooked as a glutinous vegetable, or dipped into batter and fried (Swarzwurz) - a delicious tempura dish. Leaf furriness disappears with heating and cooking. Comfrey is highly nutritious to eat, with high protein levels and even vitamin B^{12}.

But unless you have S. officinale, the medicinal species, care is needed because of toxicity due to the presence of Pyrrolizidine Alkaloids. Comfrey hybridises very easily and hybrids have sterile seeds, so if don't see seedlings growing around the place, you probably have the hybrid. Natural hybrid species, such as Russian Comfrey, are the predominant ones in cultivation.

S. officinale can be identified by the winged appearance of stems, where leaves join the stem.

Though demonised in places like Australia as too toxic to consume (I remember well how it was banned in the 1980's, when I was studying herbal medicine), scientific research since then has clarified the danger. Toxicity from ingesting Pyrrolizidine Alkaloids builds up gradually and can lead to liver damage. However, it turns out from analysis of mature leaves that little, if any, is present in them. In fact young leaves contain up to sixteen times as much, so it's best to avoid them.[14] Roots have differing amounts at different times of the year, but always have more than the leaves. Don't eat them either.

So what is a safe amount to ingest? According to Bisset and Wichtl (2000) - "a high level of consumption of leaves as a salad is five or six leaves daily." [12] So, a couple of mature leaves daily taken short term should be ok.

Grow Comfrey in sun or semi-shade in moist soil. Keep plants well fertilised and watered. They die back in winter and re-sprout early each spring. The root mass can be divided to make more plants. If any piece of root is left in the ground it will sprout. A row of Comfrey plants in the garden can act as a weed barrier. Comfrey also makes a fabulous plant fertiliser, but the Potassium levels are only around 3%, compared with around 7% for the hybrid Russian Comfrey, the variety common in cultivation.

Bocking 14, seen below, is a selected form with highest Potassium levels. Comfrey clippings can be buried under Tomatoes and Potatoes at planting time, or added to composts. Comfrey clippings also make a great mulch around Tomatoes, Potatoes and Berry bushes, but don't use it on acid lovers, as it's quite alkaline. A ring of leaves around a young plant can act as a Slug deterrent too. Use it as a liquid fertiliser - soak leaves for several weeks, then dilute with water to a pale colour.

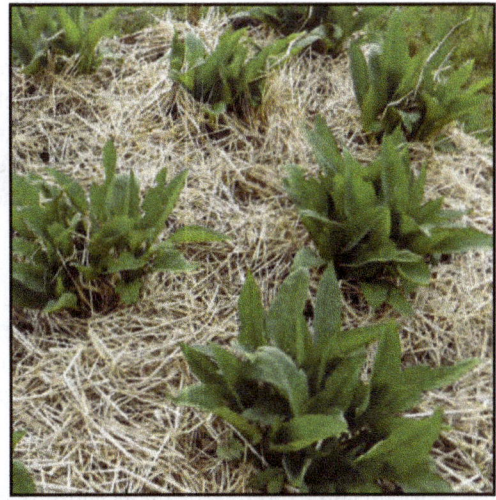

A bed of Comfrey can provide up to eight harvests per year, but only after it is established after growing two seasons. The first cut is usually made in April, when plants are some 60cm tall and before flower stalks appear. They are trimmed to about 2cm above the ground and when regrowth has reached 60cm again, about a month or so later, they are clipped again and again, until September.[24] This will stop plants from going woody and helps to keep a steady supply of fresh leaves available.

The selected variety Bocking 4 has around 35% protein, and is considered an excellent animal feed. Since Comfrey was demonised by the pharmaceutical lobby in the 1980s there has been a cover-up about how beneficial this plant is for people and animals. Tonnes of it has been fed regularly in bulk to zoo animals. My internet search failed to find any Bocking 4 for sale, also there was conflicting information about the best variety for animals and plants. So I'll just use my hybrid Russian Comfrey and Bocking 14 plants.

COWSLIP, PRIMULA VERIS
This hardy perennial native has edible leaves while the pale yellow flowers are tasty in salads or made into wine. A medicinal tea of leaves is used for relaxation or insomnia. The Saponin rich roots are edible too, but toxic if overeaten. Roots are harvested in autumn and have been used for treating whooping cough and bronchitis. But in the wild, they are not very numerous and are protected by law. So grow your own!

DANDELION, TARAXUM OFFICIANALE
This common weed of gardens is a green gold mine! The whole plant is useful as a nutritional superfood. Leaves are great in mixed salads and leaf tea, being best used before flowering starts and bitterness increases. Blanching can remove bitterness, by soaking leaves in water for a couple of hours before use. The flowers are loved by Bees and they can be harvested as young buds, or just the petals used raw in salads; or the flowers cooked as tempura (fried in batter); or briefly blanch them in boiling water, then sautée with seasonings and add Lemon juice on serving. Flowers can also be made into wine and beer. Roots can be cooked as a vegetable, being best dug in autumn, when they have the highest inulin content and the least bitterness.[14] Roots can be thinly sliced then sautéed with seasonings, or simmered in a little broth. Or wash and slice roots then dry them for storing.

Medicinally, Dandelion is traditionally used for kidney and liver problems, also for rheumatism and arthritis. It stimulates the liver, gallbladder, kidneys, pancreas and bladder. Young leaves are packed with medicinal bitter compounds and are high in vitamin A, B, C, D, plus Potassium. Roots are rich in inulin, the immune stimulating compound.

Such an ubiquitous plant and a curse to the tidy lawn grower, Dandelion was grown as a food crop until recent times in Britain. In Italy, the crop is still grown and is called Catalonia there.[14] In Ireland it was grown for food and medicine in medieval monasteries, such as the Holy Cross Abbey in Tipperary. Dandelions are grown commercially in the US, France and Japan.[15]

Planted in a humus rich garden bed with loose, deep and friable loam, Dandelions will grow large with good sized roots and provide a much improved harvest than that from the wild. Plant or thin Dandelion seedlings to be spaced around 10cm apart. Remove all flowers before they turn into seed heads or they will spread everywhere! The whole plant soaked in boiling water makes a Copper rich plant fertiliser for the garden.

DAY LILLY, HEMEROCALLIS FULVA
Not just an attractive and hardy clumping plant that thrives in a variety of situations, the flowers, shoots and roots are all edible. Use the sweet tasting flowers fresh in salads, or as a glamorous garnish, or pick them at the end of day when they've withered and add them to soups and stews for flavour and thickening, as the Chinese do.

ELAEAGNUS SPECIES
These useful shrubs were growing beautifully amongst fruit trees at the Koanga Institute in New Zealand, when I visited and Kay Baxter was waxing lyrical about these plants that I had not encountered before. They fix Nitrogen, make good companion plants and can help to increase fruit yields by some 10%, Ken Fern enthuses.[6] By trimming leaves and branches regularly, the Nitrogen they fix is shared with fruit tree roots. There are evergreen and deciduous species, and these can handle woodland shade as well as full sun, doing best on poor

to moderately fertile, well drained soil. They don't like wet soils but otherwise are tolerant of many situations. Handling the wind well, they make good screens if planted at around 75cm spacing. Evergreen varieties can be trimmed, but deciduous ones are best left untrimmed.

Providing tasty small berries early in the springtime, these must be soft and fully ripe before you eat them. They'll ripen more if put them in a warm room. Fern is very keen about this genus (so are the birds!) and recommends the best evergreen species for fruit as E. macrophylla and hybrid E. x ebbingei; while rating E. multiflora, Goumi, and E. parvifolia the best of the deciduous species. I went looking for some Elaeagnus in a local garden centre on my return to Ireland and did find a few ornamental species there, perfect to plant in my Food Forest. Fern says Eleagnus will fruit better if there are a few different cultivars nearby, such as Gilt Edge, for cross pollination.

ELECAMPANE, INULA HELENIUM

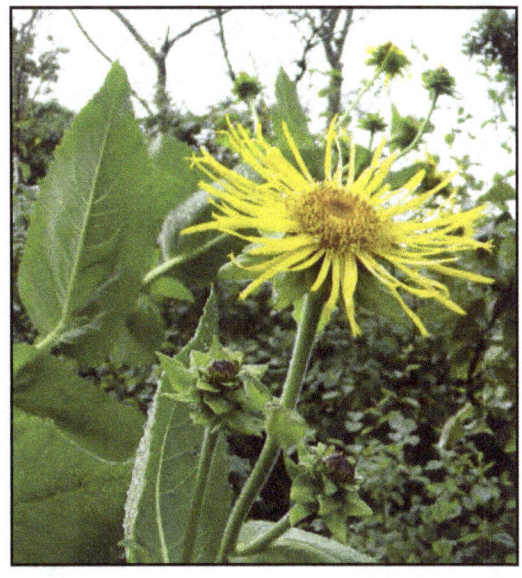

A native of Asia but now naturalised across the northern hemisphere, it yields medicine and food. The root can be candied and taken to help digestion, respiratory and chest ailments, and is specifically used for TB. It's a hardy perennial growing to a 1.5m - 2.4m height, with lovely Sunflower like flowers. The root of two or three year old plants is harvested in autumn as a vegetable or dried for medicine. A root decoction can be used for skin problems, hence another of it's names: Scabwort. Sow seeds in spring and remove offshoots in autumn for replanting, when large plants can be divided. [5]

EVENING PRIMROSE, OENOTHERA BIENNIS

This hardy biennial with attractive yellow flowers grows easily anywhere, but prefers sunny, dry situations. It self seeds prolifically, unless dead headed after flowering. All parts of the

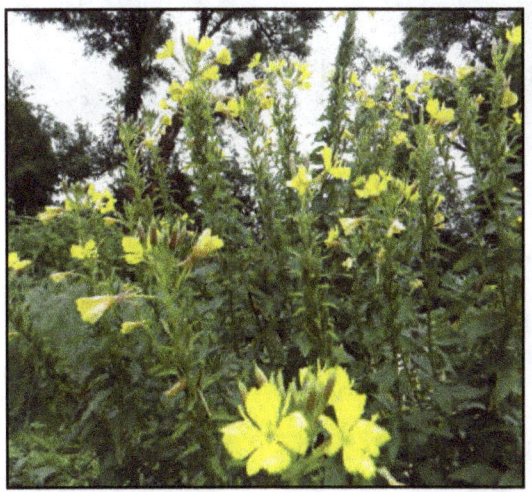

plant are edible - roots, stems, leaves and flower buds, plus the just opened flowers. Leaves are best used fresh and before flowering. In autumn, the roots of second year specimens can be boiled as a vegetable, or pickled etc. They are said to taste like Parsnip. Seed oil has fabulous medicinal qualities that has been well investigated scientifically. It's a rich source of Gama-Linolelic Acid (GLA) and has been found very useful for treating multiple sclerosis, arterial disease, rheumatoid arthritis, PMS, eczema and other conditions.[5]

FENNEL, FOENICULUM VULGARE

A hardy and attractive perennial plant that has naturalised around the world (especially common beside railway tracks in Australia). Common and Bronze Fennel has edible seeds, leaves, stems and bulbs. Bronze Fennel is a beautiful addition to the garden. Having medicinal qualities also, Fennel goes well with fish dishes and the seeds are helpful for digestion, either chewed after meals or taken as a tea. Florence Fennel / Finocchio (below) is mainly grown as an annual for it's large bulb that's great raw in salads or cooked. It can grow over winter in a polytunnel.

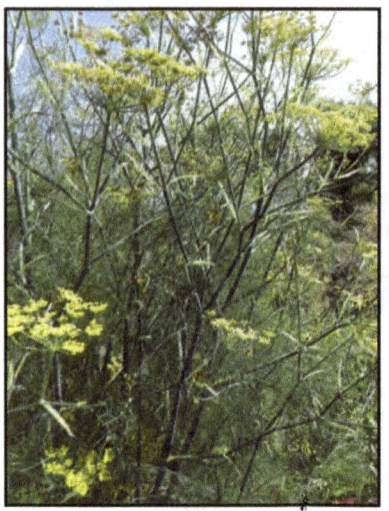

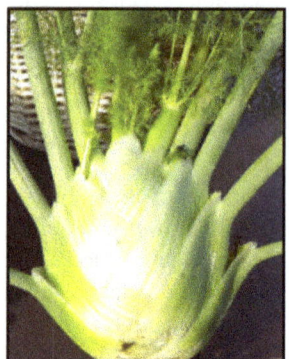

Grow Fennel in a warm, well drained, sunny spot, where they can can reach up to 2m height, though Florence Fennel will only get to half that size, or less.

FUCHSIA SPECIES

All species of this common native and domesticated garden shrub genus have berries that are edible, raw or cooked. Berries must be fully ripe, however. Ken Fern recommends F. splendens for the best fruit, though it's not the hardiest and can die right back after heavy frost, which then causes delayed fruiting later on. There are a host of cultivars available to choose from. Wild Fuchsias are often found growing in Irish hedgerows, as in the photo right, taken in County Donegal.

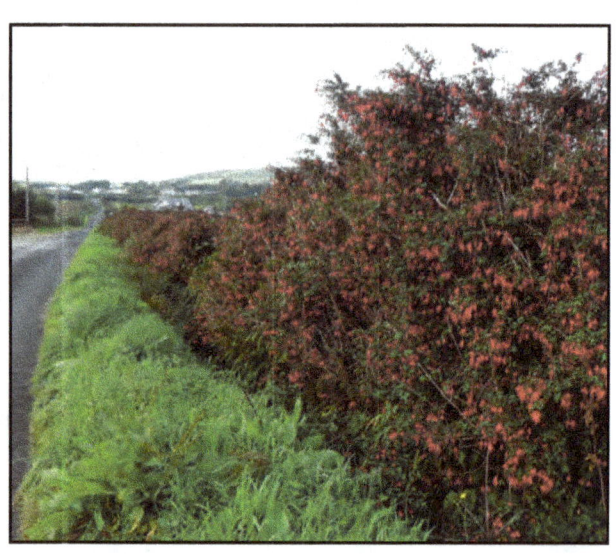

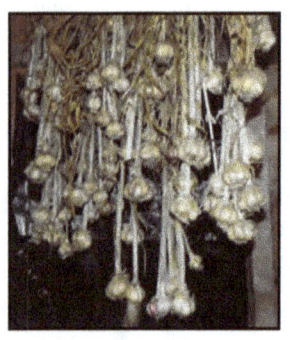

GARLIC, ALLIUM SATIVUM

Garlic grows well in Ireland, as long as soils are free draining. Grow it amongst food crops (except for Beans and Peas) and beneath Roses and fruit trees, as a good companion plant that can ward off pestilence. It does well over-wintering in a polytunnel too, where, as it matures you can keep it rather dry, as it prefers.

The flowers can be eaten[13], as can the leaves in winter and spring (use them like Chives). Garlic can be brewed to make an

insecticide and also rubbed on stings and bites to neutralise the poison. Long used as medicine, Garlic can reduce blood pressure, treat fungal problems, guard against colds and indigestion, expel worms and treat toothache (with pulp applied to teeth), TB, whooping cough (put a crushed clove in shoes), typhoid, diabetes, hepatitis and more.
5

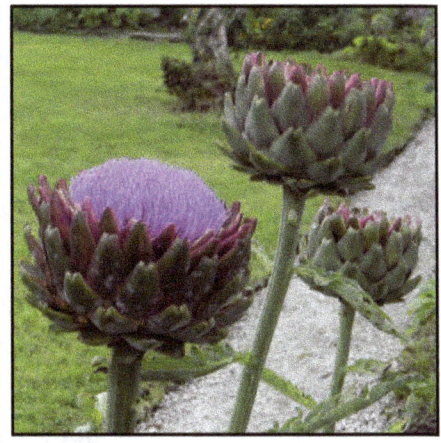

GLOBE ARTICHOKE, CYNARA SCOLYMUS
A statuesque perennial for larger gardens, it grows to about 1.5m high. Relatively low yielding, you need a few plants to make it worthwhile. A few different varieties planted can spread out the harvest. Eating the base of the bracts of the big flower buds, picked just before they open, is slow and fiddly, but rewarding when you reach the heart beneath them. Some varieties have extra big hearts, such as the Vert de Laon, that I'm growing from seed now. The Purple Artichokes I picked up from the annual local Plant Swop were a variable lot. Seedlings always are. But one plant is outstanding in its flower output, so offsets have been prised from it in springtime and these new cloned plants should also be high yielding.

Above - Flowering Artichokes in the old walled gardens at Jampa Ling Buddhist Centre, Co. Cavan.

GOJI BERRY, LYCIUM BARBARUM AND CHINENSE
Sold as a superfood, I naturally wanted to try growing my own. So, years ago I bought dried Goji berries, soaked them in water, extracted the seeds, then germinated lots of them. I planted these hardy, perennial plants on the dry rocky hillsides of my Australian farmlet and they did survive heatwaves, frosts and Rabbits. But I never saw any fruit. Moving to Ireland I bought a few plants by mail order. These grew and thrived, with long lanky branches stretching out everywhere. But years went by and I have still haven't seen fruit. So I took cuttings at pruning time and these quickly rooted. The new Gojis were planted out in the polytunnel and given trellising to climb up. They thrived even better than ever! But in summer they did develop fungus on the leaves, so it must be a bit too humid for them. Still no fruit. Hmmmm. A search online found that I was not the only one to have non fruiting Gojis, there were many others. I'm not saying that Gojis won't fruit, it may be that we have all missed something. But, just like Blueberries, I'm not excited about growing Gojis anymore.

GOLDEN BERRY, PHYSALIS PERUVIANA AKA EDULIS
This shrubby herb, a relative of Tomatoes, grows to about 1-2m high. The delicious tangy sweet yellow berries are surrounded by a lantern-like papery husk that protects them from some pests and disease. A perennial from warm climates, it's usually treated as an annual in Ireland, though they can survive a mild winter if protected. Berries are an excellent source of vitamins A, C and B-complex (Thiamine, Niacin and vitamin B12). Protein and Phosphorus are exceptionally high, but Calcium levels are low.[16]

Plants are easy to propagate from seeds or cuttings and do best grown in a polytunnel. They do tolerate some light frost, as well as heat. I was still picking berries in late December and the plants were still flowering, while Tomatoes nearby had already been killed by frost. Plants can be pruned hard after the harvest. After cutting them down I mulch over them with straw for frost protection and many come back again in spring. The green berries ripen slowly in the kitchen over several months. I wait until the yellow berry is seen glowing brightly from inside it's husk before eating it. It's at its sweetest then.

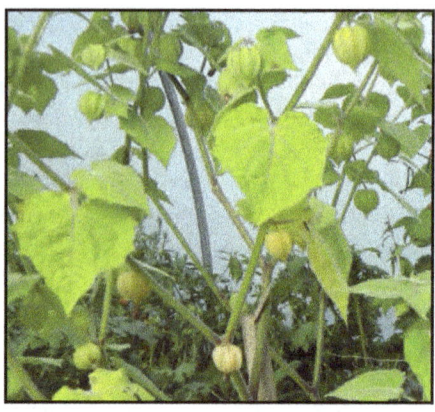

Fertile, well-drained soil is preferred, but if soil is too rich it'll gush with leaves and get straggly growth with reduced fruit production. Pests and diseases are rare, but mice and birds may take their toll. Nearly mature berries left in the husk keep well for several months in a dry place.

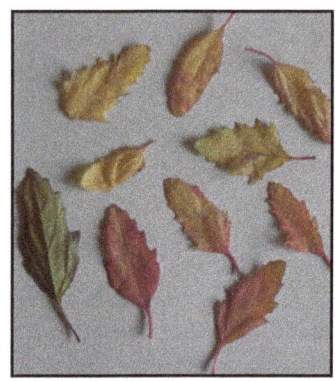

GOOD KING HENRY,
CHENOPODIUM BONUS-HENRICUS

This native perennial was once a popular leaf vegetable. A member of the Chenopod genus, its cousins include Quinoa and Fat Hen. Chenopod means 'goosefoot', you'll see the vague resemblance in the autumn leaves of Purple Topped Spinach, C. gigantum, seen left. Young leaves of all these species are edible and also the seed, but do soak seed overnight and rinse it many times before cooking or grinding for flour. Older leaves are tough and bitter due to Saponins and Oxalic Acid, but cooking reduces them. Young flower buds and shoots are also edible cooked, but fiddly to prepare. Tolerant of various conditions, plants crop best in rich soil.

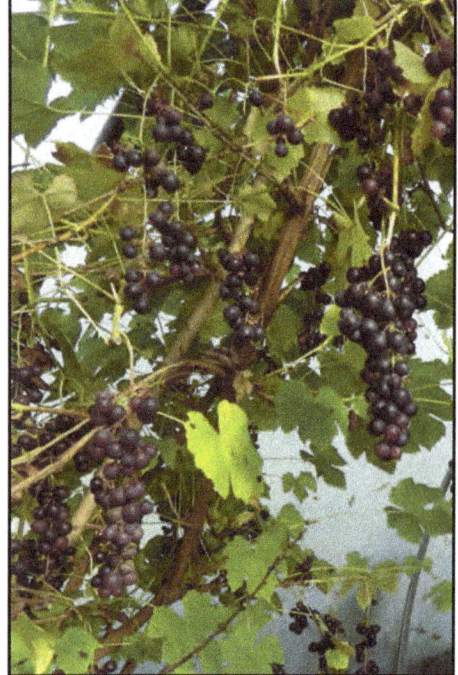

GRAPES, VITUS VINIFERA

How wonderful to feast on abundant bunches of fresh juicy dessert Grapes in summer. I also love the excellent raisins (dried Grapes) that we make for sweetening puddings over winter. Some will make Grape jelly and even the seeds are wholesome to crunch on. What is marketed as health promoting Grape Seed Extract, is just crushed seeds, it appears! As for the leaves, in spring and early summer they are used in pickling, as they help to keep preserved veggies crisp; they're also used for stuffed leaf rolls, such as the Greek dish Dolmades (which is Grape leaves stuffed with Rice and flavourings).

A polytunnel Food Forest is not complete without a Grapevine, or several. Vines can be planted near the tunnel edges, where roots can go outside for moisture, and they are best located on the north side, so as not to cast shade on the sunny parts. To extend the season, you can grow vines of early, mid and late fruiting varieties. I grow the vigorous variety most popular for polytunnels in Ireland, the Black Hamburg. (When I was in that region I was assured that no Grapes are grown that far north in Germany!) Vines are easily propagated with cuttings. Grape bunches can be stored for a while, an old French way is to hang vine-ripened bunches off hoops from the ceiling in a cool place. For best storage ability, they should be picked carefully with scissors to avoiding bruising. In a root cellar type situation they are said to keep for a month or two, if kept cool and moist in trays.

HORSERADISH, AMORACIA RUSTICANA

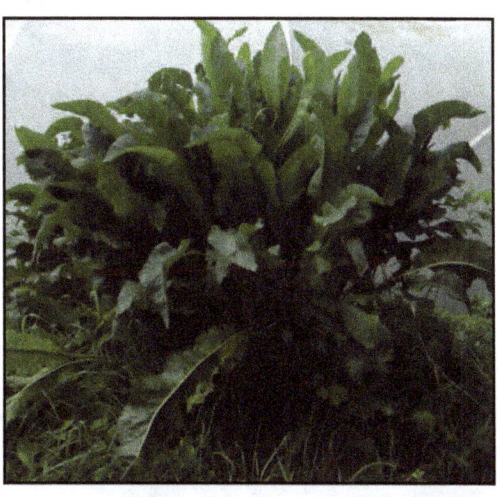

This European native is a vigorous and hardy perennial herb growing to a 1m high clump and spreading outwards indefinitely unless roots are restricted. I planted my two plants (seen right) into an old bottomless rubbish bin cut in half and each half filled with a soil and compost mix. But the roots still escaped and spread - it mustn't have been deep enough.

The long green sword-like leaves can be eaten, finely chopped in salads, when very young. The pungent roots are grated into sauces and pickles, but have your hanky ready! There's no tears if you liquidise them in a blender instead. Dig the roots, which can grow down to 60cm, from established clumps anytime, or in autumn after a spring planting. Use them fresh, before volatile oils disperse. Or keep the whole, washed root in vinegar to preserve it. Propagation from root cuttings is easy, too easy. Watch out for rampancy!

HORSETAIL, EQUISETUM ARVENSE

This perennial native herb of damp meadows is an attractive and useful 'weed' that's rich in Silica and makes a good liquid fertiliser, after boiling it up with water. Silica rich sprays such as Horsetail are used to combat fungal outbreaks in the garden. The stems and leaves also yield a yellow dye, with Alum.

HOPS, HUMULUS LUPULUS

Hops is a vigorous, hardy and attractive perennial vine, a native of northern Europe, that's mostly associated with beer making (the female flowers used for beer flavouring and preserving). Hops leaves and flowers also have decorative, culinary and medicinal uses, they yield a brown dye, and fibre can be made from the stems. As a medicine, Hops has depressant and anti-aphrodisiac effects, hence the beer drinkers' condition 'brewers droop'. The sedative effect of Hops flowers can be had from a tea or via a 'Dream Pillow' (a cloth bag filled with them), and is excellent for insomniacs; the tea is also good for indigestion. The tender young shoots are edible but slightly bitter, they can be steamed or boiled briefly, or cooked in stir fries. Young leaves, blanched briefly first, can be added to salads or soups, or sautéed.

These deep rooted plants are easy to grow in a rich, moist, well-drained soil in a sunny site, sheltered from wind. Taking three years to mature, plants will climb up to 5-6m in a season and need a stout trellis or structure to climb up, if a handy tree or hedge isn't nearby.

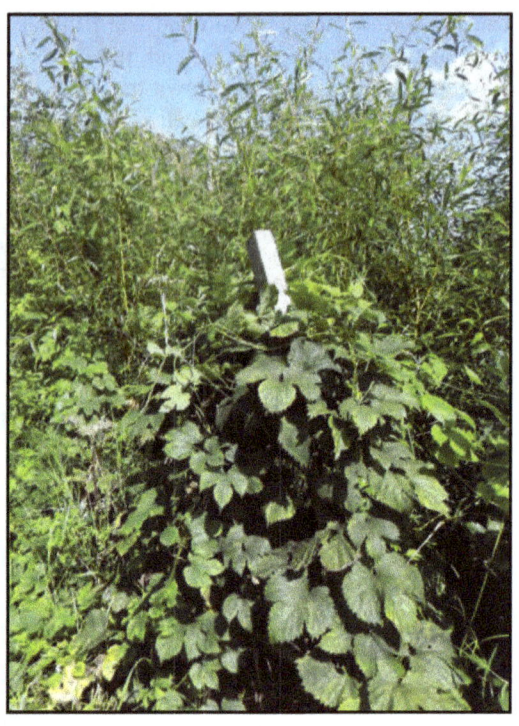

Right - Hops vines in the foreground are starting to climb up the Willows behind.

In the wild, Hops vines will typically trail up into trees, often in association with Alders. I purchased online some bare-rooted rhizomes of the popular cultivar Fuggles and planted them into mounds of good soil. No need to purchase more, I'm now digging up suckers, that pop up profusely from the established plants, and transplanting them to beside Alder trees in the Food Forest. One day it'll be a regular Irish Rainforest!

IVY, HEDERA HELIX

Ivy is very common in rural Ireland, where it's often seen smothering and killing trees with the weight of it making them rot and vulnerable to destruction from strong winds. In the past, Ivy would have been cut back regularly by the peasantry, as it was

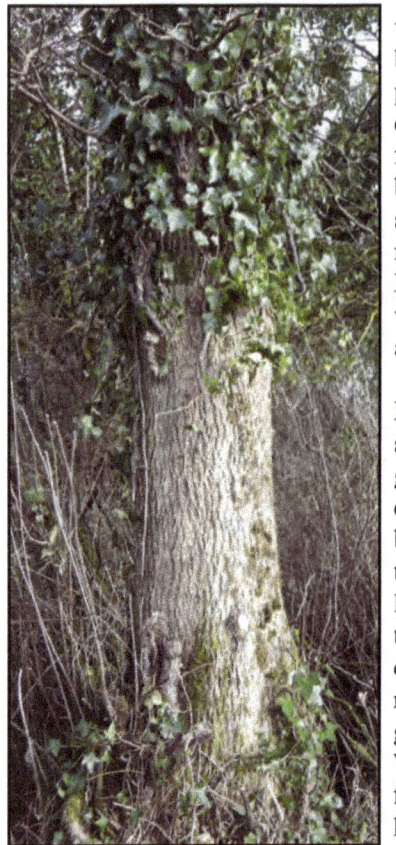

valued as a winter fodder for stock (except for Pigs), branches being cut for them to eat. The honey that Bees produce from Ivy flowers is very good too, with excellent medicinal properties. A black dye is made from boiled leaves, while twigs can yield yellow and brown dye. An important plant for wildlife, giving shelter to spiders and birds (including private nest sites), nectar for Bees and bugs, and food for Butterfly larvae; Ivy berries are a staple food for many birds in late winter and early spring, when nothing much else is around.

Indeed, the seeds get widely spread by birds and will sprout anywhere and everywhere in the garden. If Ivy grows as a ground cover where you don't want it, it's easily smothered by covering it over with old tarpaulins, black silage plastic or equivalent. To cut big stems from tree trunks you need a small saw and a pair of big loppers. I only cut Ivy that's growing up trees when the tree has become endangered by it, or when the shade cast by tonnes of it is too much for the garden. I tend to remove it from the southside of fields and leave more growing on the northside, where shading isn't an issue. When the thick stems are well dead, turning black and falling easily off the tree, they make excellent fire lighter sticks.

KALE, BRASSICA OLERACEA

Kale thrives in rich, well drained, moist soil, handles the cold and may even be sweeter when harvested after the first frost. One of the most hardy of veggies to grow, it's also fairly pest resistant. It's best for the plant if you just harvest a few well grown bottom leaves at a time, allowing new ones to be produced on the top. Generally frost hardy, if it does get extra cold you can put mulch up around the stems for protection. I grow them both outdoors and inside the polytunnels, where an autumn sown crop gives me early spring greens.

JAPANESE KNOTWEED, POLYGONUM JAPONICUM

One of the world's most invasive plants that can be difficult to kill, I'm not advocating that you plant it! But if there is an infestation of Knotweed near you, you might consider it's usefulness. Insects love the hollow stems, thus frogs and other animals find it a great source of insect food. People can also harvest it's useful bits, as one way of controlling it. The mature hollow stems are gathered by some to make into flutes, I was told in Germany. The young shoots in spring when cooked are said to have a pleasant taste and are used much like Rhubarb, in pies, jams etc. Seed can be ground and added to other flours, but it is a fiddly job. [6]

If you want to eradicate Knotweed without using chemical killers, it can be cut down, the pieces spread over the site and the area smothered with some type of light-excluding covering, such as the black silage plastic that's treated to resist UV radiation and lasts for years outside. Make sure there are no sharp bits on the ground to pierce the cover. You may want to help things rot down better by spreading a layer of manure or lawn clippings over the top, which makes a safer surface for the plastic sheet to go over. Leave it in place for as long as it takes, a year or more. On top of this, the space can be used as a weed free area for storing things, as a nursery area with pot plants, or whatever. The same smothering technique is good for eradicating other difficult-to-remove invasive plants such as Bindweed.

JERUSALEM ARTICHOKE / SUNROOT, HELIANTHOS TUBEROSUS

This North American root crop is related to Sunflowers, not Globe Artichokes. It's a perennial that can grow over 2m tall and have beautiful flowers in a hot summer. The name is a corruption from the Italian girosola, i.e. turning towards the sun. A valuable source of probiotic gut food, it is high in inulin, which does unfortunately cause flatulence, so is shunned by many, who call it 'fartichoke'. But - everything in moderation, eh? A few pieces of the root in a soup or stew will taste nutty and sweet, and is not too wind-inducing. Use it for not more than, say, 20% of a dish is my guestimation. You only need to wash the tubers, no peeling is required. It can also be finely sliced and pickled in Apple cider vinegar (see recipe on page 224), while some people ferment the starchy tubers to make fuel alcohol.

Give Sunroot a permanent position that's sheltered from the wind. Or if the wind cannot be avoided, keep stems trimmed and encourage more resilient bushy growth, by nipping out the growing tips after reaching 60cm, suggests Ken Fern.[6] It's super easy to grow, in fact, it's runners will take over the garden if not harvested. Heavy clay is not a problem for them! In spring, plant medium sized tubers about 15cm deep, selecting the least knobbly ones, at a spacing of 30cm apart, in rows that are 90cm apart, in medium fertile soil. Fuseau is the variety with least knobs and easiest to prepare. Yields can be improved by earthing up around the stems twice, suggests Klaus Laitenberger.[17] If you don't harvest all the tubers you'll end up a whole of tiny ones that are barely worth harvesting. Even small pieces can sprout, so harvesting must be thorough. But take your time with the harvest, they keep very well in the ground. They sweeten up when stored in situ over winter, as well. Or else harvest the lot and store them in damp sand. Or let Pigs root them up for food. Roots dehydrate quickly, so only remove them from storage shortly before use.

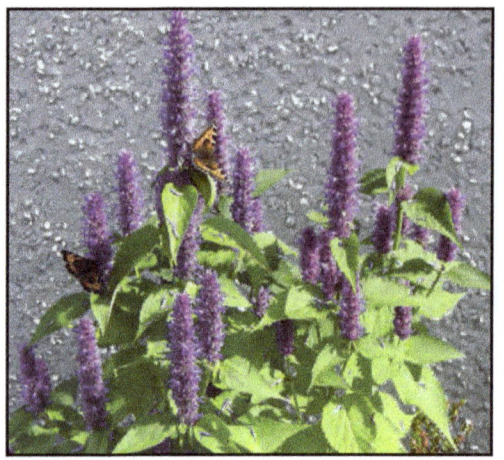

KOREAN MINT, AGASTACHE RUGOSA
A must-have plant, this hardy, short lived perennial has gorgeous purple flower spikes that last for months and are such a great magnet for Bees and Butterflies. The wonderful aromatic leaves, cut before flowering, have a minty, Anise flavour that is good for teas, salads and potpourris. Not a true mint, it's a cousin of Anise Hyssop, which has the same uses. Growing to 1m high in moderately rich soil, sunny sites and good in containers, replacements can be propagated from seed every second year or by division, or just allow it to self-seed. Only fertilise after flowering.

KOHL RABI, BRASSICA OLERACEA, GONGYLODES ACEPHALA GROUP
This wonderful vegetable is very hardy, easily grown, and stores well, but is rather unappreciated on Irish shores. Actually a swollen base that's either green, white or purple, it's lovely eaten grated raw into salads or sliced and steamed lightly, added to stews etc. Originating in northern Europe, the German name means Turnip-Cabbage. It needs a sunny site with fertile, free draining soil and plenty of moisture and nutrients to ensure steady growth, because if growth is checked or it gets too old it may go woody. Seeds can be raised in modules from April to late June and planted out a month or so later, at a spacing of 30cm by 30cm. Early sowings may bolt if weather is too cold. Store the bulbs of the later crops only. Store them somewhere cool and moist, packed in damp sand or similar, but they don't keep for too long.

LAVENDER, LAVANDULA SPECIES
This Mediterranean herb is a popular cut flower, while dried flowers go well in potpourris, herb pillows and moth repellant bags, some people even adding a few flowers to flavour culinary dishes. Lavendar's essential oil is esteemed for its calming and anti-bacterial qualities. It can also be used as a pest repellant.

Lavenders ideally need to grow in full sun and a well drained soil. There're happy in a large pot that overwinters in a polytunnel, or outdoors on top of a mound or wall. Semi-shade is ok but the aromatic oils won't be so abundant. Ireland's climate is not great for these half hardy plants. But they will thrive in a sheltered environment. Prune plants lightly in spring and early autumn to stop them from becoming woody.

LEAF BEET, CHARD AND SILVER BEET, BETA VULGARIS SUBSPECIES CICLA
This group of biennial plants are related to Beetroot. They are easier to grow and more robust and heat tolerant than true Spinach (Spinach oleracea) and can be available for most of the year. Several brightly coloured varieties of Chard are available - yellow, pink, orange and red - providing a good range of phytonutrients. Leaf Beet, aka Perpetual Beet, can keep on

producing leaves well into the second season if flower shoots are removed; if you leave a plant to seed they will happily self-sow. Fordhook Giant, a form of white stemmed Swiss Chard, is a popular cultivar that's recommended for hardiness over the winter and is regarded as having the best flavour by some.[18]

Leaves are cut as required and they are especially valued through the winter. Leaves are best cooked lightly, either by steaming, or in stir fries. Youngest leaves are used in salads. But be aware that they are high in Oxalic Acid, so restrict quantities eaten to no more than twice weekly. Stems are good cooked too, needing longer cooking than the greens, but without the Oxalic Acid.

LEMON BALM, MELISSA OFFICINALIS

This hardy, aromatic, perennial herb is very easy to grow and self seeds readily, even into concrete cracks. Plant in full sun for a stronger aroma and keep trimmed for new fresh growth. Use those fresh trimmings for tea, add leaves to salads, vinegars, cordials and cheeses, or dry them for Dream Pillows. Medicinally, Lemon Balm has a calming effect. Plants will go on producing leaves well into winter before going dormant. This is a staple tea plant! But in a dull summer, it will only produce a dull flavour.

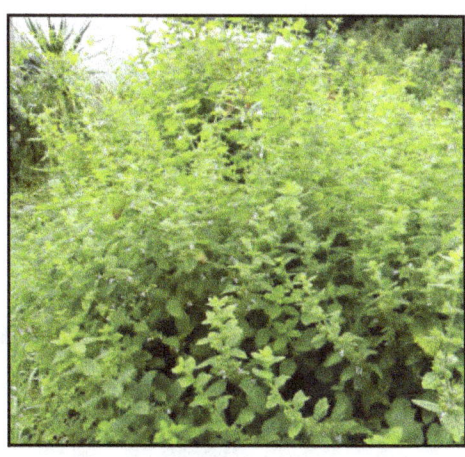

LOVAGE, LEVISTICUM OFFICINALE

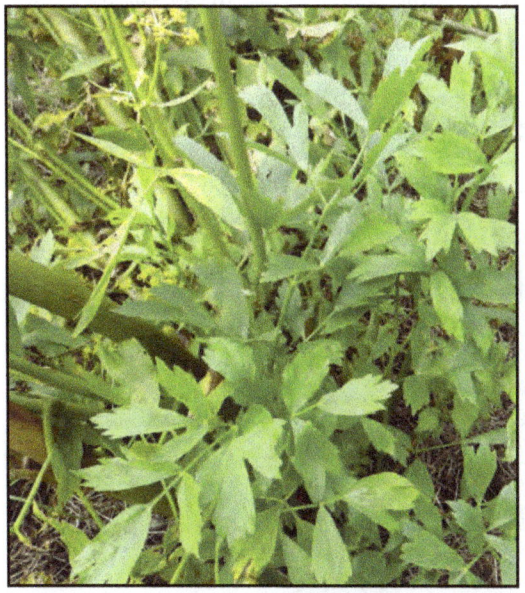

This is a great perennial herb for flavouring meals with a Celery like taste. A statuesque, hardy perennial it, grows up to 1.8m high and does best in a rich, well drained soil in sun or part shade, while it doesn't mind a heavy clay soil.

All parts have culinary and medicinal uses, aiding digestion, rheumatism and some skin problems. Young leaves and shoots/stalks in early summer are delicious in salads and soups etc. These are best harvested before flowering. Some people blanch the stems. The seeds are used for flavouring dishes and the flowers are a magnet for insects. Roots can be cooked as a vegetable, they're best when harvested after two to three years and with the bitter skin removed.

MALLOWS, MALVA SPECIES

These are several species of hardy annual and perennial small shrubs that are easy to grow, preferring well drained, fertile soil in sun or part shade. Young leaves and tender tips are used raw in salads or steamed, while older ones can be cooked like Spinach. Use leaves until flowering, then switch to harvesting the flowers. After flowering, cut Mallows back in autumn or they'll grow very straggly. A leaf decoction in a compress can treat skin problems, though Marshmallow is better. (Marshmallow is a plant of a different genera). Malva moschata, the Musk Mallow, grows to 1m tall. The Common Mallow, M. sylvestris, is a shortlived perennial that gets very straggly. Garden cultivars exist that sport more attractive flowers and good flavoured leaves, as seen right.

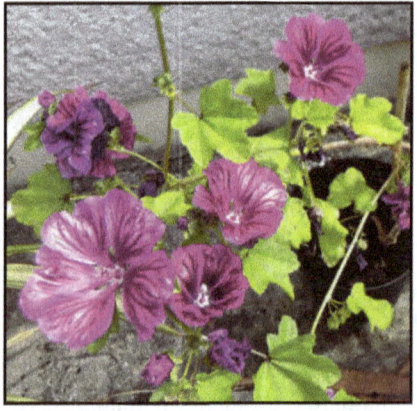

MARIGOLD, CALENDULA OFFICINALIS

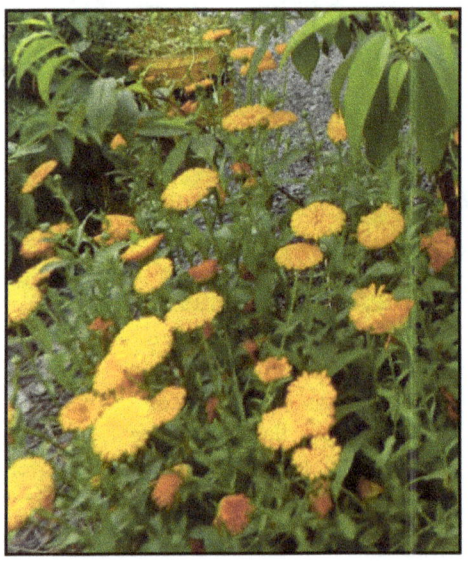

This useful and attractive annual plant is a must have in the garden! The orange-yellow flowers are lovley in salads and for garnishing also, but pick them young and only use the petals.[10] Marigold petals yield a pale yellow fabric dye (with Alum) and can colour food such as Rice ('Poor Man's Saffron'). Flowers are also used in cosmetics and skin lotions, Calendula tincture being a powerful wound healer with strong anti-bacterial and anti-fungal properties.

A hardy annual, native to the Mediterranean, Marigolds happily self-seeds and, inside a polytunnel, will flower into the winter, bringing cheery brightness. No wonder these lovely flowers are integral to the religious floral wreaths made by the Hindu people of India.

MARSHMALLOW, ALTHAEA OFFICINALIS

This attractive small shrub is a hardy perennial with mucilaginous leaves and roots, and pretty flowers that can be eaten raw in mixed salads or cooked. Butterflies love the flowers too. Its roots are the original source of confectionary marshmallows and they can be used as an egg-white substitute.

A sunny spot with a damp, fertile soil is ideal. Prune after flowering, otherwise it gets very leggy. Harvest roots in the second year in autumn, after the plant has gone dormant. Containing around 35% mucilage, roots can be made into a very soothing tea for inflammations, colds and sore throats. They can be also boiled, then fried and eaten as a vegetable.[5]

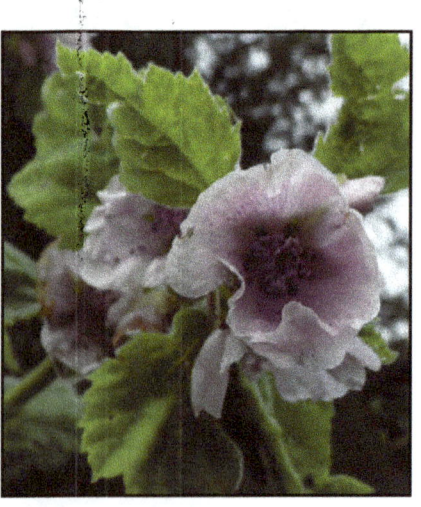

MASHUA, TROPAEOLUM TUBEROSUM

Mashua is a hardy perennial climbing plant from South America, grown where soil is too poor and wet for Potatoes, so - perfect for Ireland. It's related to the Nasturtium. Young leaves, tubers and flowers are all edible. The peppery tasting tubers contain substances that affect hormones and in their Andean homeland Mashua is shunned by men because it gives an anti-aphrodisiac effect, while they encourage their wives to eat it!

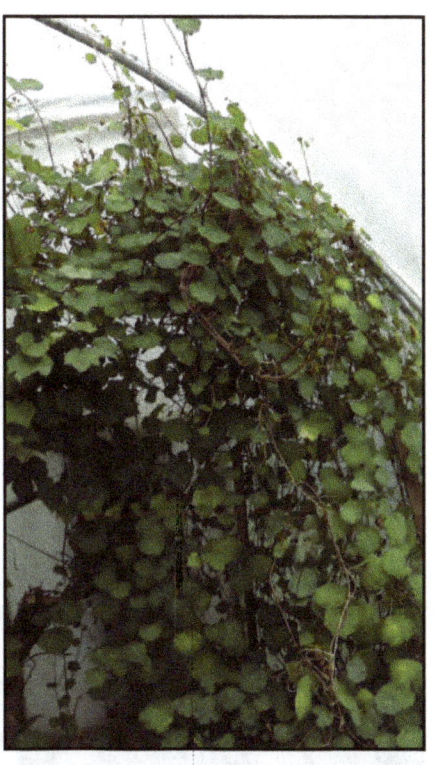

Plant tubers in April around 30cm apart and give them something to climb up. I grow mine outdoors and in the polytunnel, seen right, where they thrive and keep growing well into winter. The tubers, that come in big clusters, are larger than Ocas and develop close to the surface, so keep the plants well mulched around the stems, especially as cold weather approachs. They can handle light frosts. Harvest tubers after frost for improved flavour and store them for several months, or leave them in the ground and harvest when needed. They are very prolific and definately worthwhile growing.

MEADOWSWEET, FILIPENDULA ULMARIA

A deliciously fragrant herb of damp meadows, seen left in the foreground, the young aromatic leaves can be used for tea and to flavour cooked dishes. Flowers are also used for tea and wine making, flavouring drinks or adding to stewed fruit. As the plant is also medicinal with a mild diuretic effect, it's best not to drink too much flower or leaf tea. The roots can yield a black dye with Alum.

MINT, MENTHE SPECIES

With a wide range of varieties, from native Mints to the many cultivars, this is a perfect plant for Irish conditions. Fresh leaves are great for tea, but only use very hot, not boiling,

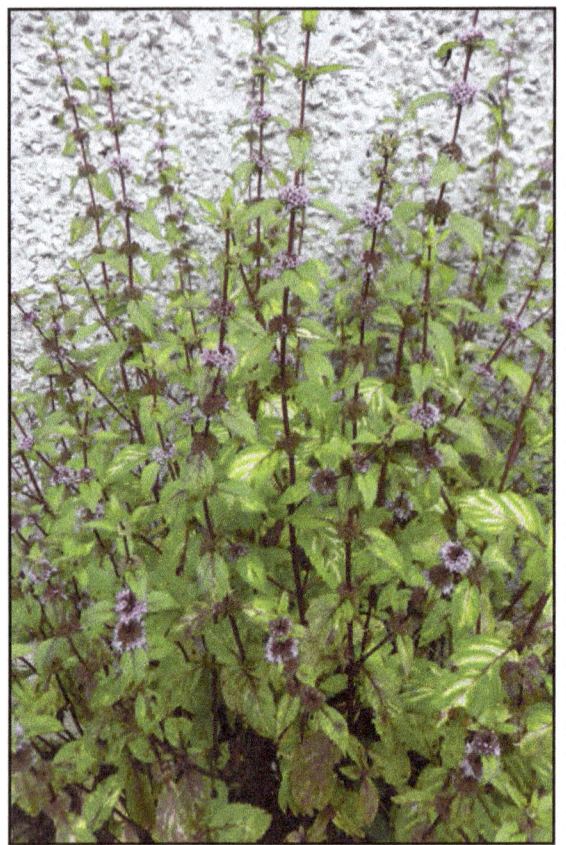

water and don't infuse Mint tea for longer than five minutes, or it goes bitter. Chopped Mint leaves can be mixed with other leaves in pestos and salads and are also good in jellies and dessert flavouring. The tea can assist digestion and headaches. In India, chutney is made from Mint leaves, see the recipe and more on page 198.

Mint is ubiquitous in Ireland and the wild Water Mint is surprisingly tasty, compared with cultivated varieties. Especially popular for tea making are the Moroccan, Curly and Chocolate Mints. (I can state this definatively, having conducted a taste testing exercise with a group at a Community Garden I helped to create in Australia.) The only non-culinary species is Eau de Cologne Mint, but this one is great in the bath, as it gets a bit soapy when soaked. Planted in moist spots, Mint will run rampantly.

I like to grow many different varieties, such as the Lemon Mint above, in 15 lt buckets, thus the spread is contained. I always keep pots 'socially distanced', otherwise their different aromas become confused if they are too close. In springtime it's good to give Mint pots a feed. In midsummer plants can handle a good haircut, chopping them down to about half their height to rejuvenate growth. Over winter, pots can be brought indoors or undercover, to give out-of-season pickings.

MITSUBA, CRYPTOTAENIA JAPONICA

This is a native Japanese vegetable, a short-lived perennial growing to 1m high. Preferring a shady, fertile and moist spot, it may die back in winter outdoors, but can survive down to -10C. Commercially it's usually grown in Japan as an annual that's produced all year round in greenhouses, the stems being blanched in special darkened beds with controlled temperature. Happy to grow in a Food Forest, or in the shade of taller vegetables, it can become a ground cover that self seeds itself. Start seeds for annual plants from spring to early autumn and protect seedlings from Slugs. Perennial plants are planted at 30cm spacing and can be picked for years, but if they get viruses, then discard them.

Leaves, roots, seeds and the blanched white stems are eaten raw or cooked very briefly, added to dishes at the end of cooking to keep the flavour, which Joy Larkcom describes as like a blend of Parsley, Celery and Angelica.[13] Pick as required the leaves and tender young stems (cut stems at ground level when 25cm high), before the plant goes to flower. Seeds can be sprouted and the young greens eaten as seedling sprouts.

MUGWORT, ARTEMISIA VULGARIS

Once known as the 'Mother of Herbs', this aromatic shrub has many uses, with young leaves used sparingly in salads. It's more known for its medicinal virtues, all parts of the plant being used. Also used as an insect repellant and yielding a yellow dye, it has a soothing effect for insomniacs when dried flowers are used in a Dream Pillow. The seeds are said to be liked by hens and may help control their lice and worms, according to Bob Flowerdew. [19]

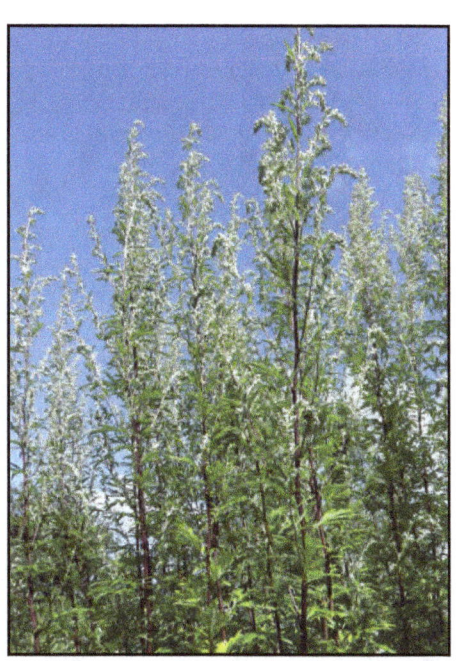

In Korean Natural Farming, Mugwort is chopped and mixed with half of its weight with brown sugar, then packed into a clay pot to ferment. The resulting Fermented Plant Juice is used to assist crops from seed germination to early vegetative growth. It's sprayed at a dilution of 1:1000 to help plants become resistant to cold and to grow fast and strong.[20]

NASTURTIUM, TROPAEOLUM MAGUS

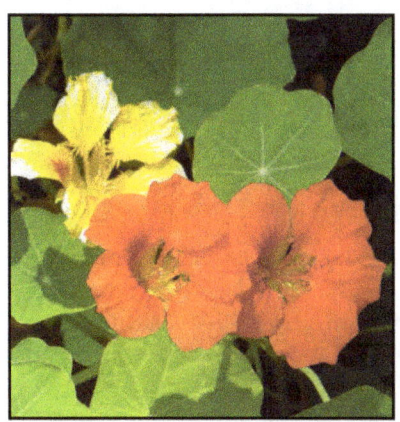

This lovely annual vine with its cheery bright flowers is a joy in the polytunnel, where it grows up trellises and trees and continues to flower well into winter. Also happy outdoors, it's not only beautiful, the edible flowers are lovely in salads, as garnishes, or even drunk as tea; while the young, peppery tasting leaves are rich in vitamin C and Iron. Toss a few young leaves into salads, or add (blended) to dips and sauces for piquancy. Plant into poor soil with good moisture to ensure lots of flowers. It will spread itself prolifically if allowed. The seeds can be pickled as a substitute for capers, picked for this while still green. It makes an ideal companion for edible garden plants, attracting beneficial insects and repelling pests.

NETTLES, STINGING, URTICA DIOICA

This worldwide herb has been a dietary staple since ancient times. Nettles kept many people alive during Ireland's Great Famine. Growing the best in moist, fertile places, the sting is neutralised by heating. Leaves are cooked lightly as an excellent Spinach substitute and also drunk as a nutritious and tasty tea. Leaves, seeds and roots are all medicinal and a great tonic. Leaves are rich in minerals, Iron and vitamin C; they are used medicinally for anaemia, skin problems and other conditions. Young leaves are best used before the plant flowers. Nettles seed freely and you'll find different aged plants everywhere. If you keep picking off the tasty young tips, you can prolong the harvest. Don't eat leaves from older plants, especially after flowering, as they can irritate the kidneys. If you get lower back pain, then stop eating them!

Young leaves can be juiced by blending them with water, then straining and taking 1-2 tablespoons two to three times daily to help with anaemia, exhaustion, hay fever and allergies, skin and joint problems, recommends Henriette Kress. She also suggests drying the leaf, powdering it and adding a heaped teaspoon to meals for general strengthening, especially good for liver and kidneys. It can lower blood pressure and blood sugar too.[8]

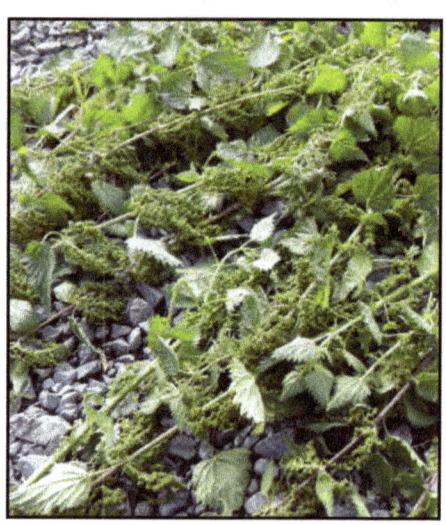

Seeds can be harvested when green, plump, and almost fully ripe, as seen right; the branches hung or laid to dry for two weeks in a dark airy place, then the dried plants are rubbed to separate the seeds and sieved to clean them. They can then be kept in a jar in a dark, dry place, or mix them with runny honey to create an electuary. Take daily, from a pinch to a tablespoonful, adding it to thick liquids and meals. Start with a small dose to see if there is any reaction, as they can cause restlessness. But the right dose will cure restlessness and help with exhaustion and lack of mojo, Kress says. In fact they are considered to have an aphrodisiac effect in herbal medicine. Which proves one of Permaculture founder Bill Mollison's maxims about gardening - that we can also "harvest pleasure".

Nettles can be used for a green dye (with Copper), for a pest repellant spray, liquid fertiliser, compost activator and hair conditioner; while the flax-like stems can be made into a tough cloth, string and paper. Plants provide valuable insect habitat too.[6] The juice of Nettles is a rennet substitute, for setting in cheesemaking, and is used traditionally to make Double Gloucester cheese.[21]

Every good gardener in the past cultivated a Nettle plot, as I do now. I need lots to dry for tea in wintertime. My plot gets a big feed of manure early in spring. I don't give it to them in summer, because Kress warns that if Nettle growth is too lush, plants will become full of toxic Nitrates for a while and are best avoided. But if you wait for a few days of sunshine to stimulate their growth before picking them, they should have assimilated it and be safe.[8]

NEW ZEALAND SPINACH, SEE TETRAGONIA

OCA, OXALIS TUBEROSA
A highland crop of the Andes, Oca is little known outside its ancestral home, where there are hundreds of varieties of many colours. The second most important root vegetable after the Potato, Ocas are a staple of the high altitudes and a principal source of carbohydrate, Calcium and Iron there. They grow and are cooked in ways similar to the Potato, but are not related. The crunchy little tubers are used in salads, or steamed, roasted, added to various dishes and also pickled. Any acidic, lemony taste (from small amounts of Oxalic Acid present) is reduced by keeping them in the light for a few days before preparing, to sweeten them up. Oca leaves are also edible amd can be added to salads, but not too many, due to Oxalic Acid. Pigs love to eat both leaves and tubers. If carefully harvested and properly handled, Ocas keep well in storage at room temperature for several months, until mid spring, when they start to sprout.

According to some, Oca is a new 'wonder crop' that's highly recommended to grow in Ireland. But on the kitchen end of things they can be very time consuming to prepare, so I'm not so sure about their acceptance. It's easy to grow small, fiddly-to-wash tubers. And if you don't harvest all of them, it can become an invasive pest. So I don't grow too many, meanwhile in New Zealand they have become a commercial crop. With the right cultural techniques, tuber size can be increased and more worthwhile growing.

The bushy plant with clover-like leaves requires little care, tolerates harsh climates and prospers in poor soils. Sow whole tubers, the bigger ones, in March or April in pots or modules in a warm, frost free spot. Then plant them in the polytunnel, or outdoors, and protect from frost. Space plants about 30cm apart, with 60cm between rows. Plants grow to about 45cm high and sprawl to some 90cm across. If soil is over fertile, top growth will be excessive, at the expense of tubers. So go easy on the Nitrogen. Don't plant them in the same place the following year, practise crop rotation so that pests or disease can't build up. They can share viruses with Potatoes, so it's best not to grow these together.

To encourage tuber formation, which starts about four months after planting and peaks at about six months, soil is mounded around the base of the plants a couple of times. Or use straw or sheet mulch materials to pack around stems. Tubers normally take another two to three months to mature, and their formation is triggered by reducing day length after the autumn equinox. While a frost will kill the plants, don't harvest immediately as tubers can keep on forming and maturing. As long as Mice or Rats don't start eating them (such happens in a dry, cosy polytunnel) and it isn't too wet, Ocas can stay in the ground over winter until you need them. Mulch thickly around them with straw or fleece to protect tubers from severe frosts. A downside of growing Ocas in a polytunnel in summer is that temperatures over 28°C can wilt or kill foliage. Such set-backs will delay tuber growth.[16]

ONIONS, ALLIUM CEPA AND OTHERS

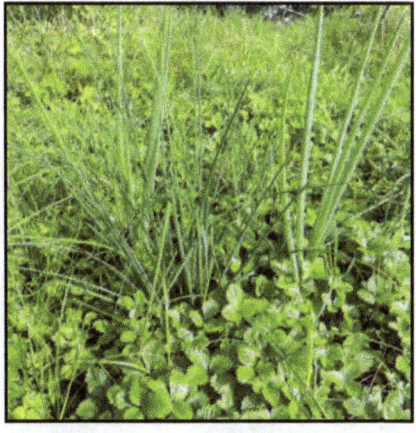

You can't grow too many Onions, but most people don't grow enough. The tiny Onion sets sold in shops in early spring or late autumn are an easy way to get plants started. Reject the ones that are either very small or large, or misshapen. These will tend to bolt easily. Little maintenance is needed, but do keep them free of weeds. Initially the new sprouts may be pulled up by curious birds (who won't eat them however), but putting an anti-bird net over the plot for a couple of weeks will stop that. Grown in a polytunnel, Onions do well over winter and as they reach maturity in early summer you cut back on watering and they'll mature and dry out nicely. Onions love urine as a fertiliser and can even handle it full strength, sprinkled over leaves that are water resistant. When pure urine is applied on hot sunny days (via a watering can), this not only fertilises them, but also kills off any weeds around them.[22]

The Welsh Onion (Allium fistulosum, actually from Siberia, seen above) and the Tree Onion are hardy perennials that are grown from seed. The leaves can be used in cooking all year round and both also have medicinal uses.[5] Strawberries are reputedly a good companion for Onions[19], as in the photo above of Welsh Onions with Wild Strawberries for groundcover.

PLANTAIN, PLANTAGO SPECIES

These ubiquitous small herbs mostly grow as 'weeds' in gardens, their value overlooked. Plantains have edible leaves, the very young ones are ok for mixed salads, or the older leaves can be cooked like Spinach; while the mucilaginous seeds, eaten raw or cooked, are high in vitamin B1 and can be either ground and added to flour, or boiled like Sago. Ripe seed stalks can be hung up for Poultry to peck at. A syrup that's good for coughs can be made from the boiled leaves. A source of dietary fibre, Psyllium husks are the seeds of Plantain species Plantago ovata.[12]

POTATOES,
SOLANUM TUBEROSUM

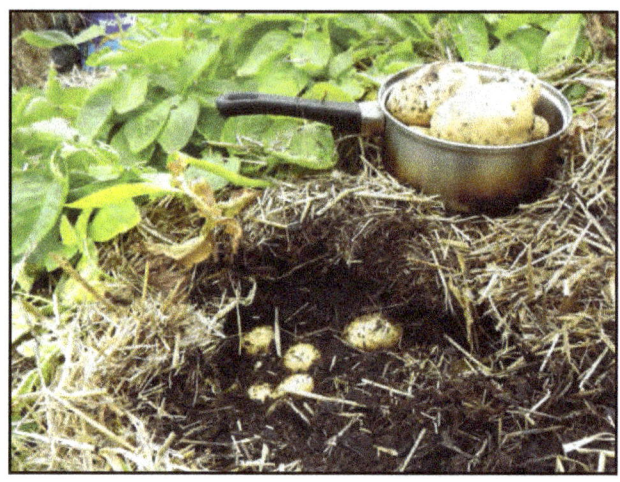

Potatoes grow well on Raised Beds and Hugel Mounds. They are often the first crop when one is breaking in new ground with no-dig growing, as seen right. As for the traditional, so-called 'Lazy Bed' style of growing, this is similar to the no-dig way - but much more work (digging up sods of soil)! Make sure that manures in Potato beds are well composted and broken down, otherwise too much Nitrogen can give strong vegetative growth at the expense of tubers, plus make plants more susceptible to Blight. Always rotate Potato crops around the garden as well, to reduce pest or disease build-up. Ideally leave a four or five year gap before growing spuds on the same spot again.

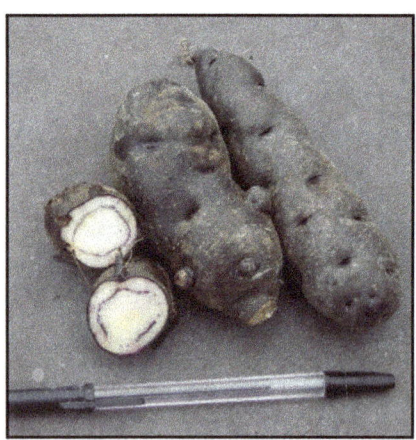

There are many Blight resistent varieties, including the Sarpo family from Hungary. I like to grow late main-season variety Sarpo Mira. The tubers grow large and abundantly, taste delicious and store well for a long time. I also plant early varieties in mid March (in the polytunnel) then mid-earlies in early April, but the early ones don't have long storage ability. Main crop varieties go in mid to late April and these store the best. A very late crop can be planted in the polytunnel in December or January, stretching the Potato season across the year. I also grow dark coloured varieties, purple-black ones from Bolivia, seen left, for the extra nutritional factors. When cooking Potatoes, soaking and boiling leaches out the Vitamin C, so it's better to wash them quickly and steam them, especially new Potatoes.

RASPBERRY, RUBUS IDAEUS

One of the easiest of soft cane fruit to grow, a range of varieties can extend the fruiting season. The leaves are used as medicine, drunk as tea, and are especially good for women in the final

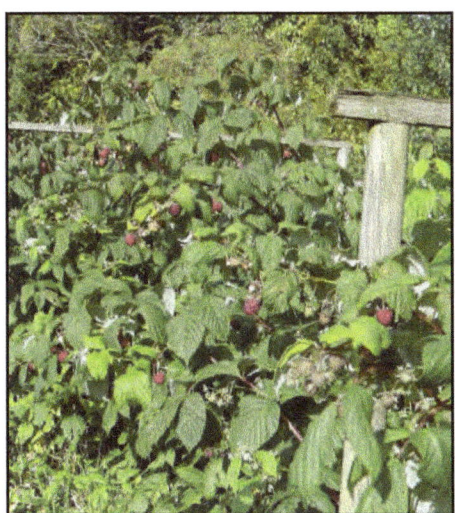

trimester of pregnancy, especially before and during labour. Many Rubus species are ideal for the Food Forest, growing well in semi-shade, or on sunny woodland edges, where they fruit better. They also provide safe places for small animals to nest and food for wildlife. Suckers will spread plants far and wide.

RHUBARB, RHEUM X HYBRIDUM

While not technically a fruit, we generally consider it as one. Rhubarb is a showy and vigorous plant that produces the earliest 'fruit' in the season. A large sunny site that's fertile, a bit acid, and well drained is perfect for growing Rhubarb. Easy to grow, it loves a raised bed, such as a Hugel Mound, with plenty of rotted manure and compost, to raise it above a heavy soil. You may be rewarded with around ten to twenty years of cropping, although plants are often replaced after only five years. Growing this perennial vegetable from seed is slow. Faster results comes from planting offsets, the crowns/divisions of mature healthy plants that are taken in winter or early spring. Three or four plants is enough for an average family's needs.

Space plants about 90cm apart and keep plants well watered and mulched to retain moisture. Feed them in autumn / winter and spring with heavy dressings of manure. Remove any young flowering stalks and remove the whole plant if viruses take hold, a plants's declining vigour being shown by mottled yellow leaves and reducing yields, or lots of only thin stalks. Replant new Rhubarb sets at a fresh new site. Harvest stems by pulling them gently off the plant base, rather than cutting them.

The cooked stems need lots of sweetener to be palatable. They are usually boiled and added to puddings, cake and tarts, or blended into sorbet. They can also be pickled, preserved and added to jams. Rhubarb is rich in antioxidants, however it does contain a lot of Oxalic Acid, so shouldn't be eaten more than about twice a week. I grow a variety that's low in Oxalic Acid, the Glaskins Perpetual, as seen above. I also grow Timperley Early, a very robust variety that starts to shoot in early December, with stems sometimes ready to harvest by March. The root can be used medicinally and the toxic leaves simmered in water for an insecticide, but beware - it kills the good bugs too!

ROSE, ROSA SPECIES

All Roses produce edible fruit (rosehips) and flower petals (but don't eat the white petal base), and these are packed with vitamins A, B, C and K. Petals are also used in oils, vinegar, syrups, drinks (infused for tea) and jams, for potpourri and baths.[12] Rosehips are best picked after frost, when they become sweeter. Below the thin layer of tasty flesh lies the hazard of fine seed hairs that need to be avoided or they'll irritate the throat.

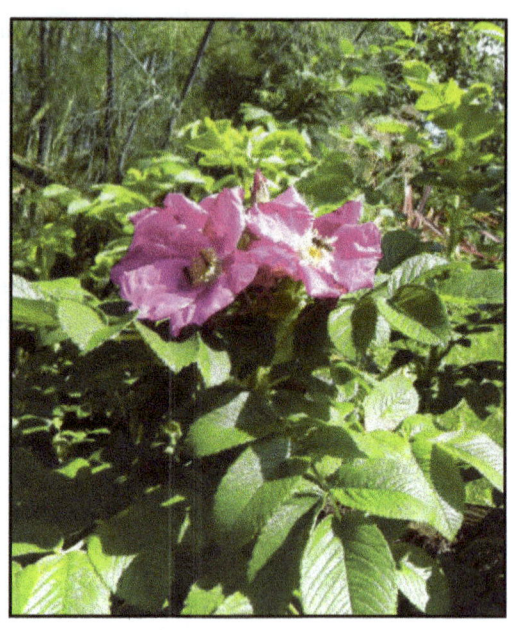

The Ramanas Rose, Rosa rugosa, seen right, is one of the best for fruit, with large rosehips that can be eaten raw or cooked, or made into tea. It also makes a good hedge, but does get rather invasive with its suckering habit. Growing to some 2m tall, the hips can be 3cm in diameter.

ROSEMARY, ROSMARINUS OFFICINALIS

This classic woody herb is an evergreen, half hardy native of the Mediterranean region, with a multitude of cultivars available. It prefers a sunny spot with well drained, not too fertile soil. It can tolerate some light frost but, if severe frost is expected, should be well mulched for protection, or brought indoors, if in a pot. Propagate with semi-hardwood cuttings, or by layering, in summertime. Cuttings grow easily from prunings.

An important component of a bouquet garni, the essential oil in leaves can also be imparted to oil for massaging sore muscles, while infusions are used as a hair tonic and mouthwash, with anti-bacterial properties and also repellant to insects. Medicinally, the tea (a teaspoon of chopped leaves infused for five minutes) is drunk for its bitter tonic quality, for improving digestion, as a circulatory and nerve tonic, for headaches, improving the memory and lifting the spirits. Flowers are edible and make a pretty garnish or salad ingredient.

SALAD BURNETT, SANGUISORBA MINOR

A hardy, small, evergreen, perennial herb, it likes any soil that's well drained, in sun or light shade, and does well in containers. Producing mildly tasty leaves year round, these are great in salads and for flavouring cooked dishes. Leaves also help assist digestion and haemorrhoids.[5] To maximise leaf production, keep cutting plants back to 15cm height, prevent them from flowering and don't over-fertilise.

SEABUCKTHORN, HIPPOPHAE RHAMNOIDES

A tall, scrawny shrub native to northern Europe, it produces the most nutritious berries of that region, rich in vitamin C and minerals. Growing rapidly to 6m tall in a sunny, well drained spot, the roots also fix Nitrogen. The small orange berry fruits are acid and tangy, somewhat like Pineapple, but they do sweeten a bit after frost. They can be made into a cordial or added to sweeter fruit juices. Birds are said to love eating them, but no birds around my plant were interested. Perhaps they'll learn. To get berries you need to have at least one male to one female, and he can fertilise up to six females. Fortunately you can buy pairs with known sex, usually clones of different varieties. Harvest when ripe with scissors, otherwise they squish easily.

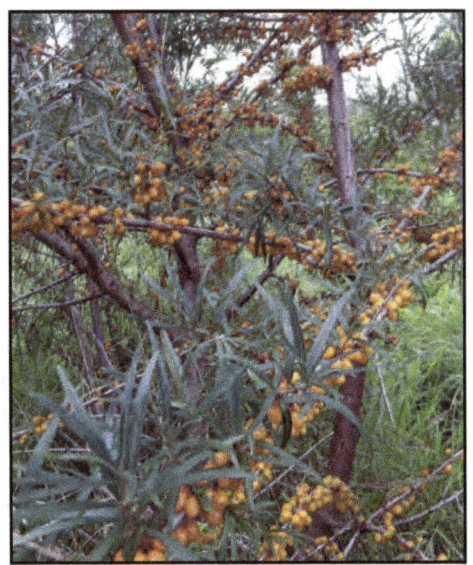

This vigorous, fast growing plant is used for stabilising coastal sand dunes, spreading by suckering. Even here on my clay soil, sucker roots like steel cables are radiating out and shoots are popping up in different places. (In the Hops bed suckers will become structural supports for the vines.) So be careful where it's planted, a dedicated hedge area or wild Food Forest may be ideal.

SHEPHERD'S PURSE, CAPSELLA BURSA-PASTORIS
This small native European herb can be recognised by its heart shaped seedpods. In Japan it's grown as a vegetable, being eaten raw and cooked. The leaves can be added to salads (picked only before flowering), while seedpods can go in soups and stews for their peppery flavour.[12]
The aromatic roots have been used as a Ginger substitute. Leaves are valued by herbalists for their styptic value (they help to stop bleeding). A fresh leaf can be crushed to put on small bleeding wounds. A tea made from the leaves can help relieve heavy menses and should not be used during pregnancy.[8]

SHUNGIKU / CHRYSANTHEMUM GREENS, GLEBIONIS CORONARIA
In China, Japan and South East Asia this attractive flowering plant, with leaves resembling the

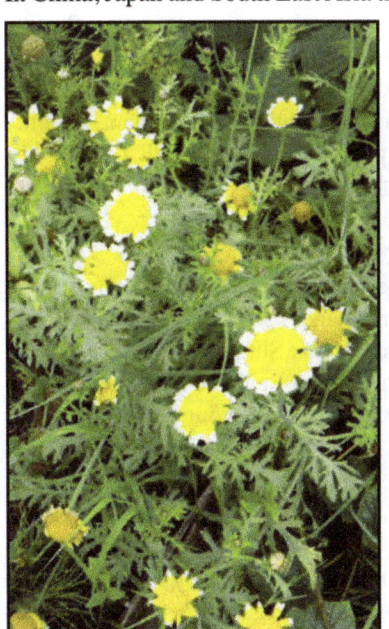

garden variety of Chrysanthemum, is popular as a spicy leaf vegetable crop. Easy to grow, both leaves and young stems as well as the yellow flower petals are eaten in salads, or cooked very lightly - incorporated into soups, stir fries and tempuras. But when going into flower, the leaves become bitter. Constant snipping of shoots can delay this. Leaf tops and flowers are used in dying, giving shades of brown or olive to orange.

Plants grow up to 60cm high, they prefer a cool climate and can handle a bit of frost. Fast growing, they'll grow in light shade over summer and happily persist over winter in an unheated polytunnel. Traditionally, they are intercropped inbetween slower growing crops in summer, and valued as winter greens. Regular clipping will keep them compact.[13]

SILVER BEET, SEE LEAF BEET

SOAPWORT, SAPONARIA OFFICINALIS
This sprawling herb is a hardy perennial with pretty pinky-white flowers. High in Saponins, this gives a soapy effect and it's traditionally used for washing delicate fabrics. Because of the Saponins, it's mildly poisonous if ingested. Soapwort is also used externally for treating skin problems.

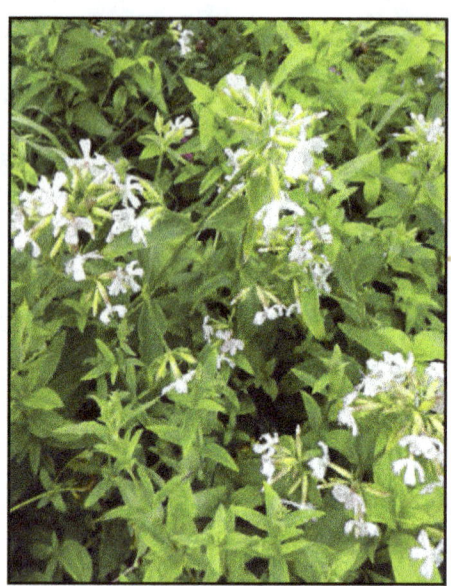

Grow in sunny, well drained locations in poor soil and away from waterways because of poisonous root exudates that could leach into them. Roots are harvested or divided for increasing in autumn. The chopped or crushed roots, when soaked overnight and boiled in a covered non metal (e.g. enamel) pan for twenty minutes and strained off, make a natural shampoo.

SORREL, RUMEX SPP

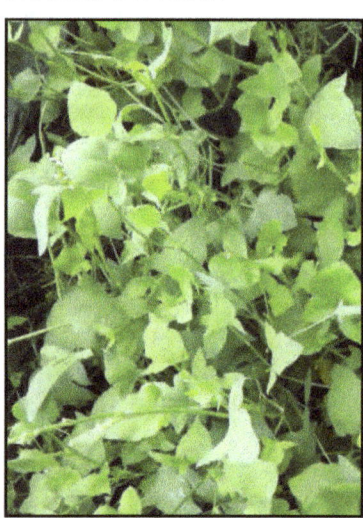

French Sorrel, Rumex acetosa, and also the smaller leaved Sheep's Sorrel (R. acetosella) and Buckler Leaved Sorrel (R.scutatus), are hardy perennial herbs, with tasty, lemony leaves. Only eat a few at a time however, because of high Oxalic Acid levels. Natives of the northern hemisphere and growing wild elsewhere, they taste best in cooler weather and get bitter when it's hot. The sour leaves are used (sparingly) in salads, soups, omelettes, etc or as a leafy vegetable cooked like Spinach. The Buckler Leaved type (seen left) is excellent for salads and does well growing in a pot. Remove flowers regularly to keep leaves tender. Also called Sour Leaves, Sorrel juice is used by Laplanders to curdle milk. The roots can yield a pink dye and the whole plant, a murky yellow dye. Sorrel prefers to grow in a rich, damp fertile soil in sun or part shade. [5]

STRAWBERRIES, FRAGARIA SPECIES
Who doesn't love to eat Strawberries? They are definitely worth growing, but being so well known, I'll concentrate on the lesser known varieties. Strawberries grow very well in Wicking Buckets, where they can be kept high enough off the ground that Slugs are less likely to find fruit, plus they're easier to pick. I grow lots and when they are most abundant I slice them up and dry them in the dehydrator, where they become long storing flavour bombs, ideal for muesli or porridge, on cakes etc. When fruiting begins, regular doses of liquid fertiliser high in Potash is recommended.

WILD STRAWBERRY, FRAGARIA VESCA
This delightful little native plant in Ireland is a hardy perennial. It spreads by runners and can be great ground cover for a Food Forest or a perennial garden bed, e.g. they combine well with

Onions, making good companions for them. Grow them in sun or shade, in fertile soil, either moist or dry. In my polytunnel they are a self-spread ground cover and give early crops, as seen right. The small fruits have great flavour and also medicinal and cosmetic uses, unlike many cultivated varieties. They can benefit anaemia, stomach and other problems. Tea from the leaf is a good tonic, but it's best to mix it with other herbs.[5] Transplant some runners from the wild and it will soon be spreading everywhere, while birds will also spread the seed.

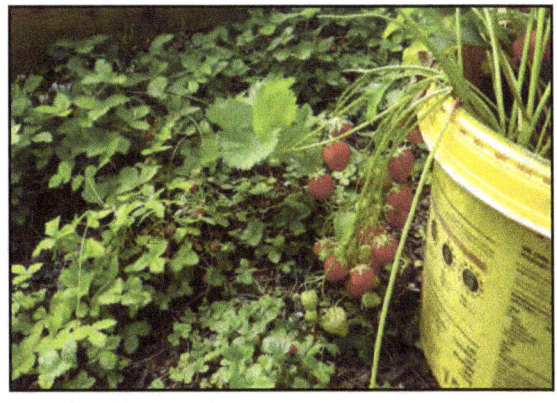

ALPINE STRAWBERRY, FRAGARIA VESCA 'SEMPERFLORENS'
One of the best plants for the garden! Unlike the closely related Wild Strawberry, this variety does not send out runners, but forms clumps. It's great planted along garden edges, for ease of harvesting, producing abundantly in summer and autumn over a few years before vigour declines. Fruit size is in-between that of wild and cultivated varieties. It's good to replace some plants every couple of years. Old, rotting fruits can be mashed up and sown where you want them growing, the birds will assist and you'll soon find it popping up everywhere.

SUMAC, RHUS TYPHINA
Stags Horn Sumac is a vigorous suckering shrub growing up to 6m height, that can become invasive when roots are disturbed. But in a spacious woodland it's worth the risk, according to Robert Hart, who was very enthusiastic about Sumac in his Food Forest gardens.[23] In the right spot it is usefully grown as a thick shelterbelt or soil stabiliser. Clusters of purple, hairy berries grow upwards from a furry branch that resembles a stags horn - hence the name.

This ornamental plant has value as a spice for flavouring food and drinks. The pinky-red flower tufts emerging in late summer are rich in Malic and Citric Acid, and these are used to make a refreshing, sweet-sour drink - 'pink lemonade'. This is made as a cold infusion, first bruising the flowers, then soaking them in cold water for a few hours and squeezing them a few times. Then strain the mix through a sieve, muslin or Coffee filter and sweeten to taste.

Or use the dried flowers for Sumac powder, a spice that's popular in the Middle East and an essential component in Morrocan spice Ras el hanaf. Make Sumac powder by rubbing the seeds from the core between gloved hands to remove seed hairs, then pulsing in a blender and sieving. Sumac leaves are high in tannin and were traditionally used for tanning leather. Autumn leaves can yield a brown dye.

SUNFLOWER, HELIANTHUS ANNUS
Easily grown with attractive flowers that enhance the beauty of the garden, the nutritious seeds are great for snacks for people and poultry. Other parts of the plant have been used for a host of applications, from seed oil for cooking and making candles, to fuel, fibre for paper and fabric from stems. When mature, dry the seedheads as they are for storage, and there's no need to hull them if you sprout the seeds or feed them to poultry.

MAXIMILIAN SUNFLOWER, HELIANTHUS MAXIMILIANI
This is a hardy perennial plant with edible tubers that can grow up to 2.5m high and 1m wide; the flowers coming late in the season (August - September), are beloved by Bees and Butterflies. Regular pruning will encourage more flowers and keep plants compact.

SWEET CICELY, MYRRHIS ODORATA
This aromatic European plant, with an Aniseed flavour and all parts edible, also has tonic qualities. A hardy perennial, the young leaves can be harvested over most of the year, finely chopped into salads or added to stewed fruits to reduce the need for sweetener. Roots can be cooked as a vegetable, made into wine or used raw, peeled and grated in salads. In summer, the aromatic, sweet seeds are used (unripe) for flavouring fruit salads. Ripe seeds are used whole or crushed and cooked with fruit dishes. Growing to 1m high in sun or light shade in moist soil, it used to grown much more extensively by food gardeners.

SWEET WOODRUFF, GALLIUM ODORATUM
This European native woodland plant is an attractive, aromatic ground cover that was once a popular strewing herb. It grows well in deep and dry shade, even right up to the trunk of trees, so is great for Food Forests. The flowers can be added to salads, while a tea made from the leaves has several medicinal uses, but don't drink too much as it can give poisoning symptoms.

SWISS CHARD, SEE LEAF BEET

TETRAGONIA / NEW ZEALAND SPINACH, TETRAGONIA EXPANSA
An edible, sprawling, perennial ground cover plant growing wild all around the Pacific region, it is frost tender. And it's only really edible if cooked properly, which is never mentioned in European books! Last century I'd sometimes harvest it from sand dunes at the back of Sydney's beaches. I'd boil the leaves for a few minutes and the water was discarded to remove the Calcium Oxalate crystals that would otherwise burn your throat! No wonder this plant has not been widely grown in Europe. No-one seems to know how to eat it safely.

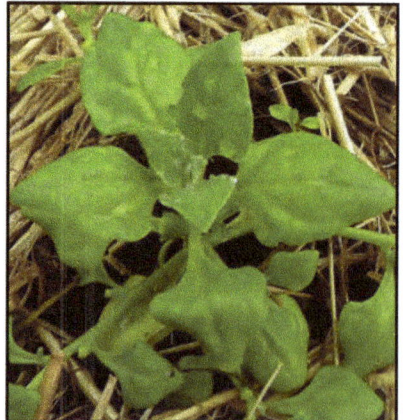

You can grow Tetragonia outdoors as an annual and it will may well self-seed and perpetuate itself. Or grow it as a ground cover in a dry sunny corner of a polytunnel. Soak the large seeds overnight and plant out after frosts have finished. Space plants 50 -70 cm apart. They don't need high fertility or much water to thrive.

Right - This young plant will soon be sprawling around.

THYME, THYMUS SPECIES
This Mediterranean herb is used for flavouring dishes and as an aid to digestion. Having antiseptic qualities, it's also used for a mouthwash, or drunk as a medicinal tea. There are a host of varieties. The main one for medicinal use is T. vulgaris, known as Common, or Garden Thyme. Wild Thyme (Thymus serpyllum) is a creeper, a good ground cover for a rockery type

situation and popular as an infusion for tea.

Grow Thyme in poor soil in a well drained spot, or in a pot or dry corner of a polytunnel, protected from extremes of cold, wind and wet. Being evergreen, it can be picked anytime. Prune after flowering.

VIOLET, VIOLA TRICOLOUR, V. ODORATA AND OTHERS

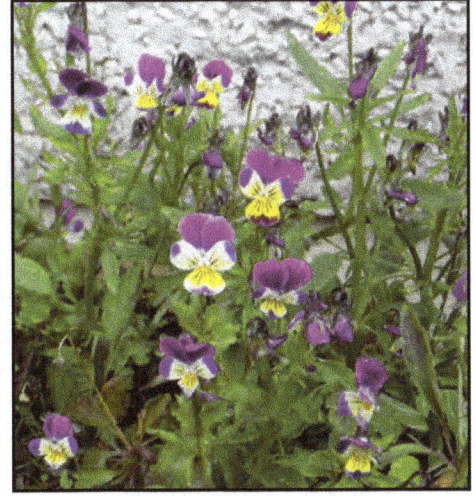

These charming small plants are European natives, hardy perennials that are not just attractive but also have various uses. V. odorata has perfumed flowers that are lovely in salads and as garnishes, also good for potpourris and perfumes; while the roots are used medicinally for soothing respiratory problems and the leaves for poultices. As for V. tricolour, it's white, yellow and purple flowers brighten up salads and sweet dishes, plus the flowers and leaves are used medicinally, as tea, or made into ointments etc, hence the name Heartsease.

Violets like to grow in semi-shady spots such as woodlands, where a rich moist soil is appreciated. Or grow them in containers.

WATERCRESS, NASTURTIUM AQUATICUM

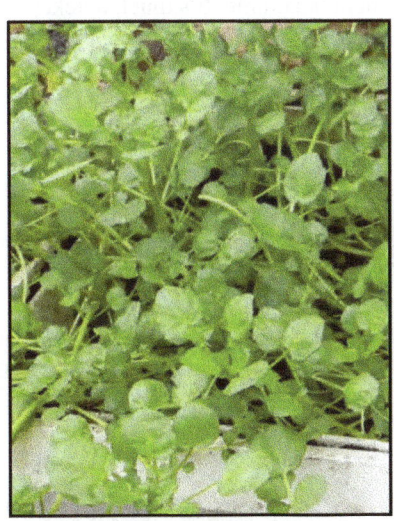

Watercress grows wild along the edges of Irish watercourses and is a great source of nutrition, especially vitamin C. However it's always best to use a garden sourced one for eating, as wild Watercress may be a host for Liver Fluke that's spread by Sheep grazing near waterways. (However cooking it sufficiently will kill the fluke.) Thriving in the cooler parts of the year, there are now varieties available (propagated by seed) that don't have to grow in water at all, as plants will happily grow in moist soil, as seen left.

Watercress is great for salads and soups. Harvest the older leaves for more flavour. They are delicious when liquidised and added to dishes such as Potato soup.

WILD GARLIC/RAMSONS, ALLIUM URSINUM

This native of northern Europe likes to form dense, Garlic smelling carpets beneath deciduous forests. Growing to a height of 50cm, Ramsons grow vigorously in early spring, before trees leaf up. All parts are edible, the sword-like leaves being harvested from March to May, before the lovely white flowers bloom. Ransoms have medicinal and culinary properties akin to cultivated Garlic. Medicinally, they are Sulphur-rich, foster our gut biota, have a cleansing

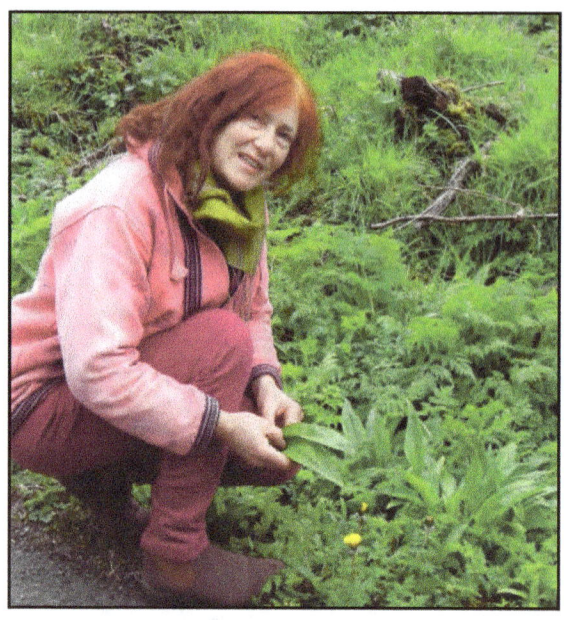

effect and can assist with heavy metal de-toxing. For out of season use they can be made into preserves, pesto and dips, or a leaf tincture (with alcohol). Leaves and flowers are best used fresh, as they don't retain their garlicky smell when dried. They can be finely chopped (also fresh green seed pods that are broken up) for eating raw in salads, also mixed with cottage cheese, or in sauces, vinegars, yoghurt salad dressing (added to a Greek Tzatziki/Indian Raita), etc. Leaves can be cooked too, e.g. sautéed with Onions, which produces a milder flavour. If you prefer them mild they can be blanched first, dipping leaves in boiling water for ten seconds, refreshing them in cold water then patting them dry.[18]

Ransom bulbs are also edible, but if over eaten can cause stomach upsets, plus eating them kills the plant.

Planted in rich, moist soil, plants die back early in summer, but re-sprout from the bulb each spring, to later drop seeds prolifically. It makes a great ground cover for a Forest Garden and can grow in semi to full shade. If growing by seed, sow them in autumn. It's much quicker to dig up an existing clump in the wild (such as the roadside above) for replanting in your garden. It takes a few years to get established and for leaves to grow large.

WINTER SAVORY, SATUREJA MONTANA

This is a hardy perennial from the Mediterranean region that is a must-have for vegetarians! It's pungent leaves stimulate the appetite, are great for flavouring and aid digestion. Known as the 'Bean Herb' (as is Summer Savory, S. hortensis, a less hardy annual plant), you add sprigs to bean dishes and it reduces the flatulence associated with eating them. A few finely chopped leaves go well in a salad in winter, although plants are only semi-evergreen.

Grow in full sun with good drainage, a big pot is ideal. Mine have seeded into concrete path cracks and they grow well there, mingled with Wild Strawberries, handily located beside the back door, as seen right.

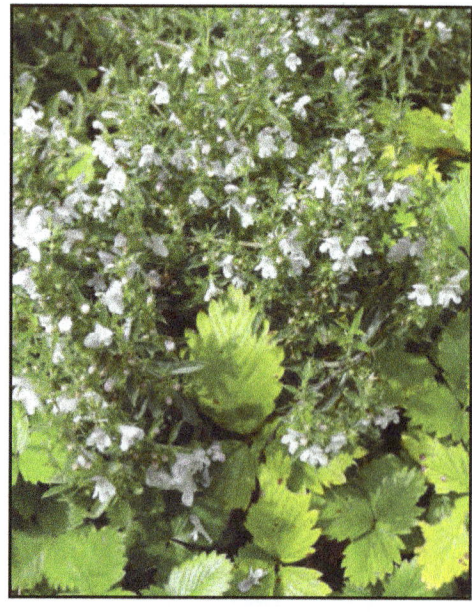

GROWING GRAINS

Cultivation of grains gave hunter gatherer people a steady source of sustenance, the dependable luxury of a nutritious and storable food crop. These cereals, that are called after the goddess Ceres, and are collectively known as 'corn', allowed them to flourish and freed up their time such that cultural development could blossom. An extraordinary megalithic monument, Gobekli Tepi in Turkey is carved with symbols of the beginning of this agricultural revolution. The extraordinary Stonehenge-like structure has been dated back to those times, around 12,000 years ago. The amazingly sophisticated cultures that arose with cereal cultivation were able to sustain themselves and their agricultural lands over millennia, unlike modern agriculture. Yet the Western mindset calls these places of cultural origins 'underdeveloped'!

Wheat thrives in a warmer, drier climate than where I live. In soggy, temperate lands Oats, Rye and Barley grow better and across northern Europe the staple peasant diet included Oatcakes and porridge, dense Rye bread and Barley beer. The gluten content of Wheat is higher than those grains, so fewer bakery goods can be made from them. Gluten aerates dough and makes bread and cakes light and fluffy. Being more versatile, Wheat was more highly valued and it was a luxury item for many. Wheat bread became a symbol of attainment, the reward of one's labours, embedded in the language: we "earn a crust", "spend our bread" and call the aristocracy "the upper crust" (the most delectable part). So sacred did corn and its associated corn gods become in Pagan spirituality, that the early Christians copied their animistic totemism, in trying to usurp them, by adopting the Wheat wafer as a symbol of the body of Jesus. They also fabricated tales of saints battling with the old gods and overcoming them. But the corn gods never went away!

Lesser known grains grow well in my gardens, I discovered. They grow vigorously in the Irish climate and have the potential to be commercial crops here. Over the dull summer of 2020, small crops of Millet, Buckwheat, Flint Corn and Quinoa thrived, both outdoors and inside the polytunnel. It was a lovely experience to watch the plants develop and prosper. These staple cereals have a powerful energetic presence that I delighted in.

What stopped me from doing this before now? Well, I'd need to grow a lot to replace grains in my diet. Then there is the problem of separating the grain from hulls and chaff - a tedious job without commercial equipment. Why would anyone bother growing backyard grains? When I looked into seed sprouting as a high nutrient food supplement for the diet, especially for wintertime, I saw that some quantity of seed would be needed. It could get costly, plus they might be imported and I try to avoid imports. So it didn't seem sustainable, if I had to buy seed. Growing small plots of grain to use for sprouting then made good sense.

OATS, AVENA SATIVA AND A. NUDA
Oats are a super food, once an Irish staple. These days Oats are more likely to be shunned by Irish people, because of bad connotations. The image of poor-house gruel seems too penitential for many. But Oats can cooked in so many other better and tastier ways than boiling it up into a gluey porridge. For my morning porridge of organic rolled Oats I don't bother with cooking, I just put a handful in a bowl and steep them in boiling water, along with Chia seeds, dried fruit, desiccated Coconut etc, for from ten minutes to an hour. The texture and taste is much better, the washing up, far less.

Unleavened Oaten bread and cakes used to be made by the Irish peasants, elsewhere in northern Europe flat breads and crispbreads were made of a mix of the flours of Oats, Barley, Rye and Wheat. Flatbread made purely of Oats was cooked on a bakestone or griddle beside the open hearth fire, or simply placed on top of embers, until crispy.

The commercial milk-like drink made of Oats is also very popular with people today, because it's a much more sustainable product compared with dairy and Almond milks. And it isn't new, people have made Oat drinks since ancient times. I recently read about such a milk substitute in a local history book about Ballinaglera Parish in north County Leitrim, where a lot of Oats used to grown and no-one is believed to have died from hunger in the Great Famine.[25] This drink was made when the Cow went dry, often in late winter or early spring, and was especially valued during famine times. It was a fermented drink, the Oatmeal being steeped in water in an earthenware crock that was normally used for milk collection for churning. The meal settled on the bottom and much of the nutritional riches dissolved in the water. The liquid was drawn off over a few days and used like milk, being humorously called 'Bull's Milk'. A woman neighbour friend confirmed to me that she also occasionally had such Oat drinks in her childhood in south Leitrim. (One of eleven children, the family was completely self-sufficient on their farm at that time.)

I imagine this is a very ancient drink, being similar to one described in a book on prehistoric English cookery. That recipe uses a mix of Oatmeal and Wheatmeal, the quantity of Wheatmeal three times that of Oats. Also made in a stoneware crock, for two kilos of meal one adds nine litres of lukewarm water and leaves it steeping for five to eight days. The liquid poured off is a sharp tasting, refreshing drink called Swats or Sowans. A second nutritious drink can be made by mixing two litres of water with the remaining creamy sludge and straining it out through a cheesecloth in a colander.[26]

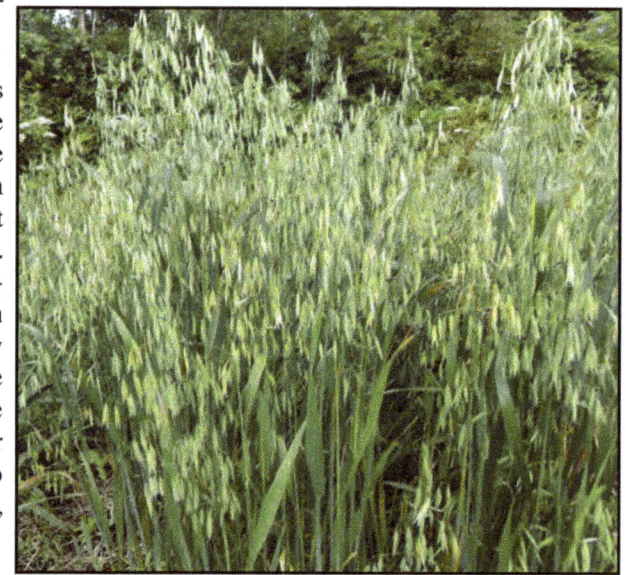

To meet demand for organic Oats in Ireland they have to be imported, yet they grow 'like weeds' here! The problem with growing your own Oats is that they are difficult to hull. However, there are now 'hull-less' varieties available. Known as Naked Oats, as seen right, they do have hulls, but these are relatively easy to remove. Whole Oats are perfectly good for sprouting and are often fed to fowl and Pigs in sprouted form, giving enhanced nutrition.

Oat straw is very useful too, great for animal bedding and for mulching soil and Potato plants. Most straw these days comes in awkwardly gigantic bales from chemical farms in other counties. In 2021 a local initiative has encouraged people to grow a small plot of Oats in Leitrim, for the straw that will be made into traditional Mummers' outfits, such as woven 'Straw Boy' costumes.

Oats grow easily just about anywhere, however well drained, moist, moderately fertile soil is best for them. Too fertile and they'll get leafy, not produce much grain and can lodge (fall over) more easily. Oats are sown in early spring or autumn, broadcast into broad bands some 30cm wide and raked to a depth of 2-5cm. A plank can be laid over the row to firm it down. Oats are ripe when they change colour from green to cream and the grains test hard to bite on. You cut the stalks when ripe, then put them somewhere dry for a few days. [27]

QUINOA, CHENOPODIUM QUINOA

This tasty South American grain, related to Beet and Chard, thrives in Ireland too. Highly nutritious, being rich in protein, Amino Acids, Calcium and Iron, it's no wonder that Quinoa is revered as the Mother of Grains by Andean people. Quinoa's growing popularity in the West has lead to unaffordable price hikes back in it's homeland.

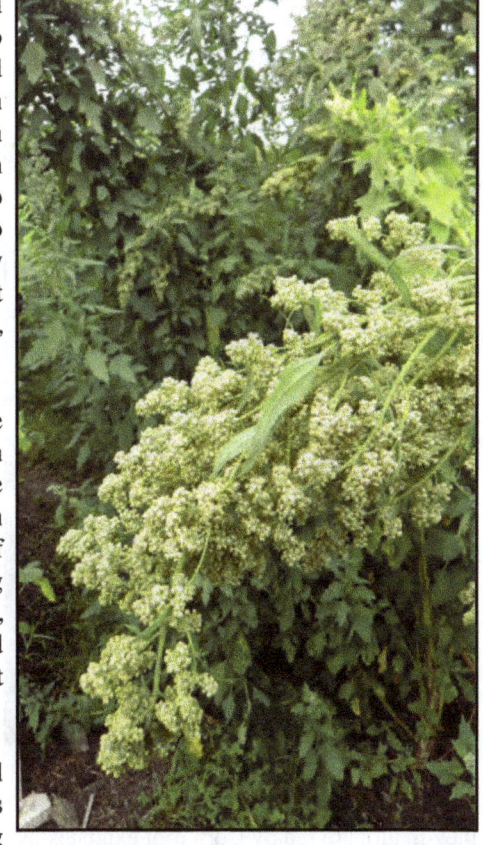

In the polytunnel in 2020 my first crop of Red Faro Quinoa grew beautifully and it also thrived outdoors, producing abundant red colourful seed heads. I first sowed the seeds in modules in the plant nursery and then transplanted seedlings in April, planting them 20cm apart, in rows 40cm apart. Seeds need to be kept moist to germinate, but then it's best to cut right back on watering. Mine grew vigorously and even rescued seedlings, that had been scratched out of the ground by birds, recovered and prospered. Tough plants!

Quinoa comes from a cool, dry climate. The crop I grew in the polytunnel, seen above in flower, was overwatered and plants grew like rockets up to the roof. The lanky stems then lodged everywhere, but they did have lots of seed heads! I didn't know I was overwatering them and they grew to over 2m tall. Outdoors, the plants were a more compact size, around 1.5m tall, which made harvesting easier, but there was less to harvest.

The seedheads didn't go unnoticed by the local birds, who got to eat a lot of them! This is despite reading in a book that Saponins coating the Quinoa seed, that are toxic and must be removed before we eat them, also act as a bird repellant! The birds hadn't read that, they took their chances. Knowing this, I'll make sure to exclude the birds next time. The outdoor Quinoa patch had many plants succumb to strong winds and lodge, so a location that's sheltered from wind would be better. Harvest happened over a few weeks as seed heads gradually all ripened. Leaves were dropping off at this point. To harvest, you either cut off the top of the stems and bring them in to dry more, or simply rub seed heads on the plants between your hands into a bucket. This is winnowed to clean it, pouring it between buckets in a good breeze outdoors, a slow and dusty job. I got bored of this and left most of it as it was, just winnowing and washing a cupful clean before cooking it. My Quinoa grain is stored in food grade plastic buckets and can keep for years, apparently.

It's imperative that, before cooking, you remove the toxic, bitter Saponins by soaking and rinsing them in several washes of water. You can also toast the grain first, before boiling it for 15 - 20 minutes and eating it like Rice. Or sprout the seeds. The young leaves are edible too, both raw and cooked. I enjoy eating the thinnings of the Quinoa plot lightly steamed.

CORN / MAIZE, ZEA MAYS

It's wonderful to eat Sweet Corn on the cob, lightly steamed in it's own paper wrapper, super fresh from the garden. In its South American homeland Flint and Flour varieties of Corn are a staple grain that's dried and ground into Cornmeal and Cornflour. A lot of Corn grown today is genetically modified and Corn starch and syrup have become universal, low grade food additives that are best avoided. (Organic Corn is GMO free.)

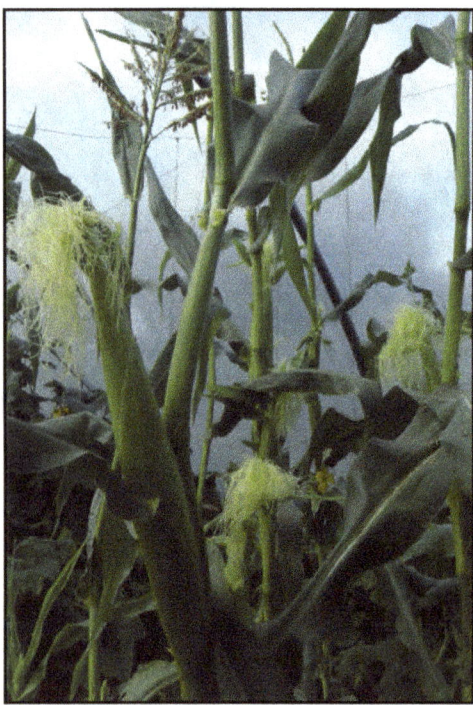

A heavy feeder and needing warmth, Maize is frost tender, so in Ireland it's safest to grow in a polytunnel. I start seeds off in the electric propagator. Plants are then potted up and later planted in the polytunnel during warm weather. Corn grows best in blocks, so plants can pollinate each other easily. Sara Pitzer recommends planting three in the centre of a 30cm square plot, at a depth of 3cm, in blocks of, say sixteen such squares (four by four). Paths can run between each block. [27]

Where it's from, a tradition is to grow Corn in a polyculture, together with Beans and Squash. They call this the 'Three Sisters' and it makes the most of the space. The beans climb up the Corn plants and Squash vines cover the ground. When grown together, the outputs are higher than if they were grown in isolation. Scientific studies have shown a 20% higher harvest than when plants are grown alone.[28] Squash shades the ground, keeping moisture in and weeds away. Bean roots, with their Nitrogen fixing bacteria, feed the Corn and they in turn are fed by Corn root exudates that provide their favourite sugar food. Cornstalks are the trellis for Bean vines to ramble up. It's a beautiful symbiosis!

I followed the 'Three Sisters' approach in the polytunnel, growing small plots of old heritage varieties of Sweet Corn and Flint Corn, seen overleaf. The Beans grew well around them and the long stems of trailing Squash plants became a bit domineering. But what an abundant and delicious crop of Squash! Though growing well, despite not much sun through the summer, the Corn crop wasn't huge, while the mice and birds took their toll.

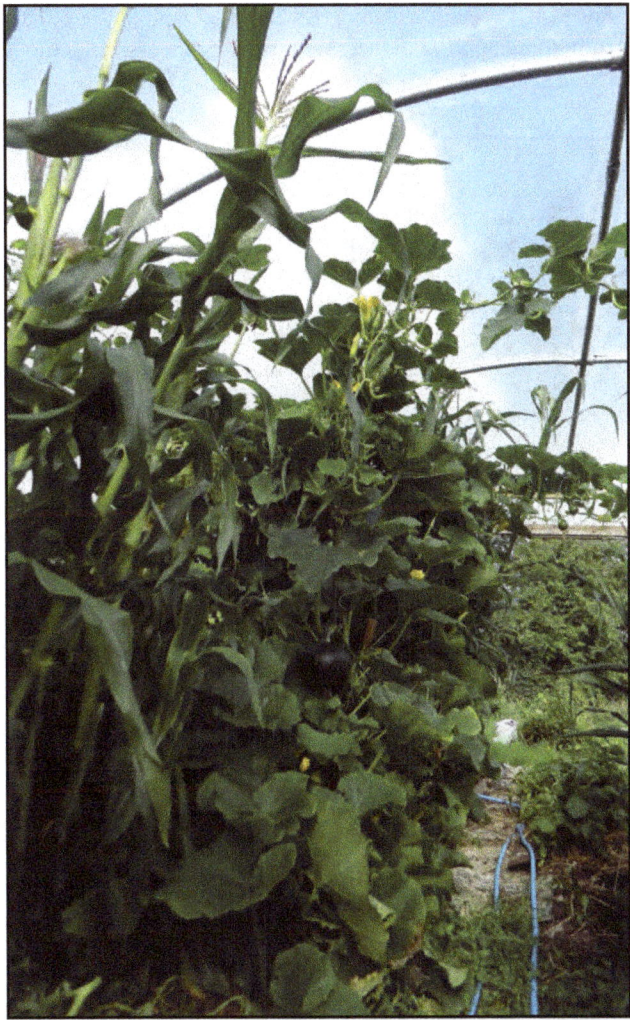

Toby Hemenway writes about a fourth plant partner for the 'Corn Guild', being the American Bee Plant that attracts the insects required for pollinating the Beans and Squash.[28] There will surely be a locally adapted insect attracting plant to grow amidst one's own Three Sisters. Corn itself is pollinated by the wind, so you may need to gently shake the top flowering male flowers to simulate wind and spread the pollen to the female flowers below. When more than one variety is grown, to avoid cross-pollination, you need to sow the different seeds at least fourteen days apart.

Timing is important to make a Corn Guild work, Hemenway explains. The Corn must go in after the last frost and it needs a head start before the other plants muscle in. He suggests making fertile planting holes at 1m spacing, into which you sow three or four Corn seeds at around 3cm depth. Native American farmers favoured multi-stemmed varieties and old heritage varieties can be bought online, as I did. After sprouting, it was traditional for baby Corn plants to have soil earthed up around the stalks, making a nutritious mound for them. A couple of weeks after sowing, a few climbing Bean seeds are sowed into each Corn mound, and a couple of vining Squash or Pumpkin seeds are sown in between the mounds. It's good to add a rich mulch around plants as it all grows, as well as a steady supply of water, plus liquid fertilisers. Pull out any weeds too.

My Corn patch gave an impressive food jungle effect, but it was also good cover for birds and mice! After tearing a small hole into several paper husked Corn cobs to check for ripeness, the birds later saw this and got a free feed, thanks to my ingress. I allowed the Flint Corn cobs to dry naturally on the plants at the end of the season, giving plenty of time for critters to find them. Live and learn!

FOXTAIL MILLET, SETERIA ITALICA
Millet is a staple grain in many parts of the world, where it's cooked like Rice and porridge,

made into flatbreads etc. The various Millet species usually grow in hot, dry climates, but my Foxtail Millet thrived both in the polytunnel and outdoors. With seed that's easy to remove from the hulls, it's well worth growing.

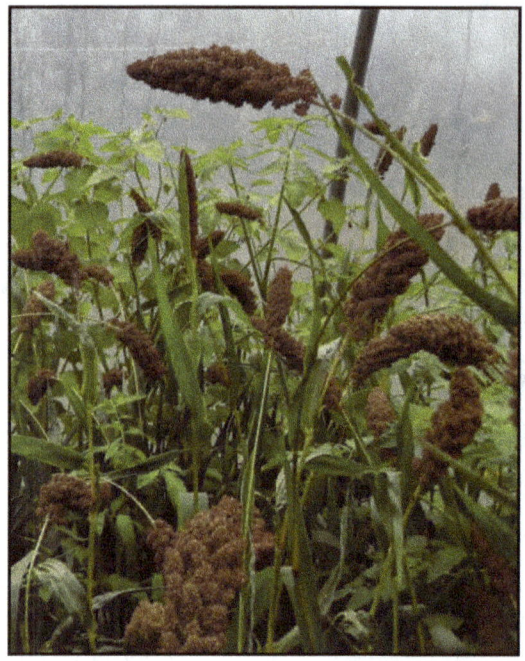

To grow a crop of Millet, a well drained, moderately fertile soil is best. Manure should have been composted for at least six months before the crop goes in. Spread it over beds in September or October, to be ready for an April-May planting. Using an age-old technique from India, I sowed seed directly into the seed bed, making furrows about 60cm apart and sprinkling the small seeds into them, at a rate of about five per 3cm. The soil was gently spread back over the furrows and firmed down with a board placed over them.[27]

Seedlings grew slowly but steadily and were thinned out to leave the best ones, spaced about 20cm apart. They grew up to 1.2m high, but they can grow higher. The attractive seed heads mature and turn brown from the top down, the bottom seeds being still green when ripening starts. Small birds perching on the large seedheads started eating them, so I cut the stalks and took them away to dry fully in a safe place. Millet is easy to de-hull, seed heads are rubbed between the hands, then winnowed to clean away the chaff. It should be stored in an airtight container in a cool dry place.

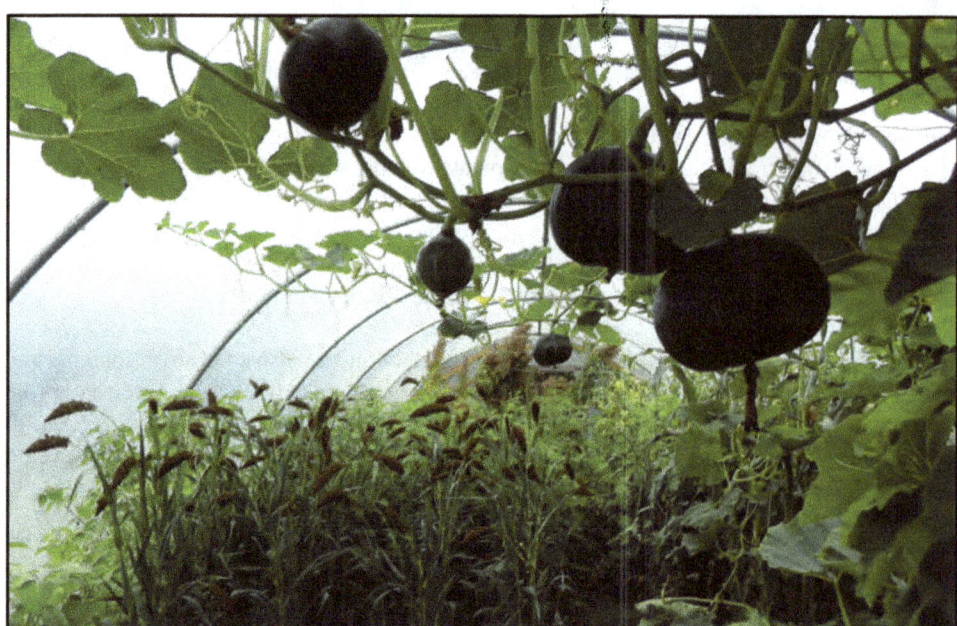

BUCKWHEAT,
FAGOPYRUM ESCULENTUM

A staple food of central Asia and Russia, Buckwheat is an unusual grain that's related to Rhubarb, while most cereals are in the Grass family. Buckwheat groats, plus the leaves, are highly nutritional and a great source of Rutin for healthy blood vessels. I sourced seed of Tartary Buckwheat online from Missouri, USA to grow in Ireland, seen right. It's a staple food in Tibet and is more frost tolerant than other varieties, with a higher level of Rutin and more strongly flavoured than common Buckwheat.

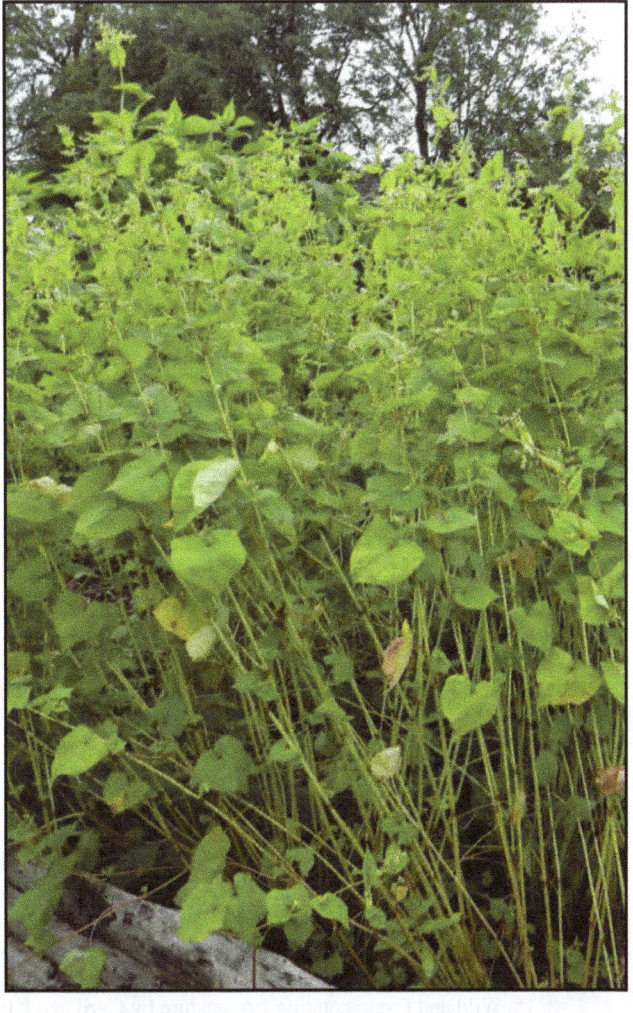

Buckwheat is a vigorous grower and is often used as a green manure crop. Dug into the ground before flowering, it's excellent for soil improvement and especially good for clay soils, while it makes Phosphorus more available. With a long flowering period, it's great for Bees, giving a strong tasting honey.

Buckwheat grows best in a sunny site with free draining, moderately fertile soil, though it can handle poor or acid soils and drought as well. Sow in warm soil after the danger of frost has passed. Scatter seed over a moist, weed-freed bed and rake it in to about 2-4cm depth. Plants grow quickly to cover the soil. They need to grow for about three months before autumn frosts kill them.

Groats should be harvested before the autumn frosts, or else seed heads can shatter. When three quarters of the seeds have gone brown, it's time to start harvesting them. I cut the stalks and left them to dry undercover. The birds and Mice took their toll, but I don't mind sharing some. When fully dry, the groats separate easily, you can rub them by hand or bang the bunches on the insides of a barrel to make them drop, then winnow to remove the chaff. Store the groats in an airtight container in a cool dry place. De-hulling Buckwheat groats is tricky, however you can use them unhulled, by grinding them into a dark, strong tasting flour, or you can sprout them. [27]

RYE, SECALE CEREALE

A staple grain of northern Europe, Rye is well suited to a short and cool growing season and it has enough gluten to make dark and heavy bread with. It's a tolerant plant, but must have well drained conditions. Rye is sown from late summer to late autumn, to overwinter and be ready by the following summer. It doesn't need to be de-hulled, just threshed and winnowed.[27] It also makes a great green manure crop and the straw is prized for animal bedding and craft weaving work. For culinary use, there is one potential hazard, the danger of Ergot fungus infecting the grain. It looks like black grains in the heads and Ergotism from eating tainted grain causes nasty hallucinations. Think I'll give this grain a miss!

BARLEY, HORDEUM VULGARE

Perhaps the earliest cultivated grain, it's a cool season crop suited to northern climates and is also adapted to be grown globally. Much of the world's Barley is fed to animals or used for malting alcoholic drinks. For the backyard, there are hull-less varieties available. (These do have a small hull, but it's easily removed by threshing and winnowing.) Barley grows best in blocks in a sunny spot with alkaline soil, though some shade is tolerated.[27] It can be baked into flat breads or added to soups. Demeter is the Greek Goddess of this grain and her sacred drink was brewed from Barley grains, a sort of beer perhaps?

REFERENCES FOR THE PLANT PROFILES

1. European Peasant Cookery, Elisabeth Luard, Grub St, London, 2004.
2. Feeding the People - Politics of the Potato, Rebecca Earle, Cambridge University Press, UK 2020
3. The Glory of the Garden (1937), Simon and Schuster, 2012, UK.
4. Bartram's Encyclopaedia of Herbal Medicine, Thomas Bartram, Robinson, London UK, 1998.
5. Jekka's Complete Herb Book, Jekka McVicar, Kyle Books, 2007, UK.
6. Plants for a Future, Ken Fern, Permanent Publications 1997, UK.
7. Food for Free, by Richard Mabey, Collins, UK, 1972.
8. Practical Herbs 1, Henriette Kress, Aeon Books, 2018, UK.
9. Complete Earth Medicine Handbook, Susanne Fischer-Rizzi, Sterling Publishing, USA, 2003.
10. Practical Herbs 1, Henriette Kress, Aeon Books, 2018, UK.
11. Grow Your Own Vegetables, Joy Larkcom, Francis Lincoln, 2002, UK.
12. Hedegerow Medicine, Julie Bruton-Seal and Matthew Seal, Merlin Unwin books, UK, 2008.
13. Oriental Vegetables, Joy Larkom, Frances Lincoln, UK, 2007.
14. The Healing Power of Celtic Plants, Angela Paine, Winchester Books, UK, 2006.
15. Wild and Free - cooking from nature by Cyril and Kit O'Ceirin, Wolf Hill, Dublin, 2013.
16. Lost Crops of the Incas: Little-Known Plants of the Andes with Promise for Worldwide Cultivation. Washington, DC: The National Academies Press, USA,1989.
17. Vegetables for the Irish Garden, Klaus Laitenberger, Milkwood Farm, Ireland, 2013.
18. Sarah Raven's Garden Cookbook, Bloomsbury, UK, 2007.
19. Companion Planting, Bob Flowerdew, Kyle Cathie Ltd, UK, 2010.
20. Dr. Cho's Global Natural Farming', by Rohini Reddy, SARRA, Karnataka, India, 2011.
21. Prehistoric Cookery Recipes and History, Jane Renfrew, English Heritage, 1985, UK.
22. Aprovecho Institute, June 1991 newsletter, USA.
23. Forest Gardening - Rediscovering Nature and Community in a Post-Industrial Age, Robert A de J Hart, Green Earth Books, UK, 1996.
24. Comfrey for Gardeners step by step guide, from www. Garden Organic. org.uk
25. Ballinaglera and Inishmagrath - history and traditions of two Leitrim Parishes, Clancy and Forde, M. Clancy, 2003, Ireland.
26. Prehistoric Cookery- recipes and history by Jane Renfrew, English Heritage, 1985, UK.
27. Homegrown Whole Grains, Sara Pitzer, Storey Publishing, USA. 2009.
28. Gaia's Garden -a guide to homescale Permaculture, Toby Hemenway, Chelsea Green, USA, 2000

"ARE YOU GOING TO HAVE ANIMALS?"

This was the question put to me by a local batchelor farmer, when I was searching the back roads by bicycle, looking for some land to buy in Ireland. I sense that unless you have animals, you won't be considered a true farmer around here. Now that I do have some animals, I'm getting a better resonance with the farming community, who just have a handful of Cows or Sheep and enjoy EU subsidies that keep this the status quo. Very few grow fruit or vegetables of any kind. But in the past, mixed farming was what everybody did.

Small, but intensive, peasant farms feature a complementary mix of plants and animals, with small animal breeds particularly suited. In old Ireland a small Cow (such as the Kerry), a Pig or Goat were kept, either tethered here and there, or ranged through tiny fields. Even with no land, animals would be kept in stone sheds and feed brought to them. You still see this in densely populated places, like Asia, where land for livestock just isn't available.

The polyfarm model offers an ecological balance with zero waste - animal waste becomes food for plants, that become food for animals, e.g. the manuring of Potato fields fertilised the staple food crop of both peasants and the animals that produced it. The Irish diet revolved around Potatoes, plus dairy products and the odd bit of Cabbage and ham. Together they gave sufficient nutrients for people to enjoy a sustainable autonomy, as long as they stayed connected to ancestral clan lands. Refusing to be workers and with no need to participate in the capitalist economy, the British plantation system in Ireland ended their sovereign freedom, by taking their land and renting it back to them, in the longest running feudal system in Europe.

Cash to pay the rent had to be generated and special crops, such as Oats, were often grown to be sold just for that purpose. Even when the Irish peasants faced starvation during the Great Famine, Oats were handed over for rent, or else they risked eviction and homelessness as well. Another mainstay of peasant income was the selling of Chicken, Duck and Goose eggs, plus their feathers and meat. This was women's business. Broody hens in cold weather were kept indoors in nests beside the hearth, while many a home also housed a Cow or two, these acting as a sort of central heating system.

Money could be made from livestock because there were no feeding costs. This is unlike my own experience of being a rare-breeds poultry micro-farmer in Australia in the 1990's. Lugging 40kg grain feed bags from the farm store regularly, as I did to feed my feathered hordes, did keep me fit. But when I meticulously tallied up the costs and income from selling eggs (for eating and hatching), chicks, breeding trios and point-of-lay pullets (nearly mature hens of around six months age) - it always showed zero profits. Except for the eggs that we ate and the satisfaction of keeping rare breeds going, there was no money to be made, even with the more pricey birds because of their rarity value. Only on a very large scale would it have been profitable, because the prices that consumers will pay is generally close to conventional mega-farm prices. People aren't used to paying the true costs of humane and sustainable production. I had to keep my prices low. But I did end up producing a bestselling book about poultry - Backyard Poultry - Naturally - so the experience wasn't for nothing!

So what did the Irish peasantry produce to feed their farm animals? They got as good as their own diet, all flourished on cooked Potatoes - of course! Supplying them with carbohydrates, vitamins and around 2% protein, Potatoes made them thrive, along with whatever could be foraged around the place, plus kitchen scraps, if there were any in peasant kitchens.

When today we look at the sustainability of commercial feeds for our pets and livestock, it's not a great picture. Feed mixes and pellets often contain genetically modified Soya beans in the EU, GMOs being allowed for animals. Fortunately the organically produced feeds don't have them.

As grass may not always be enough to feed grazing animals, you need to supplement their diet. I was warned off keeping any long ago. When grass is growing lushly all is good and we can leave them to it. But grass growth is in cycles and seasons can be hard, so it's never consistent. There will always come a time or a season when grass isn't growing and feed has to be shipped in. This can be minimised by home grown feed, as was traditional. Ideally, it can be easily stored. So what can be produced?

HOMEGROWN ANIMAL FEEDS

Buckwheat leaves & grain
Barley grain, boiled
Quinoa leaves and grain
Other grains
Potatoes, cooked
Jerusalem Artichokes
Sunflower seeds
Comfrey leaves
Stinging Nettles
Bamboo leaves
Sprouted seeds
Microgreens
Mashua
Plantain seed.

FODDER CROPS FOR POULTRY

Alfalfa
Buckwheat
Clover
Fathen
Grass, freshly cut
Kale
Mugwort seeds
Rapeseed
Rye & other grains.

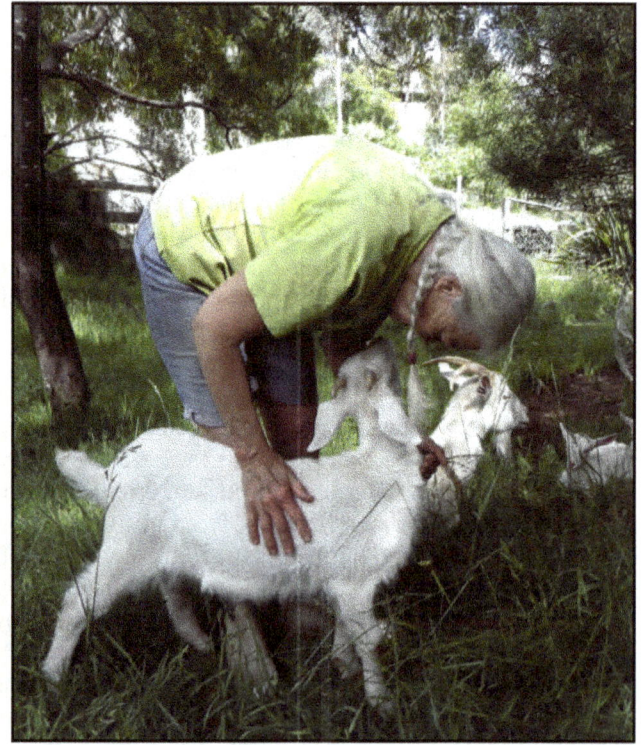

Below - Su Dennett, partner of David Holmgren, at their Permaculture paradise in central Victoria with her Goats.

HOMEGROWN ANIMAL FOODS

POTATOES
A nutritious food for both the peasantry and their livestock, Poultry, Pigs and Cows will happily eat Potatoes that are boiled and mashed. On cold days they are fed warm. Other things can be added to the mash for improved nutrition, such as wilted (dried or heated), chopped Comfrey and Nettle leaves.

JERUSALEM ARTICHOKES
Boil up the tubers and feed them mixed with other stuff. My Pigs also enjoy them raw and sprouting, plus the leaves and shoots.

PLANTAIN, PLANTAGO SPECIES
A widespread 'weed' species of small herb, the seeds are very nutritious. Hang bunches of ripe seed stalks up for poultry to reach up and peck at, then they won't be walking over it.

OATS
Whole Oats may be difficult to de-hull, but they are perfectly good for sprouting as such and are often fed to poultry and Pigs in this form, for enhanced nutritional value. Easy to grow for a staple seed crop, Naked Oats (Avena nuda) are a variety that are virtually husk free.

OTHER GRAINS
Poultry will eat any grains they can get and these don't have to come out of a commercial feed bag. The small grain plots I grew ended up with a fair bit of waste lying around at harvest time. I wished that I had some poultry to scratch around and peck it up!

As for Buckwheat, checking online I see it recommended "that poultry raised outdoors be fed a diet of no more than 30% Buckwheat". This is because it contains Fagopyrin, a substance that increases skin sensitivity to ultraviolet (UV) light, leading to sunburn.[1]

SUNFLOWERS
Easily grown, with attractive flowers, Sunflowers enhance the beauty of the garden and when seeds are mature you can dry the seed heads as they are for storage, and feed them as is. No need to process and de-hull seed, Chickens will remove the hulls themselves.

COMFREY
This fabulous herb has been an important staple green feed for animals for millenia, being packed with protein, vitamins, including B^{12}, Allantoin (the active ingredient for medicinal use), etc. It's best to wilt Comfrey in the sun for a while before feeding to Pigs or poultry, so that the prickly hairs on leaves are made palatable. Bunches can then be tied up at head height, so birds can pick off bits, rather than walking all over it on the ground. Or chop it up and add it to warm mash to wilt. Some say that up to 10% of the poultry diet can be replaced with Comfrey.

Lawrence Hills was an early researcher, breeder and promoter of Comfrey use, at Bocking, Surrey. He enthused that Pigs generally like Comfrey and that up to 30% of pig meal could be replaced with Comfrey. (They will eat the whole plant if they get a chance, so it's best to only feed cut and wilted large leaves that are brought to them.) Hill's advice was given before the problem of Pyrrolizidine Alkaloids became well known, so better to give less than 30%. Hills observed that, of twenty one cultivars tested, 'Bocking 4' was the clone yielding the most leaves, the highest amount of Potash and Allantoin, and with most resistance to Comfrey Rust. Bocking 14 was also recommended by Hills for garden fertilising and feeding to Pigs and poultry.

If kept weed free, well watered and fed with plenty of manure, Comfrey can be cut up to eight times annually. You stop cutting it in September so it can build up reserves to survive the winter. If you harvest just the large mature leaves (these have the lowest levels of Pyrrolizidine Alkaloids) over summer and dry them, you will have a store of dried leaf to feed animals over winter.[2]

STINGING NETTLES

These are another highly nutritious herb for feeding animals, if chopped and very lightly cooked or warmed, which neutralises the sting. Drying also neutralises it. Bunches of young Nettles can be hung in a protected, shady spot to dry; the leaves can then be crumbled into powder for storage, to add to other foods later, such as Potato mash. Small amounts of highly nutritious Nettle seed can also be fed in small amounts, being a great tonic.

KOREAN NATURAL FARMING APPROACH TO POULTRY FEED - USING BROWN RICE, BAMBOO LEAVES, RICE HUSKS & GREEN GRASS

Korean Natural Farming takes the self-sufficient approach and uses only what one produces oneself, including animal feed. Newly hatched chicks are fed only whole brown Rice grains in unlimited quantity for the first three days. This is to tone the digestive system, while chicks don't actually need feed over this time, being still nourished by the albumen from the egg. [3] Such a diet for gut health is completely at odds with the Western approach!

After three days for layers and one day for broilers, in the following week chicks are fed finely chopped Bamboo leaves that are mixed with mashed boiled eggs (or, as others advocate, with commercial chick feed[3]). They are fed this just once daily, two hours before sunset, before more Rice is given. Later, on day fifty, chicks have Rice husks added to feed, with the proportion of the mix gradually increasing until it's 20-25% of the total feed at six months. This lowers hens' egg laying capacity a bit, but it does increase their lifespan.

A Philipino study of the value of Bamboo leaves reported in 2015 to a World Bamboo Congress held in Korea, that:

> **"Feeding Chickens on an organic diet containing fresh Bamboo leaves results in increases in body weight by as much as 70% more than those fed on standard organic diets. The results suggest that the fibre in the Bamboo leaves enlarges the digestive tract and enables the chicks to consume more and to grow faster".** [4]

Freshly mowed green grass (ideally cut with a hand operated lawn mower) is also fed to them and can be given at a rate of up to a third of total feed for adult Chickens, according to Cho. [5]

KUNE KUNE PIGS - PERFECT PERMACULTURE PETS!

Pronounced Kunee Kunee, this small Pig breed has many admirable qualities and I'd always wanted some, but Australian law allows no Pig imports. Seeing more of them in late 2019 reignited my interest. As seen below, they were quietly grazing in the orchard of Kay Baxter and Bob Corker, at their amazing Permaculture establishment, Koanga Institute, near Wairoa in New Zealand. I was reminded that Kune Kunes are surely the most perfect Permaculture livestock and pets!

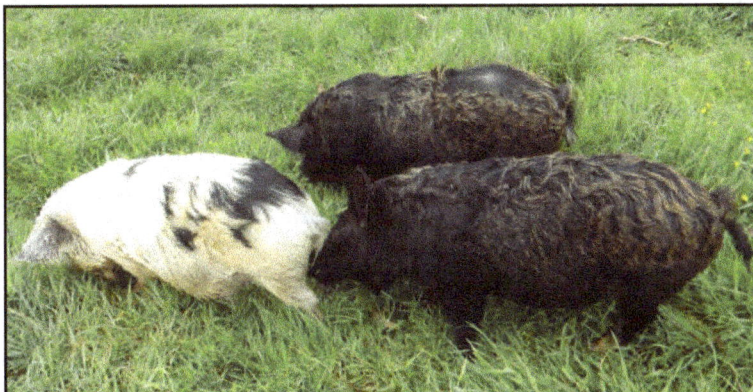

The smallest breed of domesticated Pig, Kune Kunes were taken to New Zealand with the Maori centuries ago. Their name means 'fat and round' and it is apt. But with large Pigs dominating the modern commercial breeds, numbers got to be critically low in the late 1970's. Fortunately the breed was saved and revived, and nowadays there is a New Zealand, as well as a British, Kune Kune association to promote them.

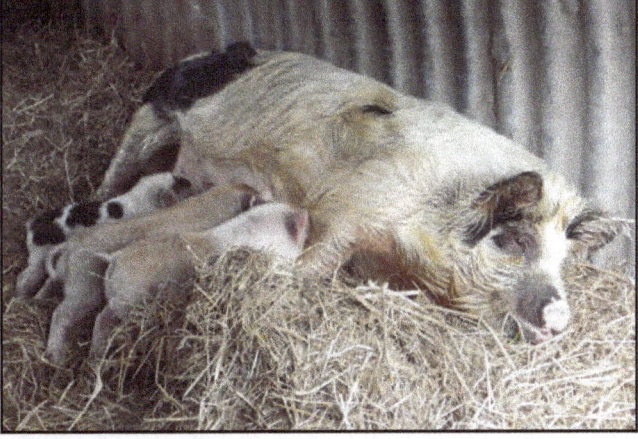

Kune Kunes typically have short, upturned snouts that are not suited to rooting up the ground as much as other breeds. They also don't challenge fences as much as European Pigs would, although Piglets can be very cunning and freedom loving! They are essentially small grass grazing Pigs that are able to thrive on low inputs. Pellets of grains, Alfalfa or the like are fed to supplement foraging, especially when grass isn't growing.

Being so docile, affectionate and easy to handle, they traditionally lived in and around Maori homes. They can apparently be trained to graze on a tether[6]. Otherwise, Pig or Sheep wire, or electric fencing will keep them in. You just have to make sure that the bottom fence wire along the ground is well pegged or tied down somehow, or they'll push the fence up and get out. I tie long thin flitches or Ash poles along the bottom wire to reinforce fences at the most tested sections.

As with other Pigs, Kune Kunes do not soil their bedding, as ruminant animals in confinement do. Living on the free range, they are very clean animals, unlike Pigs kept in confined, filthy conditions. They may occasionally need hoof trimming, tusk filing and worming, and brushing their thick coat is always welcome - they love that! Feeding them is easy because you can grow a lot of their needs. Kune Kunes enjoy a diet of grass, fresh fruit and vegetables. They only need 16% protein or less and can eat more fibre than commercial Pig breeds.

Kunes are tough in cold weather, sleeping outdoors unless it rains, when they do need dry shelter. A bundle of straw is their favourite bedding. A slow growing breed, they're fully grown after three years, by which time they can get to 60 - 70cm tall and weigh around 80 -100kg. Cross bred Pigs will not have all the Kune Kunes' admirable qualities.

WHY CHOOSE KUNE KUNES?
Having animal dependents, one loses one's freedom. So it's good to think long and hard before you take the plunge. But animals do add a wonderful emotional dimension to the landscape, they give us the joy of their touch ('contact comfort') through tactile interactions, as we exchange unconditional love. Scientists have observed that when a Dog is stroked, it's blood pressure drops and the same happens for the person stroking them. People with high anxiety enjoy decreased anxiety when interacting with their therapeutic animal friends.[7]

Pets can be chosen for multi-functionality and some will even work for their keep. Like the Jack Russell Terrier on an Australian Banana farm that I heard of, a full time ace ratter and important farm team member. With all the Poultry feed around my own Aussie small farm last century, the Rats were prolific, but Vikki the Wonderdog, my Jack Russell, hunted Rats doggedly and executed them fast and efficiently.

Milking Goats are an important part of Permaculture co-originator David Holmgren's own small farm in central Victoria, Australia. Here the Goats range through orchards (with each fruit tree individually fenced off) and they are also taken on daily walks through the bush to eat wild Brambles etc by David's partner Su Dennett, who adores them and this daily routine!

When I was travelling a lot it wasn't so good for my Dog and Llamas, so I resisted getting any more pets in Ireland. But in the pandemic lockdowns of 2020-21 I was really missing interacting with animals. Being confined to Ireland, it seemed right to take the plunge again. The decision to get any pet had to be predicated by my environment. Or rather, predator-cated. With plenty of them around, I didn't want the heartbreak of losing a small animal. I would not be a provider of live food for Pine Martens, Foxes, Crows and feral Mink. They can feed themselves elsewhere.

Some Ducks would be delightful to have in the orchard, I mused, and they're well suited to the Irish climate. Chickens would be good also, because we do eat eggs. But both make perfect Fox food, so, not those for now. I'd love to have a Donkey too, but they can be very loud at times. And, being from a dry, hot climate, Ireland is rather damp for them. Their hooves can suffer greatly in the damp and they need a fair bit of maintenance to keep well. A dairy Sheep or Goat breed would be great to have for milk and weed eating. But for feeding just the two of us, it probably wouldn't be worth the time and energy to keep and milk them. Plus, I'd need a bit more land for these larger animals that have strong herding instincts and should not be kept on their own.

I wanted a friendly and intelligent pet that doesn't want to bite the postman or attack little kids. Kunes are gentle and docile, happy little herbivores, as smart as any Dog. I could train them up for the Permaculture lifestyle. I didn't want another Cat or Dog - predatory carnivores that find it sporty to harass and eat wild life, despite being well fed. And, as a vegetarian, I didn't want to be feeding meat to an animal. One of the shocking realities of food inequity is that while many people in the world are starving, one-fifth of all the world's fish harvest and meat production goes to feeding people's pets![8] A vegan pet was the go and Kune Kunes are so.

Having plenty of suitable plants growing already, I could produce their food on-site. And also reduce lawn mower use and hoeing, harnessing their urge to root plants up and employing them as 'Pig Tractors', clearing rough bits of land and fertilising it with their manure. In a worst case scenario, if I had to get rid of a Kune Kune for some reason, somebody would no doubt take it off my hands and even eat it. Their meat is said to be delicious. Meanwhile, other pets that are unwanted are a big problem, with many abandoned and starving in the wild, while dumped Cats and Dogs hasten the extinction of wildlife they hunt.

Discovering that Kune Kunes are bred in Ireland, I had to get some! I picked up my two castrated male pedigree piglets from Mayo in May 2021 and I wasn't disappointed. The fun had begun!

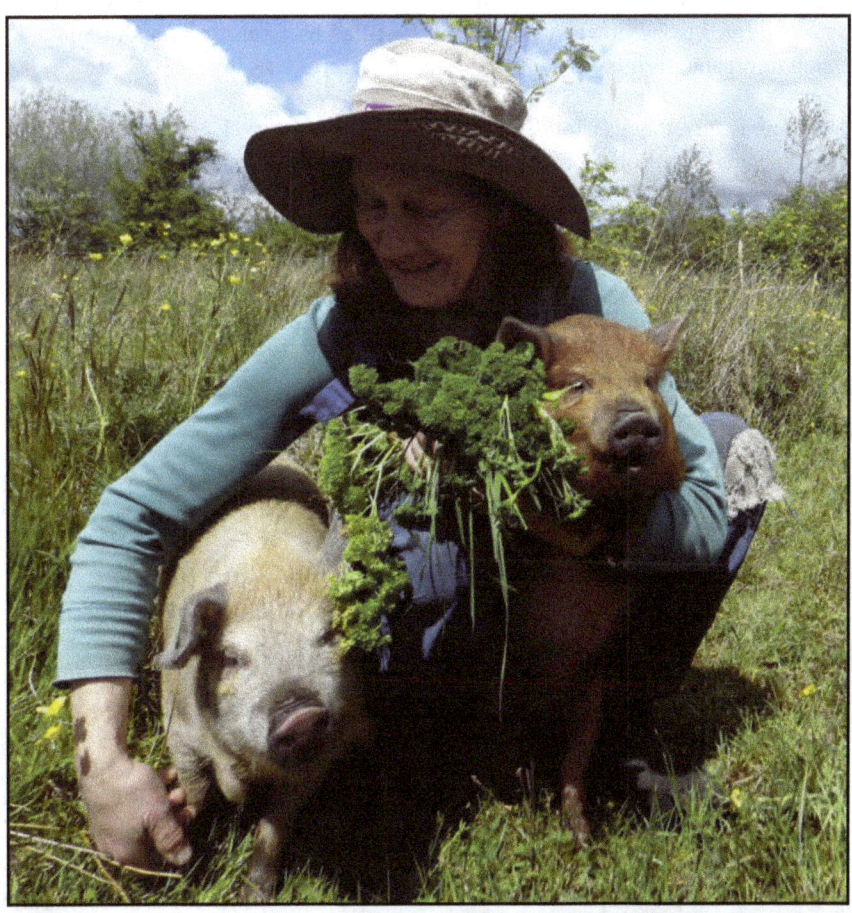

TO BEE OR NOT TO BEE?

Bees are exquisite jewels of the insect world, sacred to ancient societies and fundamental to food security - with their essential pollination services for crop production and the delectable and healing elixir that their honey provides us. Perfect as micro-livestock for the micro-farmer, I haven't yet taken up Beekeeping myself. However, if and when I do, it will be native Bees that I keep, for sure!

Watching a film about Honey Bees a while ago we were taken aback to learn that honey comes at such a high cost to the Bees. Their foraging travails take them the equivalent of flying around the whole planet just to produce a small jar full! Truly, Honey is a luxury food and not to be quaffed! We did cut down on consumption after that, finding sweetness in other forms. But we still buy it.

It would certainly make logical sense to keep Bees in the orchard and I've pondered on the pros and cons of it. On the plus side I could be eating honey with less food miles, the Bees would have plenty of scope in the lush gardens and I'd probably achieve a higher fruit yield from the enhanced pollination. Over the last few years a massive drop in insect numbers, like a shocking 90% decline in parts of Germany, means that a lot of crops are not getting much pollination and yields are down. This gap can be filled by Beekeepers and, of course, mass conversion to organic farming!

But on the minus side, there's a lot of learning needed to get started, plus expensive equipment and time required. With global Bee problems such as Colony Collapse, would it be successful? And would it be sustainable for my personal economy?

Fortunately, I have a neighbour Beekeeper and he assures me that his Bees already forage in my orchards. Bees have a big territory, flying daily around 2km for their food. The neighbours don't use chemicals much around here, there are probably plenty of native Black Bees, Bumblebees and other bugs providing free pollination services in my gardens tool. But what is the bigger picture of the Honey Bee today?

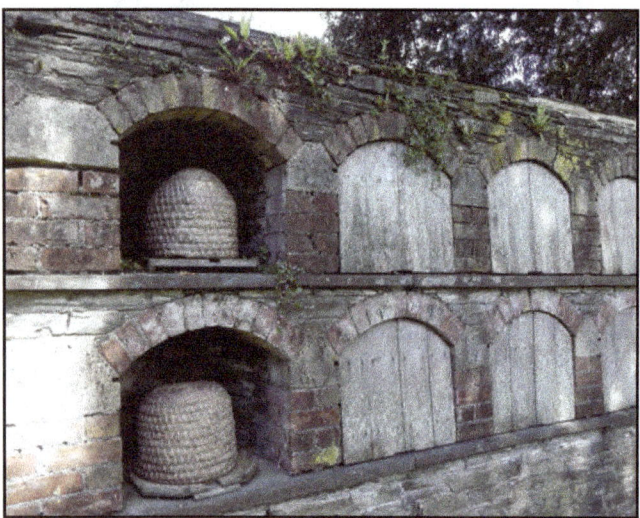

Left - Old Bee hives at the 'Lost Gardens of Heligan' in Cornwall. UK.

BIG BEE

Globally, Bees are big business. Not just for honey, but for pollinating farmer's crops. Queen Bee rearing and Bee colony trading is also big business, with new Bees installed every year to fill the constant demand by mega-orchardists. The service they provide is so essential. But

Bees don't like to be in a chemical drenched environment. Killed or weakened by farm pesticides, especially the ones based on Tobacco, Bees are also highly sensitive to electromagnetic radiation and tend to swarm to avoid strong fields. Around 5G and other antennas they drop dead and their bodies litter the ground. It's hardly a surprise then, that instead of Bee colonies thriving over several years, they grow weak and become vulnerable to disease, or they disappear and die after just one season.

Australia is the world's biggest exporter of queen Bees, with a continuing Varroa-mite-free status. It's the only country in the world without this awful Bee pest that has affected almost every colony in Europe since the late 1970s. (Asian Bees have developed resistance to Varroa mites, but their honey production is not as high as European Honey Bees.) If Varroa took hold in Australia, would this lead to a global famine? Potentially - yes!

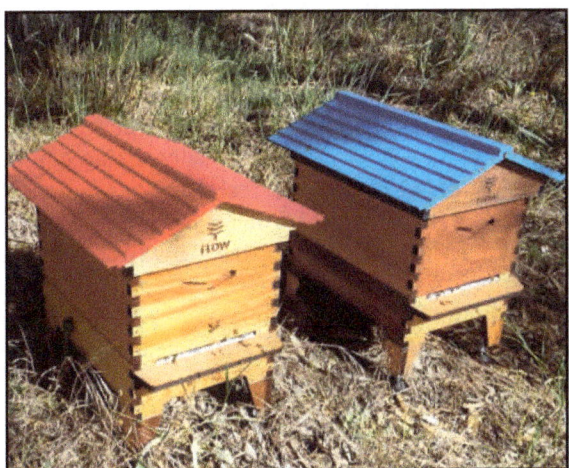

To avoid a global Bee catastrophe, the world needs to have more backyard Beekeepers, people who value health, use no chemical toxins and breed for Varroa resistance, while maintaining the local native Bee varieties that are best adapted to the local environment.

Left - A friend sent me me this photo of her Flow Hives, a revolution in honey production developed in Australia recently. The honey is super easy to harvest.

WHICH BEE IS BEST?
Ireland has it's own native Honey Bee, known as the Black Bee, Apis mellifera mellifera, (though its colour can vary). Recognised as a very pure and genetically diverse regional strain of European Honey Bee, incoming foreign Bee strains threaten it's continuing purity, as well as potentially importing new pests and diseases. In 2012 a society to promote the Irish Bee was set up. At the annual conference of the Native Irish Honey Bee Society (NIHBS) in March 2018 it was reported that members "were shocked to learn of the amounts of queens and colonies of Bees that were imported into the country in the last year. The numbers are startling and cannot be allowed to continue. With those figures comes a question: why do some Beekeepers need to import all those Bees on a yearly basis? Very simple answer - they do not survive here. They are brought in every year with little regard for the damage they are doing to our native Honey Bee. The Bees we have on this island are superior to any Bee that is imported...superior because they have adapted to our climate over a long period of time. If imports continue at this rate it may soon be too late [from the threat of hybridisation]. ...If we do not protect them they will dwindle and die out." [9]

The Irish Black Bee can fly around at lower temperatures and still produce good amounts of honey even in poor weather conditions, compared to other varieties. They are also relatively long lived, docile and have a low swarming tendency. The NIHBS is educating the public about native queen Bee rearing and encourages individual beekeepers to successfully breed them. They also support research projects into the Black Bee and scientific monitoring of them for Varroa resistance, as well as promoting conservation of the species across the island of Ireland.

THERAPEUTIC HONEYS

Kiwi entrepreneurs in New Zealand are brilliant at marketing and their Manuka honey is a jewel in their crown. With its well attested, globally recognised anti-bacterial properties, this product can command top dollar! When I discussed this last century with Australian Tea Tree oil pioneer, Christopher Dean of Thursday Plantation, he told me that there are many species of related trees whose honey could potentially give therapeutic effects similar to Manuka honey. Bees make it from flowers of Melaleuca scoparium, a species of Tea Tree related to Melaleuca alternifolia, the therapeutic oil species. (While Tea Tree is a subtropical species, Manuka is from more temperate climes and could possibly grow in Ireland.) Other unrelated plant honeys would no doubt also have therapeutic potentials. Many have long been renowned for their anti-bacterial properties and used for dressing burns and wounds with.

In Ireland native Bees survive the relatively mild winters and over the cold months they are able to thrive on the flowers of Ivy. Irish monofloral honeys are commercially produced from Ivy and Heather. Recently members of the Athlone Institute of Technology undertook a preliminary study that looked into the medicinal properties of Ivy honey, as compared with Manuka. They focussed on both the anti-microbial and anti-inflammatory activity of both non heat-treated honeys and were able to confirm anti-microbial activity with them, plus the ability to reduce recovery times for burns, etc. Antibiotic resistant strains of bacteria were also reduced by these honeys. The researchers concluded that "initial indications are that Ivy honey has potential as a wound healing agent." [9]

KEEPING BEES HEALTHY NATURALLY

So what is a natural approach to Bee keeping? I have picked up a few tips from Beekeepers. Some twenty years ago a fellow dowser in New Zealand told me about an ancient European observation that Bees are less stressed, more vigorous and more likely to produce extra amounts of honey when hives are placed over the course of an underground water stream. His dowsing rods detected these zones of intense energy that give the Bees a real buzz. Not only did they Bees become more productive than Bees in randomly placed hives, but they were also afforded protection against Varroa mites. The mites were absent in any hives correctly placed according to dowsing.

I told this to a woman in Germany years later, but she was not impressed and felt that this was an exploitation of the Bees. She's a member of an esoteric Bee keeping group who do interesting things like positioning hives in groups of six in a hexagonal arrangement. I don't have any more details about that and I'll take her comments on board. We live in a world of give and take and need to find the best balance. I'll leave it to the reader to decide on the best ethics here!

Bees are happiest and healthiest when hives are kept as far from electromagnetic fields as possible, avoiding 'smart meters', phone masts, high voltage electricity lines and the like. If you want to check how sensitive they are, just switch on a mobile phone, place it on top of a Bee hive and see what happens. (Or take my word for it and leave them in peace!)

I feel the assertion, that global insect decline is due to a combination of toxic chemical saturation of farmland, plus the intensification of electromagnetic fields over the last couple of decades, must be correct. (The smaller the animal, the worse the effects of radiation on it.)

A non-toxic solution to Varroa mites has been developed by Biodynamic agriculture researchers. They create a 'pepper' to deal with them, a natural pesticide made by burning Varroa mites at certain times and sprinkling the ash between the honeycombs. This is mainly done in summer and whenever inspections are made. Biodynamic researchers Maria and Matthias Thun wrote that "Following a number of comparative trials we recommend burning and making an ash of the Varroa mite in the usual way…The ash should be made and sprinkled when the Sun and Moon are in Taurus (May/June)." [10]

ANIMAL REFERENCES

1. https://www.heritageacresmarket.com/fodder-for-chickens/
2. Comfrey: Past, Present and Future, Lawrence Hills, Henry Doubleday Research Association, UK, 1976.
3. An Introduction to Natural Farming Poultry Production in Hawai'i, the Wave of the Future Michael W. DuPonte, Kiersten Akahoshi, Keala Cowell, and Lehua Wall CTAHR Cooperative Extension Service, Hilo, HI, July 2016 College of Tropical Agriculture and Human Resourcs, University of Hawaii at Manoa, USA.
4. Bamboo Leaves as Chicken Feed and Fodder, Carmelita B. Bersalona, 10th World Bamboo Congress, Korea 2015.
5. Dr. Cho's Global Natural Farming, by Rohini Reddy, South Asia Rural Reconstruction Association, Karnataka, India, 2011. Available as a free pdf download online.
6. //www.blockhill.co.nz/pigs
7. The Wisdom of Donkeys, Andy Merrifield, Short Books, UK, 2008.
8. Little Green Book - 100 Ways to Tread Softly on the Planet part 2, Sunday Independent, 22/9/2019.
9. The Four Seasons, issue 69, spring 2018. www.nihbs.org
10. The Maria Thun Biodynamic Calendar 2021, Floris Books, UK.

PEASANT IN PARADISE

CHAPTER FIVE

WINTERTIME

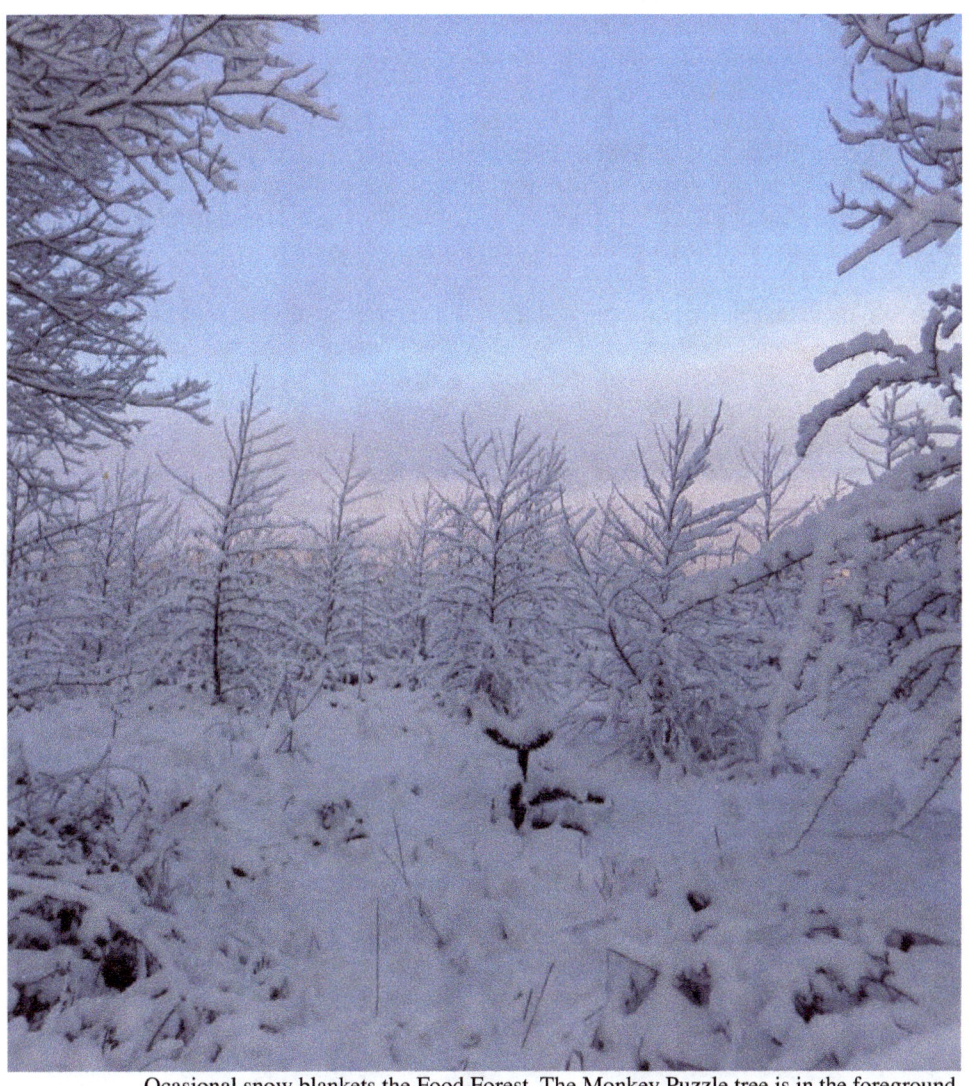

Ocasional snow blankets the Food Forest. The Monkey Puzzle tree is in the foreground.

WINTERTIME

> "Abundance is strictly seasonal and must be preserved for those times when the fields and woods are bare. The store cupboard is of the utmost importance - stocking requires judgement, patience and skill." [1] **Elisabeth Luard**

The traditional Celtic year begins on November 1st, the first day of winter, when people honoured their ancestors, looked to their origins, feasted on surplus animals and rejoiced in the turning of the wheel of the year. The Christian equivalent of this festive time, the Eve of All Saints, better known today as Halloween, is a faint echo, but in its ghastly commercial aspect - stripped of the dignity and reverence that was once bestowed on the dead. This survey of a year of eco-living also connects back to past times, to the old ways that are now proving the way of the future. Winter is the season when rest and recreation lead us to contemplation, while we also prepare the foundations for another year of abundant growth.

Wintertime is revealing. The leafless trees become skeletal architecture, exposing farther views. Hidden places become visible. Ancient archeologies stand out. We explore the fields around us where the remains of farmsteads of ancient vintage might be found. Weedy bumps in the landscape harking back from the Iron Age to medieval times, these enduring earthworks are often protected by the fear of upsetting fairy presences (once referred to as 'the gentry').

Wintertime can reveal shy or nocturnal creatures that are normally not seen. Walking up my road, all white with a light carpet of snow, footprints announce the presence of Foxes and Pine Martens, reminding me why I don't keep poultry. Winter exposes these hidden realities and the bare essence of place.

Wintertime means spending more time in the Great Indoors. Finally, one has time for thoughtful reflection, unhurried contemplation, immersion in the inner worlds. It's time for creating intangible cultural wealth, the season most suited for writing, developing recipes or singing. It's certainly not hibernation time! Plenty of eco-activities to keep me occupied and fit.

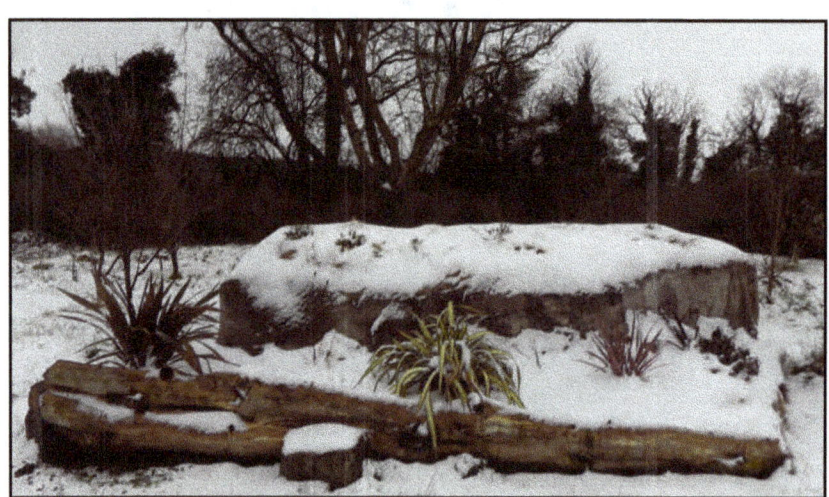

Left - Snowfall brightens the backyard landscape. The clamp shelters bins full of root vegetables.

WINTER GARDEN ACTIVITIES

* Bringing tender pot plants indoors.
* Checking fruit and veggies in storage and removing anything rotten; anything withering can be made into preserves to extend shelf life.
* Harvesting outdoors Brussel Sprouts, Leeks, Cabbages and Kale.
* Harvesting root crops left in the ground and mulching them for frost protection.
* Harvesting salad greens and the last Tomatoes etc in the polytunnel.
* Cleaning out garden beds and mulching them.
* Gathering materials for making big compost heaps.
* Going through seed and plant catalogues and ordering what's needed.
* Planting bare-rooted deciduous fruit and nut trees, and berries.
* Any plants needing to be re-located or divided, this is also done in their dormancy.
* Cleaning up under fruit trees, removing any diseased bits, e.g. leaves with scab.
* Pruning fruit trees: Apples, Mulberries, Pears, Quinces and Medlars.

When the short winter days are inclement, it's time to contract into the cosy kitchen and keep the fire blazing. I make the most of the long hours spent there with a range of activities. As well as preparing meals and creative pursuits, I'll be working on my businesses, making pickles and ferments, watching birds and clouds out the big picture window, sewing/mending/repairing things, listening to music and drying things around the fire. A bit of yoga thrown in, gives the perfect "stretch in the day".

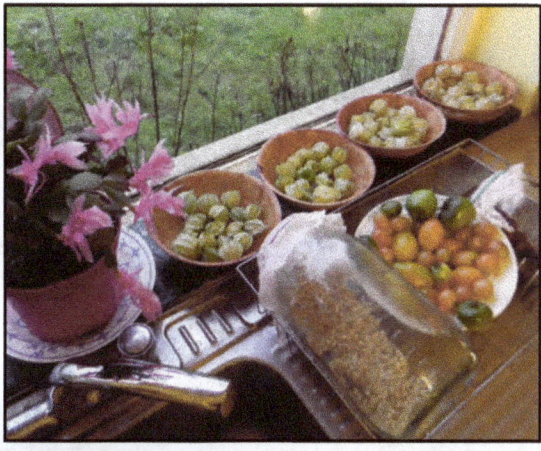

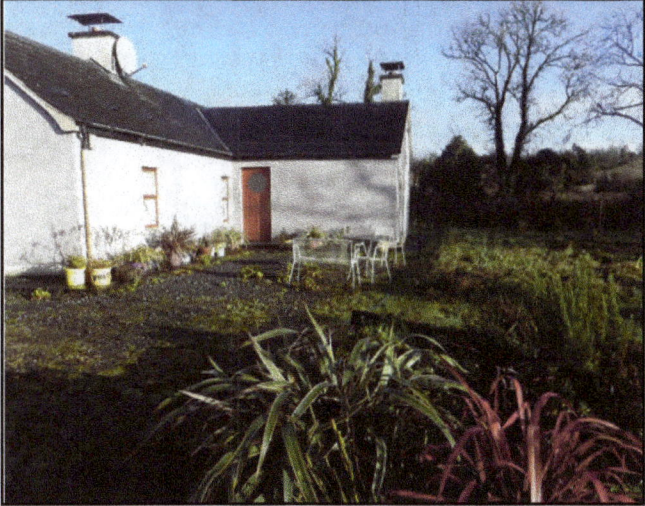

Above - December harvest of Tomatoes, Golden Berries, sprouting seeds and Christman Cactus flowers. Left - The low angle of winter solstice sunshine goes into the cottage for healthy, natural lighting.

With winter's long hours of darkness, we can get exposed to a lot of artificial lighting. It can be a curse as much as a boon. Light bulbs must be carefully chosen to avoid adverse health affects. For example, fluorescent lighting has well known ill effects. They flicker and disturb our brains, while modern compact fluorescents bulbs are not much better, plus they contain Mercury and really don't fit in an eco ethos. I guess it was the old fluoro strip lighting in school classrooms that caused my regular migraines, that only stopped when I left school at sixteen and moved to the countryside to pursue the peasant life. That lighting probably set me up for developing greater electro-sensitivity later on in the wifi age (the effects of electro-stress being cumulative and additive).

With all the exposure to unnatural indoor lighting and especially when weather is dull, it's no wonder that seasonal, wintertime depression (SAD syndrome) is common in temperate zones. A great antidote and preventative is natural light, so time is well spent in the polytunnel where, even on a cold windy winter's day, one can enjoy the sunlight, warmth and green beauty, while getting meaningful exercise with gardening. There's no need to get SAD!

1. European Peasant Cookery, Elisabeth Luard, Grub Street, London, UK, 1986.

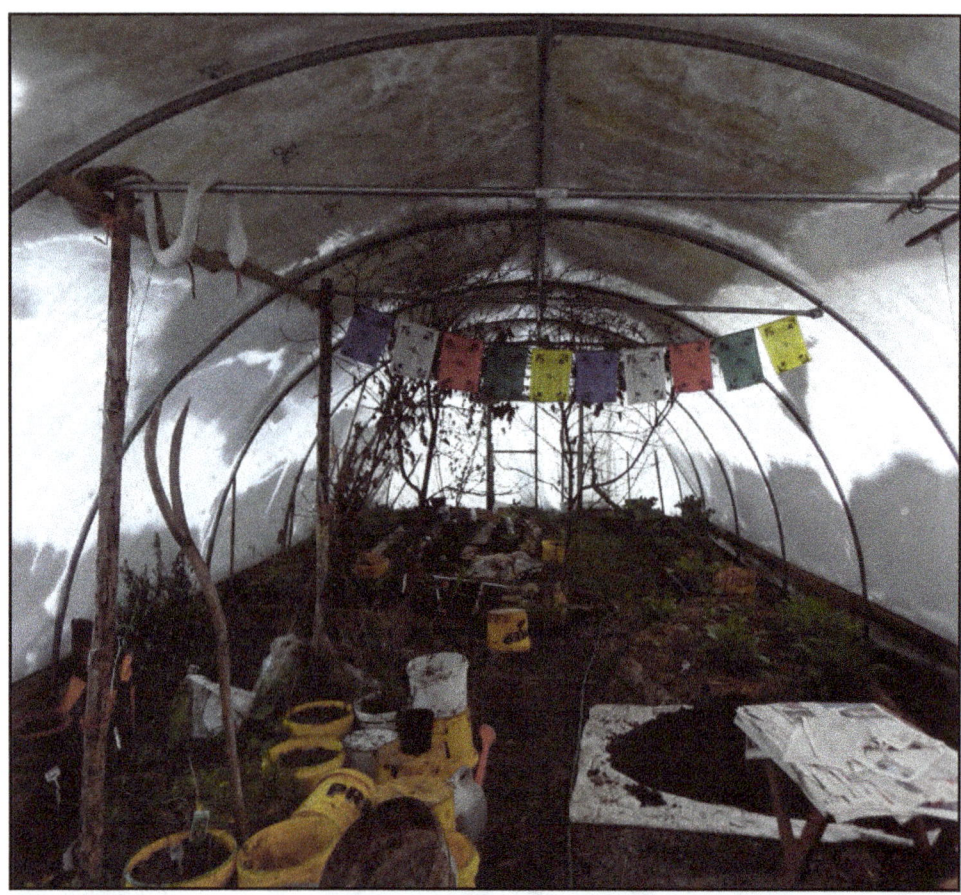

Above- Snow sits heavily on top of the winter polytunnel as I gather materials for re-potting Strawberry plants in early spring. Gentle tapping with a soft broom on the plastic membrane above me sends snow sliding down off the sides. Doors at each end are always left a bit open through the winter to allow for air flow, otherwise heavy frosts will be more severe inside the polytunnel.

SACRED HEARTH OF THE HOME

Brisk weather and the chopping of firewood makes for a great appetiser. And there's plenty of indoor time for cooking delicious meals that would never be so good from a restaurant. A trip to various larders and my basket is brimming with root vegetables, dried beans and pickles. It's a highly satisfying bounty, once so fundamental to life that the home hearth and larder were considered sacrosanct. The hearth, providing cooking and warmth, was the very heart of the home, developing deep mythic qualities.

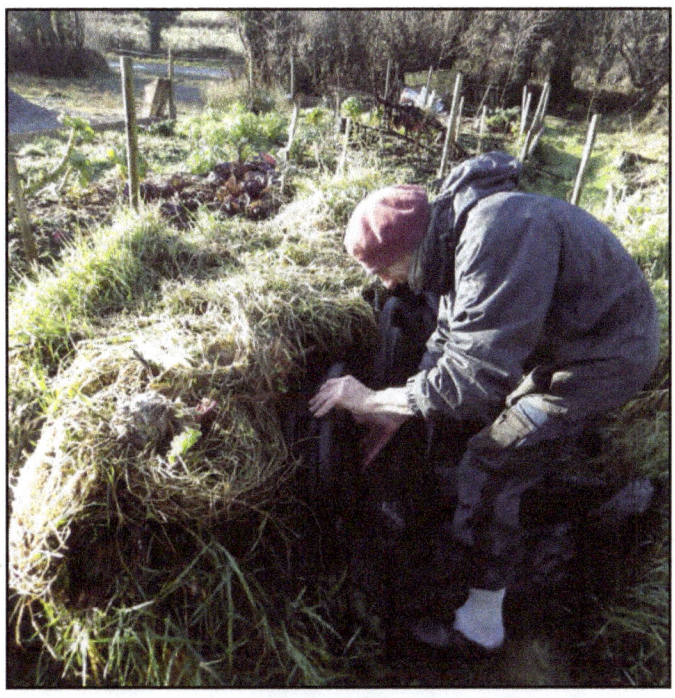

Above - Clamp experiment - Potatoes are stored in damp sand in plastic garbage bins laid on their sides and covered with soil and mulch. It worked fine, but the bins were not really rigid enough for the job, metal ones would be better. All good permaculture is experimental.

The theme of the sacred hearth seems to be universal. The ancient Greeks had their hearth goddess Hestia, while the Romans sanctified domesticity, with goddess Vesta the divine keeper of every Roman's hearth. Vesta, one of the most ancient and popular of all the Roman deities, was accorded the honour of a full time clergy devoted solely to her rites, with Vestal virgin priestesses tending Her perpetual temple fire until Christianity ended this in the year 394 CE. In each Roman home the head woman prepared offerings to Vesta that she cast into the fire at family meal times. Vesta presided over lesser spirits called the Penates, symbolised by a penis, and also Lars familaris, and these were also given food offerings tossed into the fire. The Lares spirit, originally associated with the land surrounding the home and its guardianship, was strongly linked to the family and concerned for its protection. Meanwhile, people in Silesia buried pots of offerings to the Stetewaldiu, 'The Masters of the Premises' behind the stove or hearth in new buildings and beneath its corners, and they'd regularly toss food offerings into the flames to keep The Masters friendly.

In Ireland early Christianity continued the theme, with St Brigit the divine guardian of every hearth, with a perpetual fire kept at Kildare. Across Europe there are traditions that the hearth was a place for divination and rituals of healing and protection. Spirits of the underworld might be contacted there too. The accessories of the hearth had spiritual associations and ritual uses. Pokers, tongs and brushes had sacred significance, while the chimney hook even had legal significance in some regions. [1]

My old stone cottage is typical of many in Ireland, with its (originally) three rooms. The main hearth was located under the chimney in the central room, providing both heat and cooking. This was the living room, the dining room and kitchen combined. But it was referred to, in last century Leitrim at least, as "the kitchen". [2] Smaller, single room mud cottages often just had a fire on the flat flagstone floor, its smoke slowly escaping through the thatched roof. The elders in the home would have the privilege of a seat up close to the fire. They might sit on a stone with a cushion on top, or on a wood and woven straw rope ('sugan') chair, and they often slept beside the fire as well, cosy in a 'settle bed' (forerunner of the sofa bed).

Traditions in Europe have it that the hearth is the favourite haunt of ancestral spirits and, from experience, I can concur with this. From professional dowsing surveys of peoples' homes in Ireland, especially in old farm houses of multiple generations of family, I've encountered it myself. The atmosphere can be thick with ancestral spirits and they are often found stationed beside the fire, sitting in their old favourite seat, fondly watching over their descendants.

Ancient traditions of the sacred hearth in Ireland have been unearthed by archeological discoveries. In County Fermanagh archeologists were able to excavate an Iron Age settlement on a crannog (a man-made lake island used in times of danger), because the lake had dried up. The crannog homes were in use from around 2,000 years ago. The remains of several homesteads were investigated and beneath the hearth of each were found carefully placed bone combs. These highly valued possessions were symbolic of divine female power and they were probably ritually placed as an offering to the female spirit of sovereignty, to garner protection of the home.

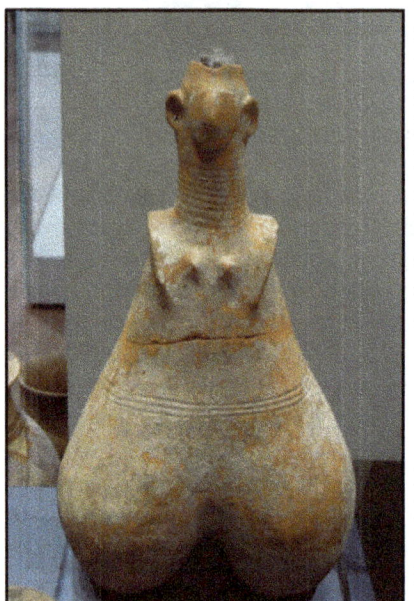

The larder has likewise been considered a magical, feminine domain. It receives the bounty of Earth's womb and acts as a surrogate for that chalice of nourishment. The Russians call it the kladovaia and klad means treasure. Larders are treasure stores. The Roman Penates were guardian spirits that watched over larders. Penates were originally honoured at Vesta temple's inner sanctums. A Roman's kitchen and larder were the household equivalents of Vesta's sacred domain. These days, kitchens mostly everywhere remain strongly female territory.

Left - A ceramic figure in the British Museum.
We might call her Earth Larder Mother.

In Elizabethan England, households kept several larders, with at least one wet and one dry one. The wet one was for pickles and salting fish; the dry one for dry goods only. There might also have been separate game and pastry pantries too, each with different environmental conditions.[3] I appreciated the need for this, when the smell of jars of pickled Garlic was rather overpowering amongst my otherwise fragrant dried fruits. I have several different types of food storages now. A similar concept applies to kitchens in other parts of the world. In the steamy tropics of Malaysia, where I often visit, it's quite normal to have a wet and a dry kitchen, for example.

1. The Tradition of Household Spirits, Ancestral Lore and Practises, Claude Lecouteux, Inner Traditions, Canada, 2000.
2. Ballinaglera and Inishmagrath - the history and traditions of two Leitrim parishes, Clancy and Forde, Maura Clancy, 2003, Ireland.
3. Winter Vegetarian by Darra Goldstein, Harper Perennial, 1996, USA.

WINTER HARVEST

Many vegetables can be left in the ground over winter, as long as it's not too freezing or wet, while thickly mulching around them can protect them somewhat. Veggies and herbs that can be left in the ground, or that keep growing over winter, include the following.

Beetroot
Broccoli
(Purple Sprouting)
Brussel Sprouts
Cabbages
Celeriac
Celery Leaf
Chard
Chicory
Chinese Artichoke
Corn Salad
Green in the Snow
Jerusalem Artichoke
Kale
Kohl rabi
Leeks
Mashua
Mizuna
Mustard
Oca
Onions
Pak choi
Parsley
Parsnips
Potatoes
Rosemary
Sage
Salsify
Scorzonera
Spinach
Swiss Chard
Turnips
Thyme
Welsh Onion
Winter Savoury

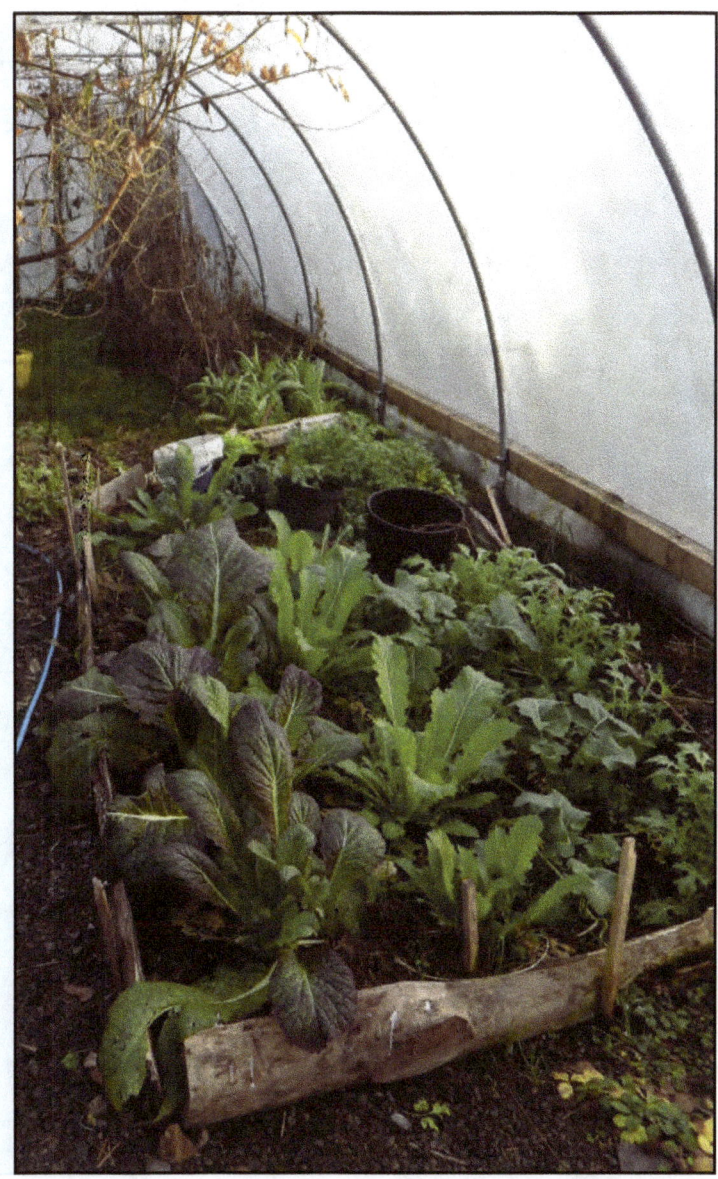

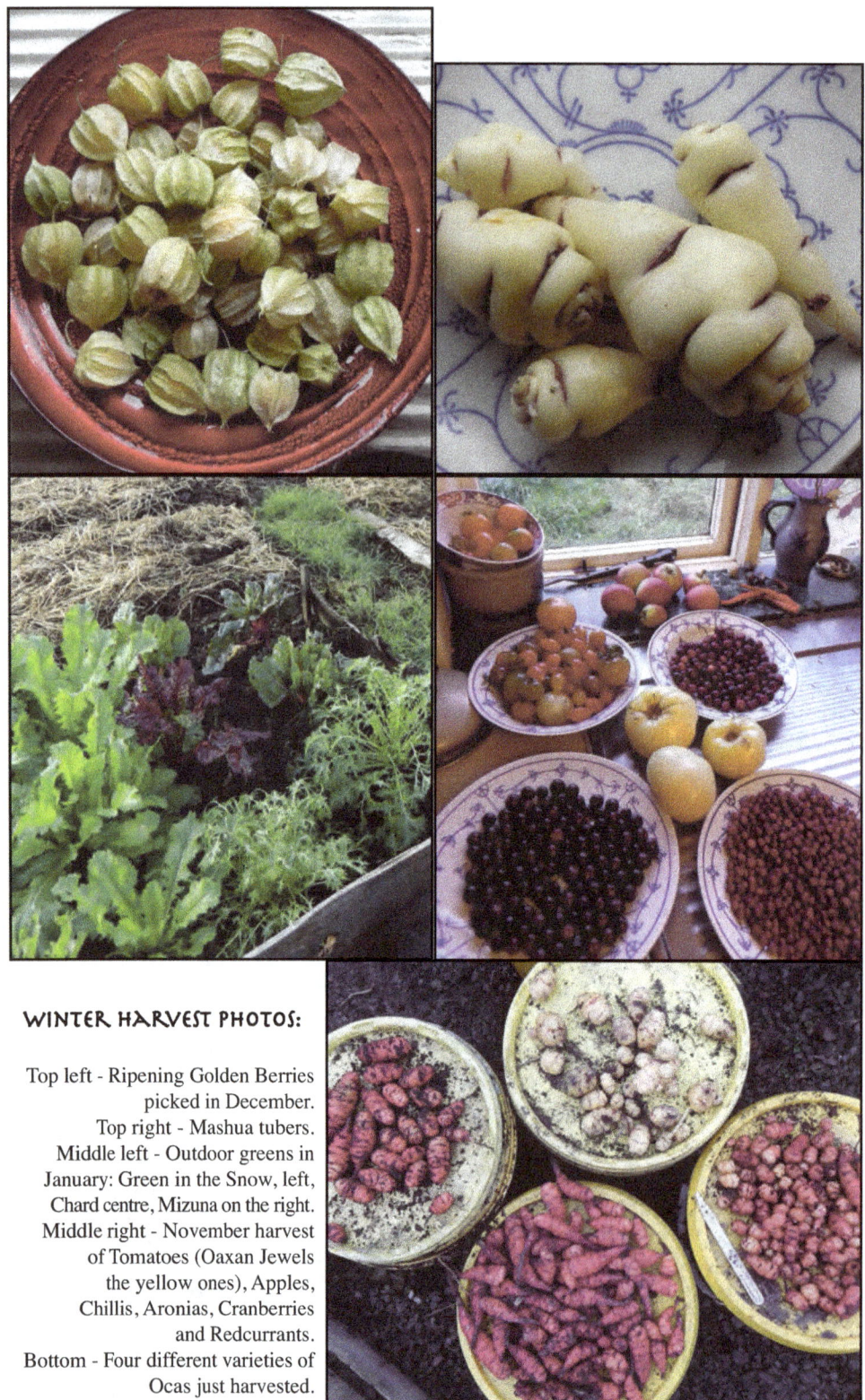

WINTER HARVEST PHOTOS:

Top left - Ripening Golden Berries picked in December.
Top right - Mashua tubers.
Middle left - Outdoor greens in January: Green in the Snow, left, Chard centre, Mizuna on the right.
Middle right - November harvest of Tomatoes (Oaxan Jewels the yellow ones), Apples, Chillis, Aronias, Cranberries and Redcurrants.
Bottom - Four different varieties of Ocas just harvested.

WINTER COMPOSTING

Winter is the season for making bulk compost. Conveniently, nature provides plenty of suitable materials at this time. I enjoy raking the fallen leaves from roadside Oaks (right) and Chestnut trees that blow down the road and deposit thickly in some spots. Oak leaves are particularly wonderful to use, nutrient dense and the tannins in them a repellant for Slugs and Snails. Too much tannin can harm the soil, which is why you need to wait until the weather has half rotted them and leached it mostly away, or give them time to compost in the heap, before using them.

Where animals are shedded in the winter, manure can be easily available to gardeners. We collect small trolley loads of the neighbour's

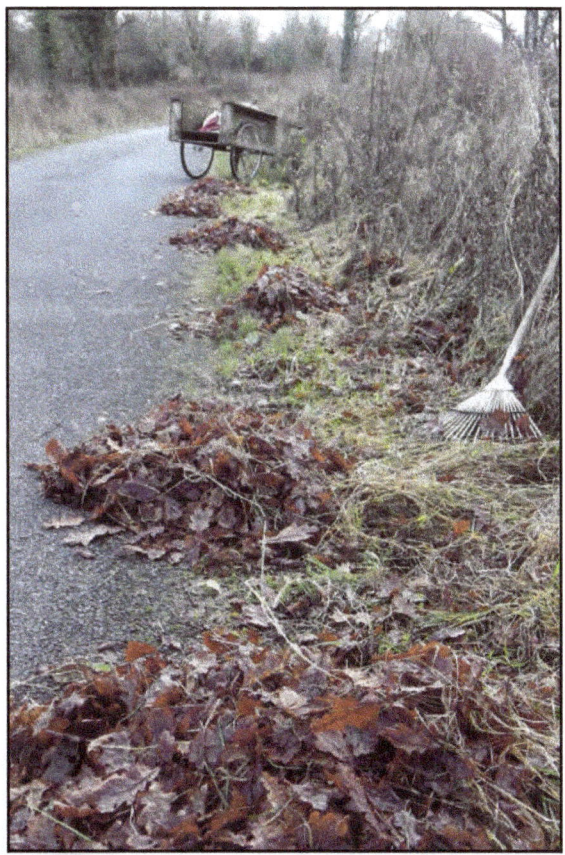

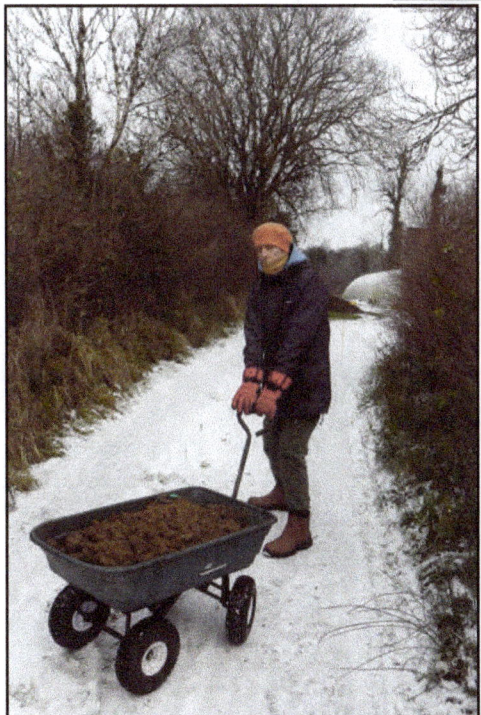

horse manure every day, as seen left. To balance all the Nitrogen in the manure you need a thick layer of Carbon, such as tree leaves. A clear out of the finished veggies in the polytunnel provides much Carbon rich matter for the heap. Leaf and stick filled house gutters are a treasure trove of rot too, well worth the trouble of cleaning them!

The cosy winter house fire provides lots of ash from wood and peat and this is great for sprinkling over manure, acid soil and the compost heap, adding a fine mineral rich layer, with some 5-15% Potassium, 10-25% Calcium 1-4% Magnesium, and 1-3% Phosphorus. But if it's too thick a layer it becomes toxic, a highly alkaline lye. Keep the ash dry and use it for a host of other things, e.g. as a Slug repellant, sprinkled in a ring around plants.

There's much hacking down of vegetation this season too, so wood chips are often available in winter. For most people a pile of wood chips is just another form of waste to get rid of. Because wood needs loads of Nitrogen to help break it down, it isn't popular in the garden usually, unless you just spread it on pathways as a weed suppressant. However when it does break down it makes very good mulch around fruit and other trees. Wood chips and urine are a perfect combination! I sprinkle it over the heap from the watering can over the winter, when garden plants don't need it.

Another boon for the composter is to get some giant bales of spoiled silage. The huge plastic wrapped bales are ubiquitous here. I'm told that some people plant their veggies straight into the spoiled silage after unrolling the bale, and that it's also valuable as a thick weed mat. I've been adding layers of it to compost heaps and mulching under trees with it.

It's a great feeling of satisfaction when the annual big compost heap is finished, after weeks of building it up as high as I can, then covering it over. I can leave the microorganisms to take over the work and celebrate!

Below - Our neighbour's Horse manure is spread on the surface of spent beds each winter. Winter veggies, such as Black (Tuscan) Kale left and centre, are still thriving.

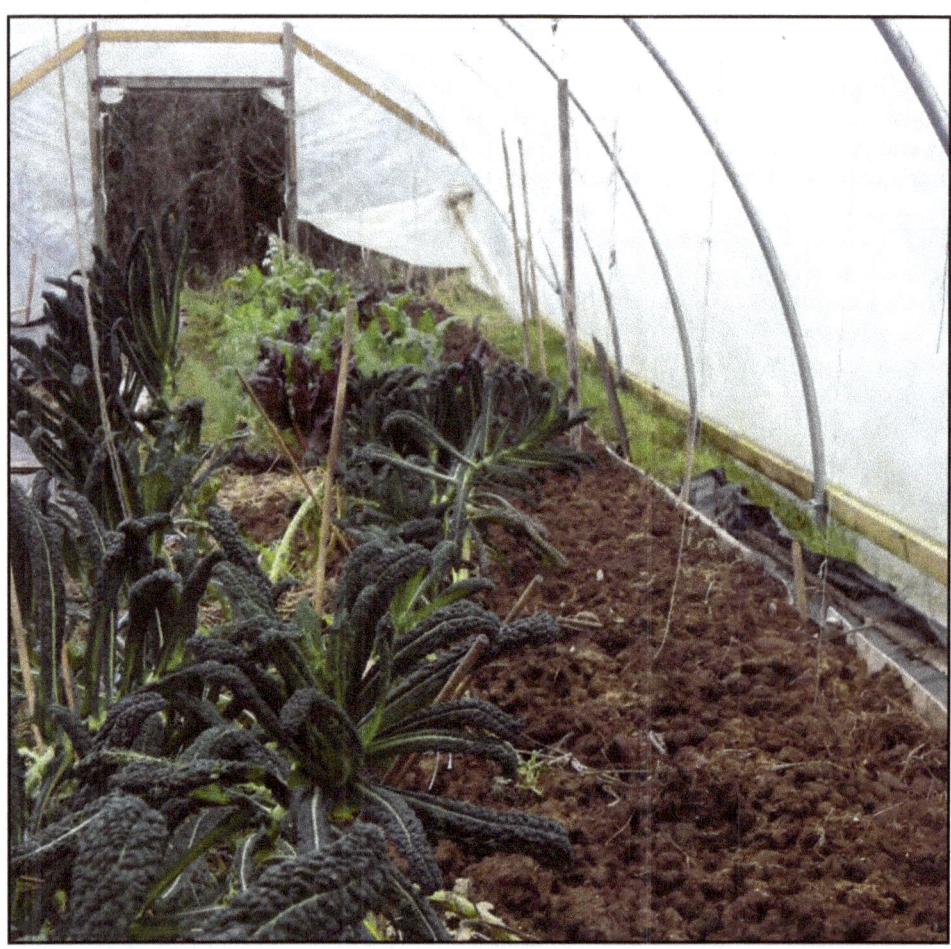

SEED SPROUTING

> "To sprout a seed is to let nature convert it into a perfect food.
> No man-made process can match the way in which
> the plant enzymes effortlessly change all the inert proteins,
> fats and starches into amino acids, essential fatty acids and simple sugars.
> It's one of nature's true miracles." [1] Edward Cairney

Plants seed abundantly to ensure their survival and this is a wonderful resource for us. If we always grow non-hybrid, heirloom plants we can save the seeds of annuals and grow them on indefinitely; while seeds are a food source themselves when they are sprouted. The transformative process that fires germination enhances the nutritional value of seeds, to supercharge plant growth and enrich our diet. Sprouted seeds are especially rich in vitamins C and B, while Carotene levels can increase eightfold.

The general method is to soak seeds, depending on their size, for from several hours to overnight, in a large glass jar with a piece of muslin/cheesecloth tied over the mouth. They are then given a good rinsing with warmish water and drained, the jar being kept in a warm place such as on top of a kitchen worktop. Each day they ideally get rinsed twice, or more times in hot weather. When ready to eat, sprout growth can be slowed by moving them to a cool place in darkness (and still keep up the rinsing). The time it takes will depend on temperature and other factors. It's slower in winter.

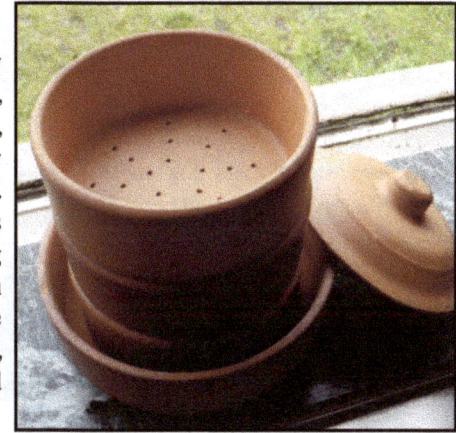

Small batches at a time are ideal, otherwise any excess ones will grow on to become too tough, stringy, bitter or rotten. As for quantities required, with large seeds like grains and beans you may need a cup full or so each time you sprout them. For the smaller seeds, just a few tablespoons should do. The books I consulted all had varying instructions, some very different! So the main thing is to just have a go at sprouting and see what works best, adjusting quantities, times, rinsing regimes etc to your own preferences and rhythms.

Above - A ceramic sprouter is a way to avoid plastic.

Sprouts and micro-greens are generally eaten raw ideally - as garnishes, in salads, dips and on sandwiches. They are great feed for other animals too.

MICRO-GREENS

Sprouts can be grown on for a longer time in trays, then it's the greens, rather than the seeds, that are eaten as 'micro-greens' (aka seedling sprouts, salad greens and sprout greens). These greens are much more nutritious than normal salad leaves and especially rich in chlorophyll. It's a good method to use for larger seeds, Cairney recommends Sunflower and Buckwheat.[1]

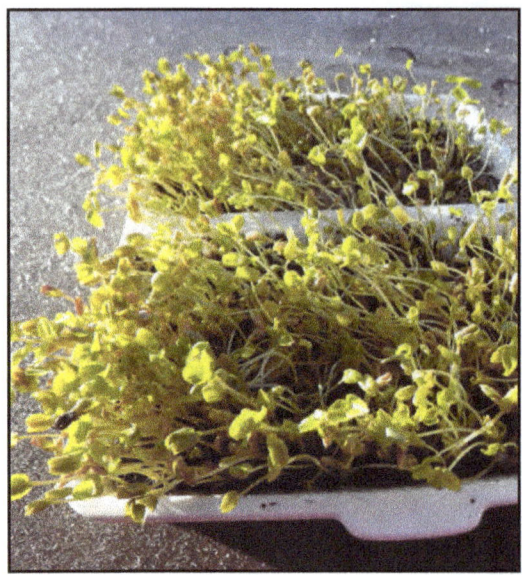

An easy method is to soak them overnight in a sprouting jar, rinse, then sow them on top of a layer of some 2cm depth of compost or good soil, with a sprinkle of compost over the top of them. Or leave them in the jar to start sprouting for one more day before sowing. Then the seed is spread evenly across the tray, with only one layer of seeds ideally.

Watering only needs to be done once daily, or spray them a few times daily. Adding a little liquid seaweed to the water makes a great fertiliser. Leaves should be ready to harvest in a week or so, they are cut off at the base with scissors. Some sprouts, such as Wheatgrass will then grow back and you can have another cut.

I got some ceramic baking dishes for sprouting micro-greens, as with the Sunflower sprouts seen above, thus avoiding having seeds in contact with plastic. I also experimented with a winter sprouting system where two or three such dishes were stacked inside a plastic storage box, to keep them cosy. I kept the dishes apart with rings of clear plastic, which allows light in. The box sat on my sunny bathroom window, as seen right, and I had a lovely series of winter micro-harvests.

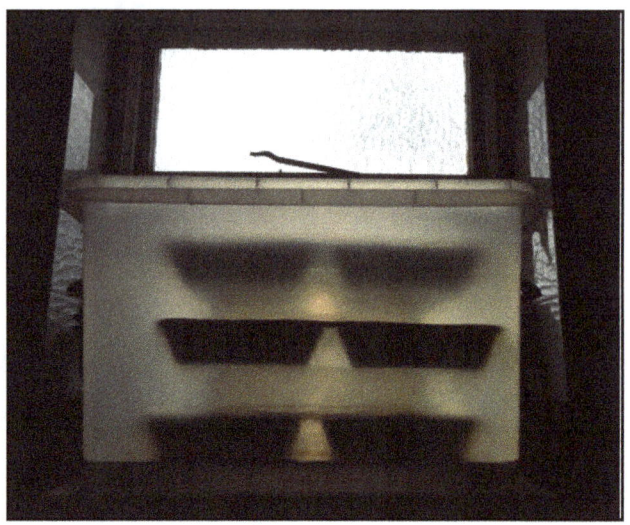

WHAT CAN BE SPROUTED?
Just about all our food plant seeds are edible as sprouts or micro-greens. But not the Nightshade/ Solanacea family, including Potatoes, Tomatoes and Peppers - these are toxic.

ALFALFA
These classic sprouts are rich in protein, a range of vitamins including B^{12}, as well as Calcium, Magnesium, Potassium, Iron, Selenium and Zinc. Soak time can be just a few hours or overnight, harvest when 1-2cm long, when they have bulked up quite a lot.

ALMONDS
These are eaten before the shoot emerges, when they have initially swollen. High in protein

and vitamins, E in particular, as well as Calcium, Potassium, Phosphorus, Magnesium. (Unfortunately, the Almond industry is a very heavy water user and is not very sustainable in it's production.) You can make a vegan seed 'yoghurt' with Almond sprouts, writes Cairney. A cupful is blended with a cupful of Rejuvelac (see under Wheat sprouting below) until smooth. These are left to ferment in a warm spot overnight.[1]

BEANS

The various pulses are great sources of protein, vitamins and minerals. Puy Lentil sprouts are tasty and as for the Mung Bean sprouts of Chinese cuisine, these are produced in a specialised way to make them plump, involving darkness and pressure.[2]

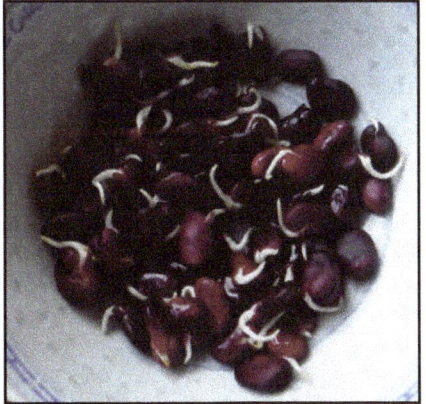

Legumes contain varying amounts of an anti-digestive factor that prevents premature germination of the seed. This Trypsin inhibitor causes abdominal discomfort and flatulence when we eat them, but it is reduced by sufficient soaking and cooking. Heating also destroys beneficial nutritional factors such as plant enzymes. Fortunately the sprouting process neutralises these toxins so that the beans can be enjoyed raw, with extra nutrition as well. Mung and Soya beans have less of such toxicity than do French and Broad beans, says Larkcom.[2]

Right - sprouted Black Russian Fava Beans

Ancient Chinese wisdom says that people with delicate digestive systems should always cook sprouted beans. In China's northern regions sprouted Horse Beans (aka Broad beans / Favas) have been an important fresh vegetable in the icy depths of winter. See a recipe for such on page 229. Kidney beans are best avoided for sprouting, warns Daphne Lambert.[3]

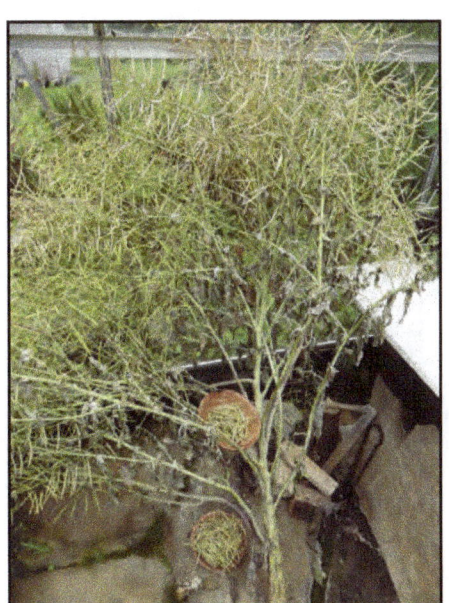

BUCKWHEAT

This is rich in Rutin (great for maintaining capillary health), also Lecithin, Calcium and vitamins A and C particularly. Sprouted either whole with their hulls on, or the de-hulled grain, they are ready in two to three days, being harvested when just around 1.5cm (a half inch) long. Or grow them on larger as micro-greens.[4]

CABBAGE FAMILY

All members of this family produce seeds that are suitable for sprouting and are packed with vitamins A, C and U plus Iodine and Sulphur[1]. Mainly grown as micro-greens, sprouts can be strong tasting, so are best eaten mixed with milder sprouts. Soak overnight, harvest a few days later.

Left - John's Kale seed drying.

In autumn I harvested a large old John's Kale for seeds, a big shrub covered in pods. After letting it fully dry in the Bath House, then stripping the pods off and twisting and scrunching them to release the seeds, I was happy to get a harvest of 200 grams of seed! Only a couple of spoons full are needed at a time, so it shall go a long way.

CLOVERS
Red or White Clover seeds need only a few hours of soaking and they are ready when 2.5 - 5cm long, after a few days sprouting. They are rich in vitamins A and C plus trace elements.

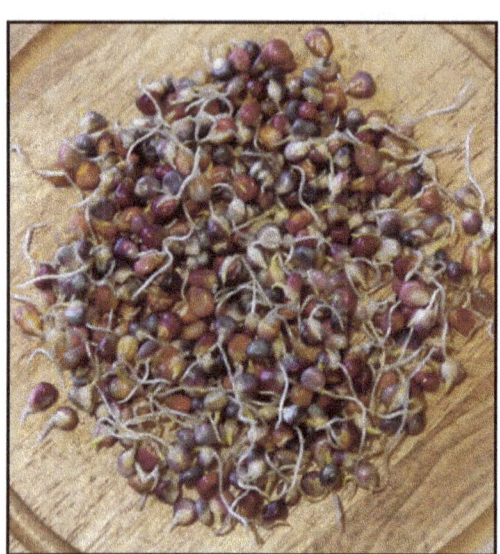

CORN
Corn sprouts are rich in vitamins A, B and E, as well as Magnesium, Phosphorus and Potassium. Soak overnight and harvest sprouts when they around 1cm long.[4]

Left - Sprouts of the beautiful, many coloured heirloom Corn variety Glass Gem.

CRESS
Ready in four to five days, Cress sprouts are packed with vitamins A and C, plus minerals. They are used for garnishes, salads and sandwiches.

GARLIC CHIVES
These sprouted seeds have some of the medicinal benefits that Garlic has.

LETTUCE
Just a few spoonfuls of seed are needed and soak time is minimal, from three to seven hours.

LINSEED (FLAX)
This is a good seed sprout for poultry.

MILLET
These are harvested after a few days, when around 0.5cm (a quarter inch) long.[4]

MITSUBA
A Japanese perennial herb that handles cool conditions, Larkom describes the dark green seedling sprouts as having a "pleasant, Angelica-like flavour".[2]

MUSTARD
Ready in four to five days, these spicy sprouts are rich in Mustard oil, Vitamins A and C and minerals. Use in juices, salads, sandwiches and soups.

OATS
Whole Oat sprouts are rich in vitamins B, E plus minerals. Soak overnight, then harvest after a day or two, when they are as long as the seed.[4]

Photo previous page - Naked Oats drying in the polytunnel.

ONION
Popular as sprouted seed in China and also in Japan, where they are harvested as seedling sprouts when some 5cm high. Larkom found them rather slow growing.[2]

PEAS
All types can be sprouted until the first leaves show. Start them in the dark at around 25°C. They can be ready in six to eight days, tasting just like raw Peas.[2] They are quite a delicious delicacy, also at the Pea shoot stage. Pea shoots are the tips of young plants, a very tender delicacy. Use in salads raw, with a dash of Lemon juice, or very lightly steamed or stir fried. Seeds can be sown in the ground or in a tray of compost and closely packed together. Start them in the trays in darkness, says Larkom, then give them light to green up when 15cm tall.[2]

PERILLA
"The quintessential Japanese herb for seasoning and garnishing", according to Joy Larkom, Perilla has a unique flavour which is also apparent in its sprouted seeds and seedling sprouts. She finds them slow growing compared with most micro-greens.[2]

PLANTAIN
A garden 'weed' with nutritious seed for sprouting, rich in protein, vitamin B[1] and minerals.

PUMPKINS AND SQUASH
These seeds need just a day of sprouting to swell them and are harvested before the shoot emerges. They are rich in vitamins B and E, as well as Phosphorus and Zinc.

QUINOA
After soaking for three to five hours, they are a very fast growing sprout, ready in just a day or so. The sprouted seeds are rich in protein, plus vitamins B and E. Harvest them when they are around 0.5 - 1cm long or more.[4]

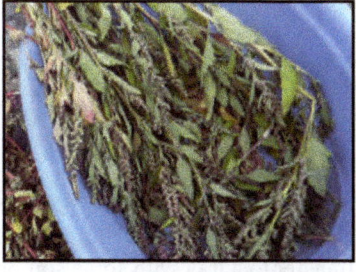

Right - Quinoa seedheads drying.

RADISH
Rich in Potassium and vitamin C, Radish sprouts are spicy hot, so need to be eaten mixed with others. After overnight soaking, they grow fast and are ready in two to five days. Larkom starts them in the dark and she praises the large winter 'China Rose' Radish variety for sprouting.[2] The larger the variety of Radish seed, the bigger the sprout.

RICE, WHOLE BROWN
Ready in two to four days, they're harvested when sprouts are the same length as the seed.[4]

RYE
Ready in two to four days, they're harvested when the sprout is the same length as the seed.[4]

SHUNGIKU
In China, Japan and south east Asia this attractive flowering plant is popular as a spicy leaf vegetable crop and sprouted seeds are also spicy. The seedling sprouts are ready within about two weeks, says Joy Larkom.[2]

SUNFLOWER (UNHULLED)
When soaked for a few hours or overnight, rinsed, then sprouted for two or three days (if longer, they become bitter), these delicious sprouts are rich in a range of vitamins, minerals, amino acids, essential fatty acids etc. When grown as micro-greens, they also give us Chlorophyll. When soaking, seeds tend to float on top of the water, so weigh them down with something or soak them in a full jar with the lid on.[1]

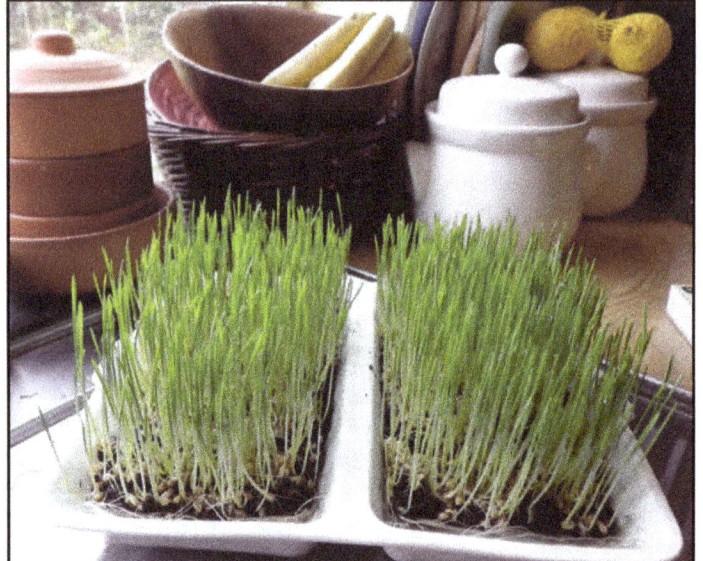

WATERCRESS
These sprouts are spicy hot, while rich in vitamins A and C, plus minerals and Chlorophyll.

WHEAT
Eaten when the sweet sprouts are around 1cm, they're rich in vitamins B and E, plus Magnesium and Phosphorus. Extracted juice of the first leaves is a powerful nutritional supplement. As well as putting them in salads and dips, you can also use Wheat sprouts to make healthy breads, the sprouts being first blended to a smooth dough with added water. Soak overnight and sprout for a few days. For Wheatgrass, as above, soak then sprout in a jar for a day, then transfer to a tray with some soil or kitchen paper and leave in indirect light for a week or so. Cut grass at the base and it will grow a second batch.

The health drink 'Rejuvelac' is a digestive tonic made from by fermenting Wheat sprouts. To a half cupful of sprouts is added fresh, pure water to three quarter fill a quart (2 litre) size jar. This is left in a warm place for 24 hours and the liquid is then strained off and is ready to drink, with a pleasant slightly sharp taste. It will keep a few days in a cool place. Meanwhile the sprouted Wheat grains can be used again and possibly a third time, by adding water again and leaving it to ferment more. Rejuvelac can also be used to make vegan 'yoghurts' and 'cheeses'. For example a cupful of Almonds sprouted for one day can be blended with a cupful of Rejuvelac until smooth. This is left to stand in a jar in a warm place overnight.[1]

1. The Sprouters Handbook, Edward Cairney, Argyll Publishing, 2011, UK.
2. Oriental Vegetables, Joy Larkcom, 1991, Frances Lincoln Ltd, UK.
3. Living Food, Daphne Lambert, Unbound, UK, 2016.
4. Homegrown Whole Grains, Sara Pitzer, Storey Publishing, USA, 2009.

WINTER RECIPES

The modern peasant with a brimming larder welcomes the winter diet with its delicious fruits of much labour, carefully saved over the previous growing season. There're a multitude of ways to prepare the staple foods and every meal can be different. Here are some favourite recipes for winter staples that I've tried and tested, tweaked and invented over the years. Some are my vegan versions of traditional recipes. Like all good peasant dishes, they don't always specify exact amounts, so use your common sense and intuition to work out the best proportions of ingredients.

CATALAN SOUP

An excellent traditional Spanish recipe from Catalonia.[1] Perfect peasant food, simplicity itself, the greatest part of this hearty soup comes out of my gardens. Just revel in the natural earthiness of it!

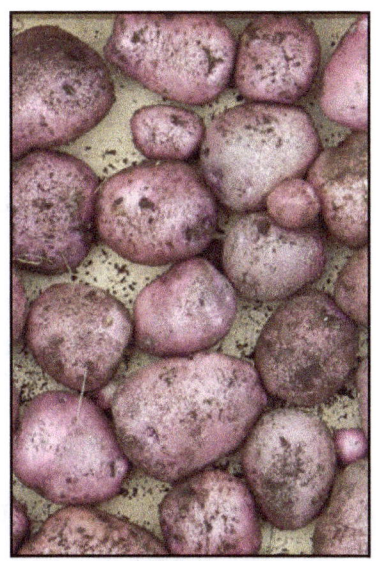

Broad Beans, fresh or dried
Potatoes, floury are best, diced
(twice the quality of beans)
Onions and Garlic, chopped
Stock, optional
Bay leaf, Thyme and the like
Salt and Pepper.
Yoghurt or Coconut milk
Parsley, a handful (optional)

Soak dried Broad Beans overnight and discard soak water before cooking briefly first. Shelling them is optional. Fry Onions and Garlic for a few minutes until soft. Add the other stuff and simmer ten or so minutes. Allow it to cool a little, then process in a blender or puree somehow. (This will pulverise the tough outer skins of the beans, though there will be a few inedible bits left. But it does save you from having to peel them!)

You may want to separately blend the beans and just roughly mash the Potatoes by hand, otherwise they can go gluey when liquidised, not a great texture. Reheat gently for a short time before serving and add a dollop of dairy or the like and chopped Parsley.

TWO VARIATIONS -

1. A green variation on this soup makes excellent use of the Mustard leaves that grow so well through the winter (especially in the polytunnel). Finely chop a bunch of Mustard greens. Then briefly stir fry them with a little oil and add them to the soup just before serving. Joy

Larkom suggests adding a pinch of Nutmeg to the leaves as they cook.[2]

2. Another variation calls for Fermented Green Beans (see page 212), cut into short lengths, added to the soup just before serving.[3] (Don't cook them, as overheating destroys the lactic ferment enzymes.)

PINK HUMMUS DIP

This classic dip is usually made with Chickpeas, but Broad Beans are also great, or a mix of the two. (Chickpeas are now being grown in Ireland.)

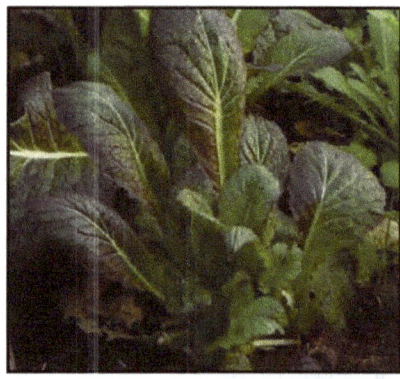

Broad Beans, soaked overnight and rinsed
Beetroot, deep red variety
Lemon juice
Tahini, a tablespoon or two
Olive oil, a tablespoon or two
Garlic to taste
Salt and Cayenne Pepper

Cook Beetroot with beans until tender and allow to cool. Then blend together in a food processor, finally adding other ingredients, adjusting to taste, of course!

GREEN HUMMUS DIP

As above, but instead of Beetroot, briefly stir fry a bunch of chopped Mustard greens (seen right) then blend these in together with the bean mix at the end.

LEEK, POTATO AND SUNROOT SOUP

Garlic
Two Onions, sliced
Two Leeks, sliced
400gm Potatoes, cubed
400gm Sunroot/Jerusalem Artichoke sliced
200gm Broad Beans soaked overnight and rinsed
Stock, optional
Spices - Bay leaves, Tumeric etc
Coconut oil or butter
Coconut cream/milk or yoghurt

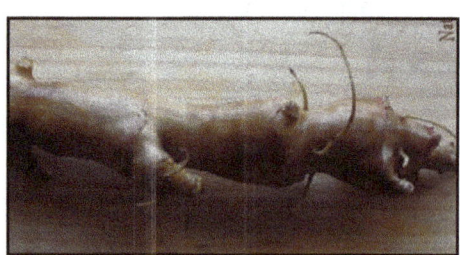

Above - Sunroot tuber, Fuseau variety.

A simply delicious combination! Sweat Onions in oil until soft. Add veggies and Garlic and fry a more few minutes. Add water or stock and simmer until cooked. Cool, mash or liquidise, then re-heat and serve with a dash of the dairy or equivalent.

FERMENTED GREEN BEAN SALAD

Cauliflower or Broccoli chunks, steamed and cooled
Potatoes, chopped slices steamed and cooled
Fermented Green Beans, chopped (see page 212)
Mustard Green leaves, finely chopped
Yoghurt dressing
- thick yoghurt + Olive oil + Lemon juice
or vinegar + Garlic + salt
      Mix and serve.

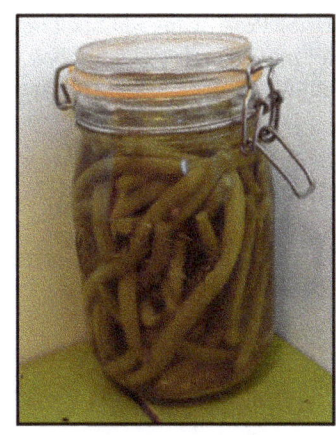

POLISH PEASANT SOUP

Based on a traditional recipe, this soup can be produced mostly from one's garden and larder stores but I've added some extra exotic ingredients, which can, of course, be substituted.

Three big Beetroot, diced
Two Onions, chopped
Garlic to taste
Red Cabbage, shredded
Stock (optional)
Coconut cream
Salt and Spices - Bay leaves, Cummin,
  Thyme, Rosemary, Lovage, Oregano etc
Apple cider vinegar, a dash
Coconut oil for frying
Cream or yoghurt

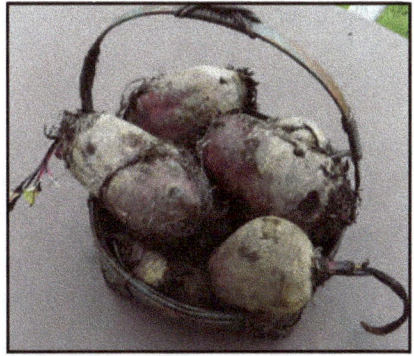

Fry Onions and Garlic a few minutes. Add Beetroot and stir for two minutes. Add stock and Coconut cream, simmer until tender. Add vinegar, cool then liquidise in a food processor. Return to pot, add spices and Cabbage and simmer five minutes, let it still be a bit crunchy. Serve with a dollop of dairy or equivalent.

WINE DARK SEA SOUP

My own recipe. When stirred, it resembles frothing ocean waves indeed.

Dried Peas or Broad Beans, half a cup
Spelt grain or Brown Rice, half a cup
Two Onions, chopped
Four Beetroot, chopped
Carrageen, a handful soaked ten minutes,
  with stalks and rough bits removed.
Lemon, the juice of one
Chillis chopped fine
Salt and Spices e.g. Garam masala, Ras el Hanouf
Coconut milk, thick yoghurt or cream for serving.

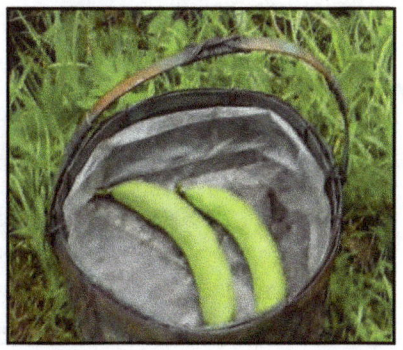

Dried Peas/Beans and Spelt or Rice are soaked overnight and soak water is drained off. Throw all into a single pot and cook until soft. Cool then liquidise. Re-heat, add powdered spices, adjust flavours. Turn off heat then add Lemon juice. Serve with a dollop of creamy stuff.

BROAD BEAN SOUP, SICILIAN STYLE

Maccu di favi, meaning Crushed Fava Beans, is a traditional dish from southern Italy.[4] It's perfect for slow cooking on the wood heater top or in a slow cooker.

Broad beans dried, two cups soaked overnight and drained
Fennel tops, a handful chopped
Chillis and salt to taste

Simmer lightly in a heavy bottomed saucepan and stir occasionally for three hours. After two hours, stir more and add the Chilli and Fennel. Crush beans with big wooden spoon into a coarse puree as you stir. Add more water if too thick and, only when finished, season to taste with salt. Serve garnished with some Fennel leaf.

RECIPE REFERENCES

1. Potato - the definitive guide to Potatoes and Potato Cooking, Alex Barker and Sally Mansfield, Anness Publishing, 2002, UK.
2. Oriental Vegetables, Joy Larkom, Frances Lincoln, UK, 2007.
3. Preserving Food without Freezing or Canning, by the Gardeners and Farmers of Terre Vivante, Chelsea green Publishing, Vermont, USA, 1999.
4. Flavours of Sicily, Mariapaola Dettore, McRae Books, 2005, Italy.

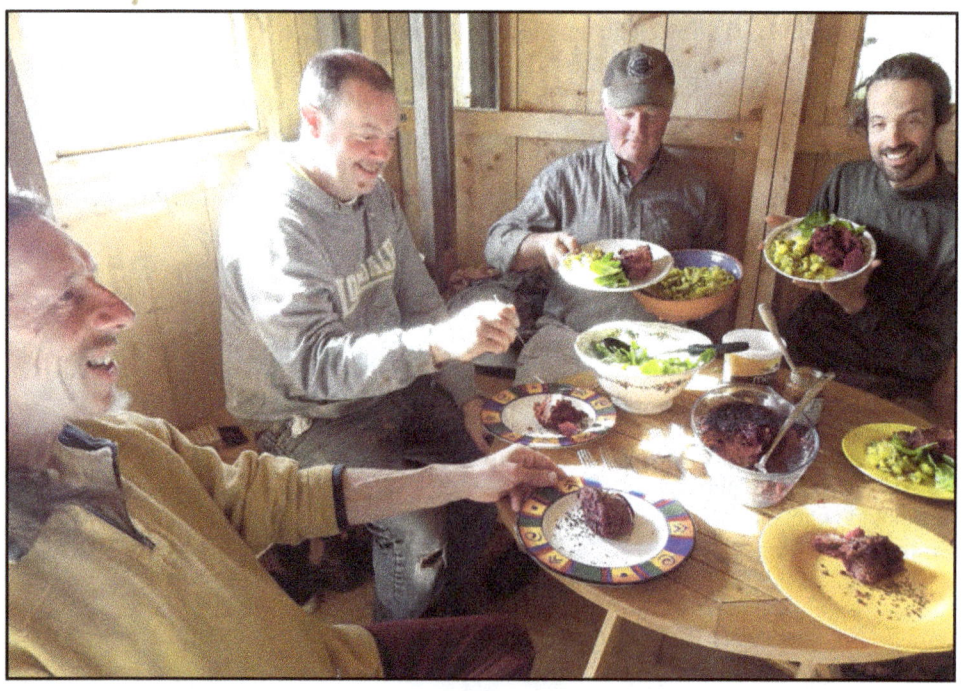

CHAPTER SIX

SPRINGTIME

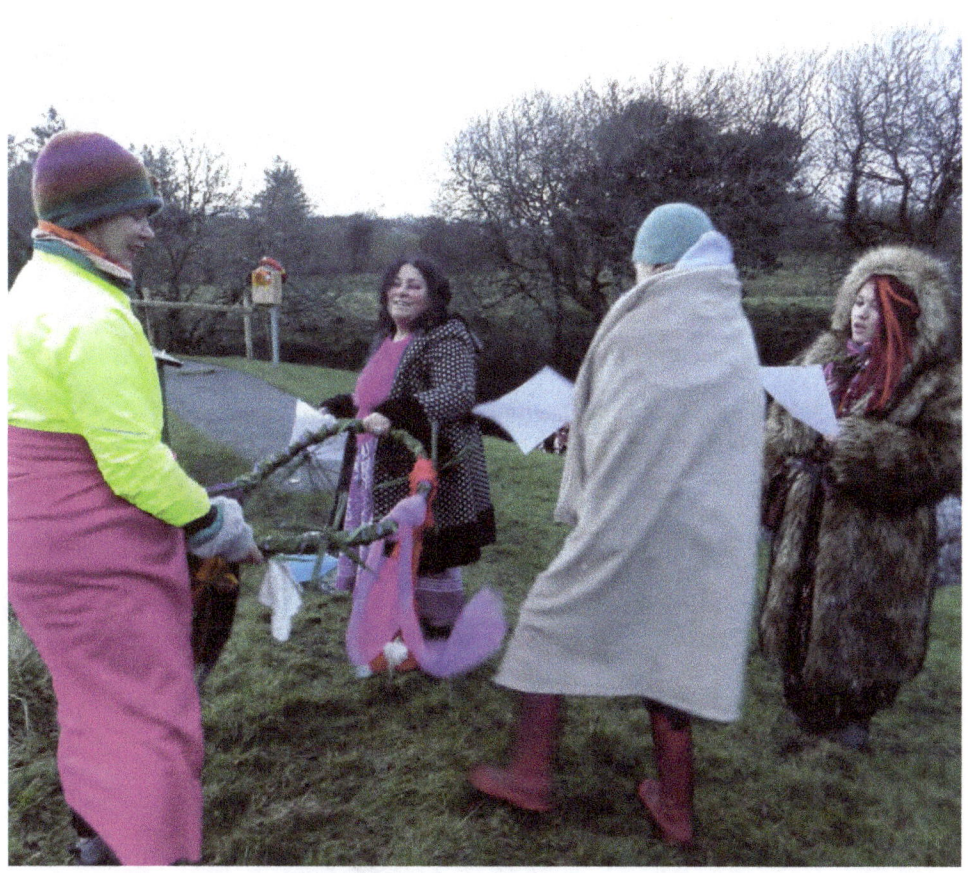

Celebrating Imbolc, the start of spring - a ceremony with renowned Irish shaman Simone ni Chinneide (centre) at the Shannon Pot, source of the River Shannon. At the open air ritual, at a place of watery beginnings, we passed through the ceremonial hoop, resonating with the rebirth of nature in springtime.

SPRINGTIME

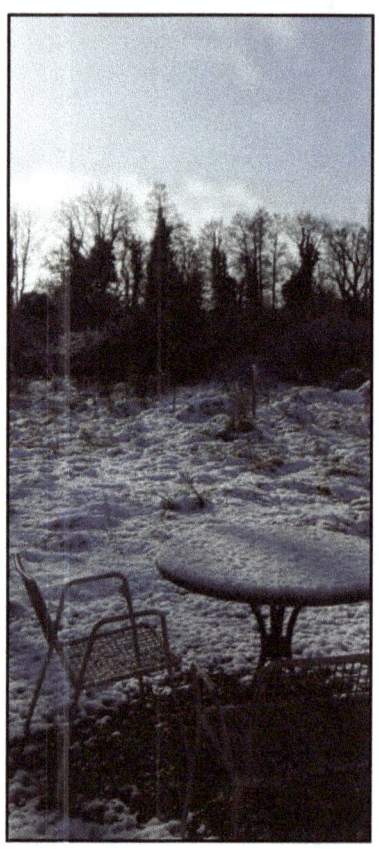

In Ireland springtime comes slowly and softly, noticed more by the birds than us. It may be the coldest time of year, with occasional snow storms and frost. It's hard to see that winter is ending. But there are tiny buds on bare branches that are pulsing to a cosmic beat and starting to awaken, while daffodils peep their green tips skywards.

Spring may creep in slowly here, but in tradition it begins on February 1st, with the festival of Imbolc, named for when sheep milk starts to flow and the lambing season begins. This early date, half way between the winter and summer solstices and what's known as a cross quarter day, can feel more like winter. Some think it reflects on a different climate in the past, when spring came earlier.

In Asia spring is celebrated around now too, but it hinges on the time of the first new Moon in spring, while ceremonies encourage the awakening of dragon spirits that slumber underground, calling on them to rise up and enliven life. At this time of year in Ireland, most would still be hibernating! However there can be much activity in peasant gardens now, as one prepares for the sowing and planting of staple crops.

PEASANT ACTIVITIES IN SPRINGTIME

* Planting deciduous trees and shrubs.
* Pruning Apples, Pears, Quinces, Plums, Cherries, Apricots, Peaches, Nectarines, Figs and Medlars.
* Pruning hedges.
* Feeding and mulching fruit trees and berries.
* Preparing garden beds.
* Sowing Broad Beans, Peas, Onions and Garlic directly into their beds.
* Cleaning polytunnel plastic to allow more light in.
* Wild food foraging in late spring.
* Chitting Potatoes (sprouting them) in the light, for planting late spring.
* Growing sprouts and micro-greens in the house.
* Checking food stores and removing anything rotten.
If Garlic is sprouting, making pickles with them. See recipe, page 197.
* Sowing seeds of Tomatoes, Basil, Peppers, Chillis, French beans, Aubergine, Squash, Sweet Corn and early greens undercover or with heat.
* Sowing summer crops from March.
* Hand pollinating blossoms of Peaches, Nectarines and Apricots and cover them if frost threatens.

TREE PLANTING TIME

It might seem that the land and nature is asleep, but this makes it an ideal time to be planting bare rooted deciduous trees and shrubs. You need to get them into the ground by May ideally, with planting spots made ready in advance.

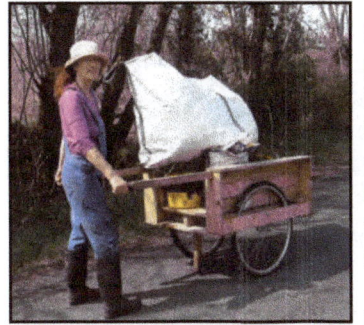

I planted an orchard as the very first act of rooting myself to my new home in Ireland, in late spring of 2015. A dozen fruit trees were bought in winter and they waited with their bare roots nested into some moist soil and wrapped in a sheet of plastic so they didn't dry out. Finally, with their buds starting to burst open, I took them in the handcart from Peter's place the short distance up the road to their new home.

Being new to the place, I had no compost at the ready to plant fruit trees with. I had dreams of planting them on small mounds to improve the poor drainage. But without any spare soil or compost I had to just plant them into the heavy soil. The trees didn't seem to mind too much and the clay soil is rich, but I didn't have any comparisons until a few years later.

When I later planted a second orchard in an adjacent field, with various heritage varieties of fruit trees, this time I was better organised and planted all of them on a mound. No hole was dug. Clods of soil that were leftover from earthworks were the basis of each mound. For each tree a donut shaped ring of clods was put around where it was to grow. The hole in the centre was half filled with a free draining soil and compost mix.

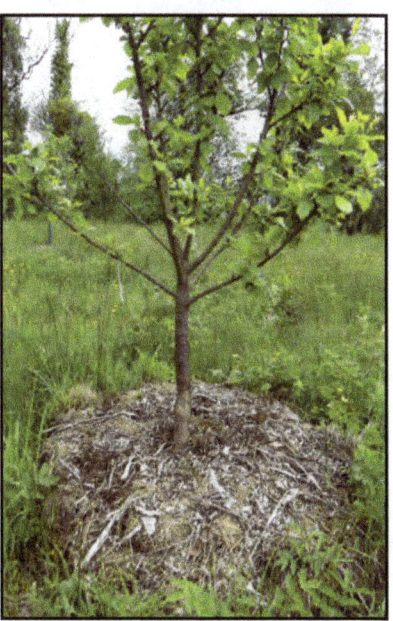

At planting time the tree roots were nestled into the central hole and covered with more soil and compost that was gently well packed in to avoid air pockets, and then mulched over with straw. The trees thrived on neglect and they did grow more vigorously than the ones in the older orchard.

SEED SOWING

February may be cold, but it's the month to start seed propagation, so you need to do it indoors on a warm windowsill, or in a heated propagator unit. I have a small electrically heated propagator box that fits enough seed trays for our needs. I put on a new batch every fortnight or so and get loads of lovely seedlings. On a larger scale, electric heating mats can be used on propagating tables to heat seeds and seedlings.

An alternative and more natural version can be made with a large composting pile of manure - at least one cubic metre volume - with seed trays placed on top to gain some of the heat that is produced. This heap would ideally be enclosed somehow, such as boxed in by square straw bales with an old window over the top. The top would need covering on cold nights too. I'm getting tired just thinking about making this set-up, so I'll stick to the small box from Aldi.

In February Broad Beans will be my main seeds to sow, putting seed into small pots and modules to germinate, and protecting them from critters that love to excavate and eat them. Once the tough, cold hardy plants have grown on a bit they are usually safe to plant. Broad Beans are so fabulous because they produce the earliest beans, delicious for eating both young in the pod or mature. Slugs might enjoy them too.

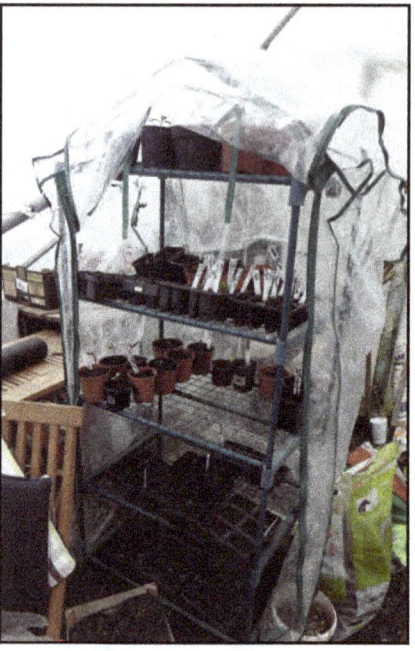

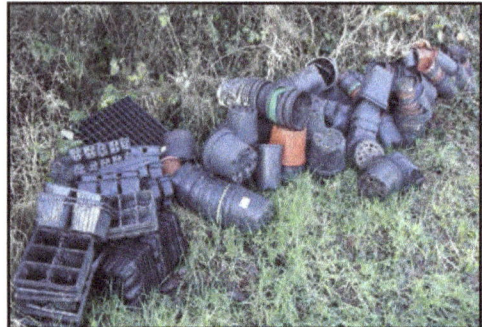

Above - The propagating unit works well, but the plastic covers are short lived.
Left - Buying in seedlings and plants results in a lot of waste plastic. But mine do get re-used over and over, while I dont bother washing them and still get good results.
Below - Chitting early Potatoes.

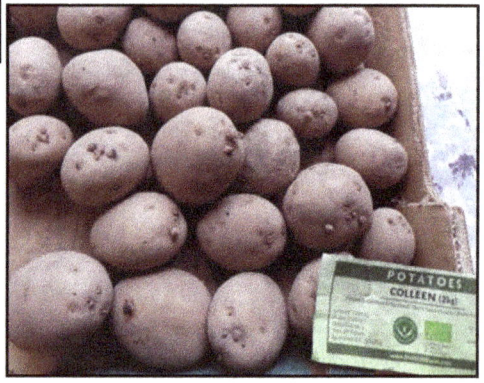

Meanwhile, the polytunnel greens keep us going with small amounts of salad veggies and perennial herbs, but growth may well be slow until late spring. Plants like Parsley, Watercress, Claytonia, Green in the Snow and Kale persist. It's time to let more light in to them and scrub clean the polytunnel plastic where it's dirty and green with algae.

Spring is the time to finish weeding, feeding, pruning and mulching all the perennial plants. Ground can be cleared more easily in early spring, when you can see where tenacious perennial weeds are rooted and remove them. Annual plant weeds can simply be mown over or smothered with sheet mulch each year.

Early spring is the time for controlling invasive plants that want to dominate others, like the boring Snowberries (inedible) and prickly Brambles of the hedgerows. To maintain social harmony in plant world I prune them back. Hedge trimming has to be done before the birds begin to nest, so this is the season to finish the job.

Late Spring can feel like an Irish summer, with bright, warm spells. This can trick Mother Nature into a growth phase and young shoots of plants might be frozen by any frosts. Flowers of fruit trees may also be affected and the crop ruined. To protect them from frosts, vulnerable plants can be given an overnight covering, or bring those in pots indoors at night if necessary. But it's worth it, because those delicate babies that you carefully tend grow all the better and they'll be flying before you know it.

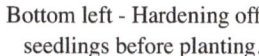

Right - Crab Apple blooms.

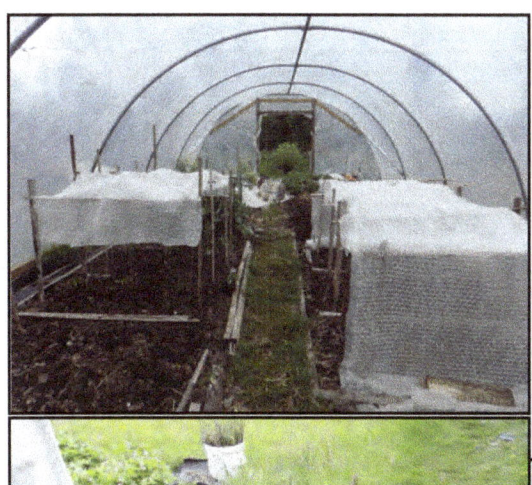

Left - Protecting seedlings with bubblewrap and below, with 'fleece'.

Bottom left - Hardening off seedlings before planting.

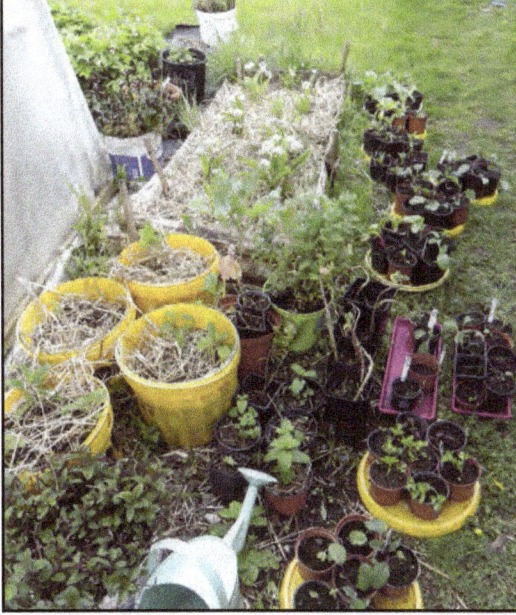

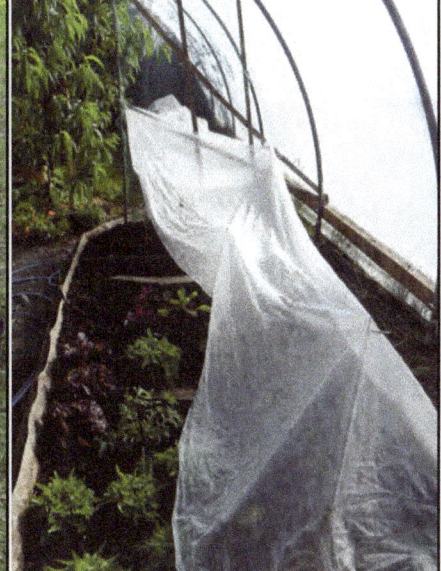

SPRING FORAGING

Come springtime and the buds on native trees start to burst open. It's a time when fields and hedgerows can be foraged for their tender young leaves that can be eaten fresh or dried. In Vermont (USA) foresters and farmers would snack on the new leaves of many species, including Beech, Maple, Elm, Willow, Apple, Poplar and Birch being the most popular, while Elm was the favourite.[1] This was paralleled in Europe too.

Native Americans also harvested the inner bark of many species of trees in springtime, as the sap started to rise, when it's easiest to harvest. They extracted the inner bark from Poplar, Pine, Spruce, Willow and Birch trees, and it was dried and ground as a flour and soup thickener. The best bark was harvested from the sunny side of young trees. But it was mostly resorted to as famine survival food. The inner bark of Scotch Pine was reported to be a famine food in 1732 in Lapland too, the best bits said to be found near the base of large trees. The inner bark of Oak was also eaten in north America, but it was first leached of its tannins and boiled in several changes of water, before being dried and ground for flour.

The buds of Pine trees are edible, as are the pollen rich, male flowers of White Pine. Pine needle leaf tea is medicinal and much richer in vitamin C than Oranges, you simply fill a cup with young needles and add boiling water to steep them. Tea from Pine twigs and needles together is even healthier. You simmer the bare, chopped twig pieces for about fifteen minutes, then pour the liquid into a teapot with fresh Pine needles, steeping it for another fifteen minutes. Or make it into storable syrup, with sugar added, that's popularly used for respiratory problems.

Pine bark extract has been found to be powerfully antioxidant, a brain booster that gives multiple benefits for heart, skin, joint health and more. The edible inner bark is rich in vitamins C and A, as well as flavonoids, sugar and starch.[1]

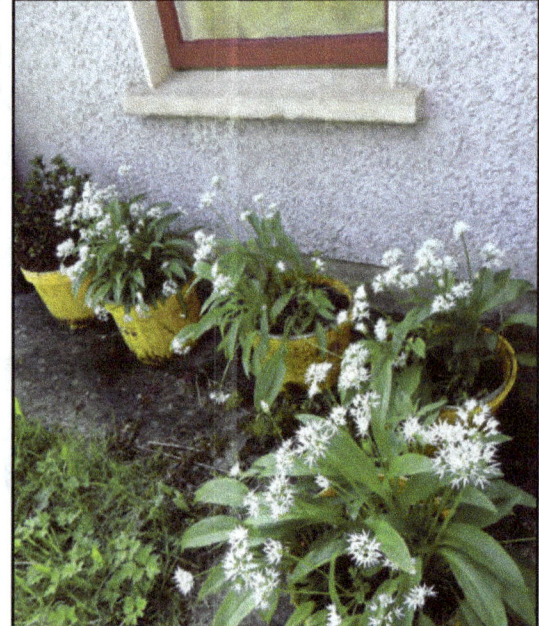

Right - Wild Garlic flowering in a shady north facing corner.

SPRINGTIME WILD FOODS
Birch
Beech
Maple
Elm
Willow
Poplar
Spruce
Hawthorn
Lime/Linden
Nettles
Wild Garlic

SPRING FORAGE PLANTS

SILVER BIRCH
The fresh bright green leaves of Birch trees in spring and early summer can be eaten in salads. Or make a tea from them, with a half teaspoonful of dried leaves per cup of boiling water steeped for ten minutes. For a fresh leaf tea, you need four or five leaves per cup.

Birch sap can be tapped from the trunk in springtime. You might drill a hole 5cm deep at a 45 degree angle into the trunk, insert a tube and plug it with something like plasticine. Only drain off half a litre of sap maximum, then plug the hole up. The sap is boiled down to thicken it into a naturally sweet syrup, or made into wine.

BEECH
Beech leaves, when very young only, are nice to eat in salads and soups.

HAWTHORN
Young leaves in small amounts can be eaten raw between April and May. Eat them straight from the tree, or in salads or on sandwiches. Make a heart-strengthening tea from two teaspoons of leaves and/or flowering twigs, infusing it for ten minutes and taking two cups daily for at least three months as a general heart tonic.

Young shoots can be added to salads, the flowers added to fruit salads or made into wine. Consuming the leaves imparts a calming effect and helps with concentration, says Kress.[2]

Below - Fairy Hawthorn on farmland in County Leitrim in springtime.
Where industrial scale farms predominate, you don't see these scenes anymore.

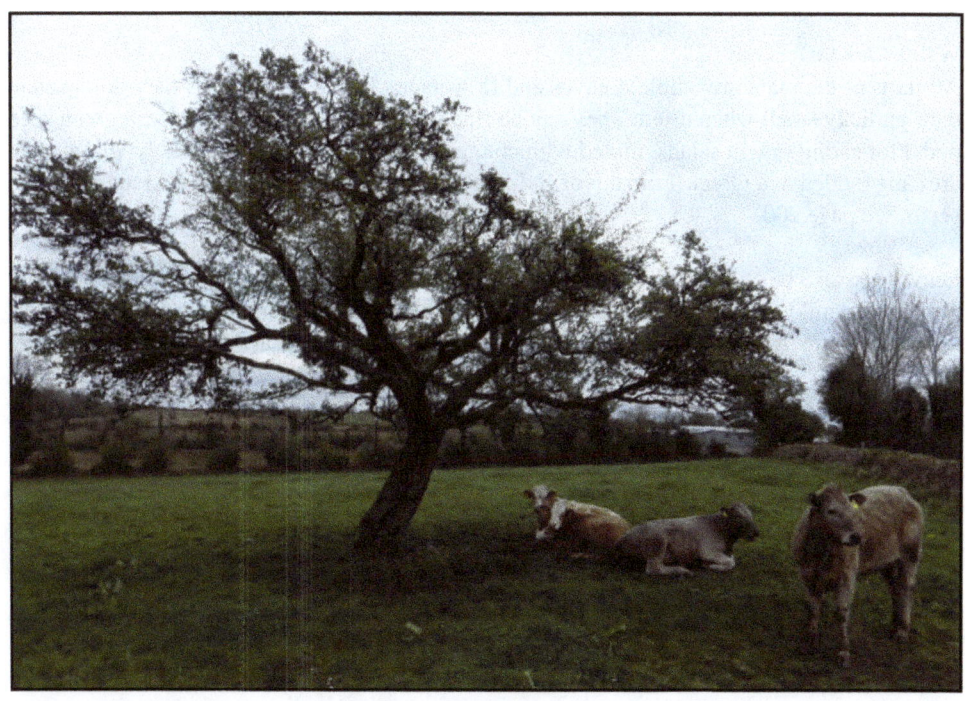

LIME / LINDEN
Eat young Lime leaves, that are sweet but mucilaginous, in salads, sandwiches and soups.

NETTLES
When Nettles are tender and young in spring it's good to gather as much as possible, for cooking them fresh as a vegetable and for fresh leaf tea, and more for drying and storing. Pick stems before the plants flower and make small bunches of Nettles for hanging in shady dry places, or put one layer of them on newspaper indoors on shelves and turn them over after a week. In a fortnight or so they should be crispy and dry enough to store. Crumble the dry leaves into powder to add to other foods and for storage. Or dry whole leaves for tea.

SPRUCE TREES
Spruce Syrup, a traditional cough remedy that's also used to flavour desserts, is made in northern Europe using new spring shoots of Spruce trees (and also mixed with Pine and Fir shoots for a 'forest flavour' syrup). Kress says to rinse the shoots, cover them in water and leave them overnight, then boil for an hour or two and leave overnight again. The liquid is then strained off, measured and a half quantity of sugar added. This is simmered until it clears and when a few drops are dropped onto a cold surface they stop flowing when a spoon is pulled through them. Store in sterilised jars and enjoy on pancakes, she suggests.[3]

Spruce needle tea, made from needles harvested from the sunny side of the tree, is rich in vitamin C and is a good respiratory medicine also. A few teaspoons of needles are steeped in boiling water for five minutes.

All Spruces have inner bark that is edible raw. It was dried and ground into flour by native Americans, who also made a favourite alcoholic drink by boiling young Spruce twigs in water, adding Maple syrup, honey or molasses, and allowing it to ferment. [1]

WILD GARLIC
All parts of the plant are edible. Leaves and flowers are best used fresh, as they don't retain their garlicky smell when dried. They can be finely chopped (as well as the fresh green seed pods) for eating raw in salads, mixed with cottage cheese, in sauces, vinegars, yoghurt salad dressing (added to a Greek Tzatziki or Indian Raita), etc. The fresh leaves also make a great pesto, see page 200.

Leaves can also be cooked, e.g. sautéed with onions, which produces a milder flavour. If you prefer them mild they can be blanched first, dipping leaves in boiling water for ten seconds, refreshing them in cold water, then patting them dry. Ransom bulbs are also edible, but if over eaten can cause stomach upsets, plus eating them kills the plant.

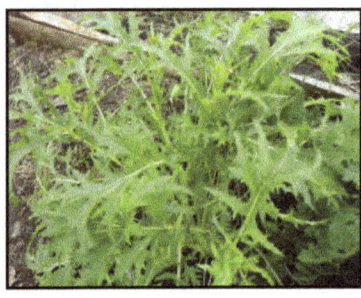

1. The Healing Trees - the edible and herbal qualities of northeastern woodland trees, Robbie Hanna Anderman, Burnstown Publishing, 2017, ON, Canada.
2. Practical Herbs 2, Henriette Kress, Aeon Books, 2018, UK.
3. Practical Herbs 1, Henriette Kress, Aeon Books, 2018, UK.

Left - This Mizuna in the polytunnel in April is starting to bolt.

SPRING LEAVES, STEMS, BULBS AND SHOOTS

Angelica
Asparagus
Bay
Beetroot
Cabbage
Celery Leaf
Chickweed
Chives
Claytonia
Chard
Comfrey
Dandelion
Docks
Endive
Fennel bulbs
Kale
Lemon balm
Lettuce
Lovage
Mallows
Marigold
Marshmallow
Meadowsweet
Mint
Mizuna
Mugwort
Mustards
Plantains
Primrose
Raspberry
Reedmace
Rhubarb
Sage
Sorrel
Spinach
Sweet Cicely
Thyme
Parsley
Watercress

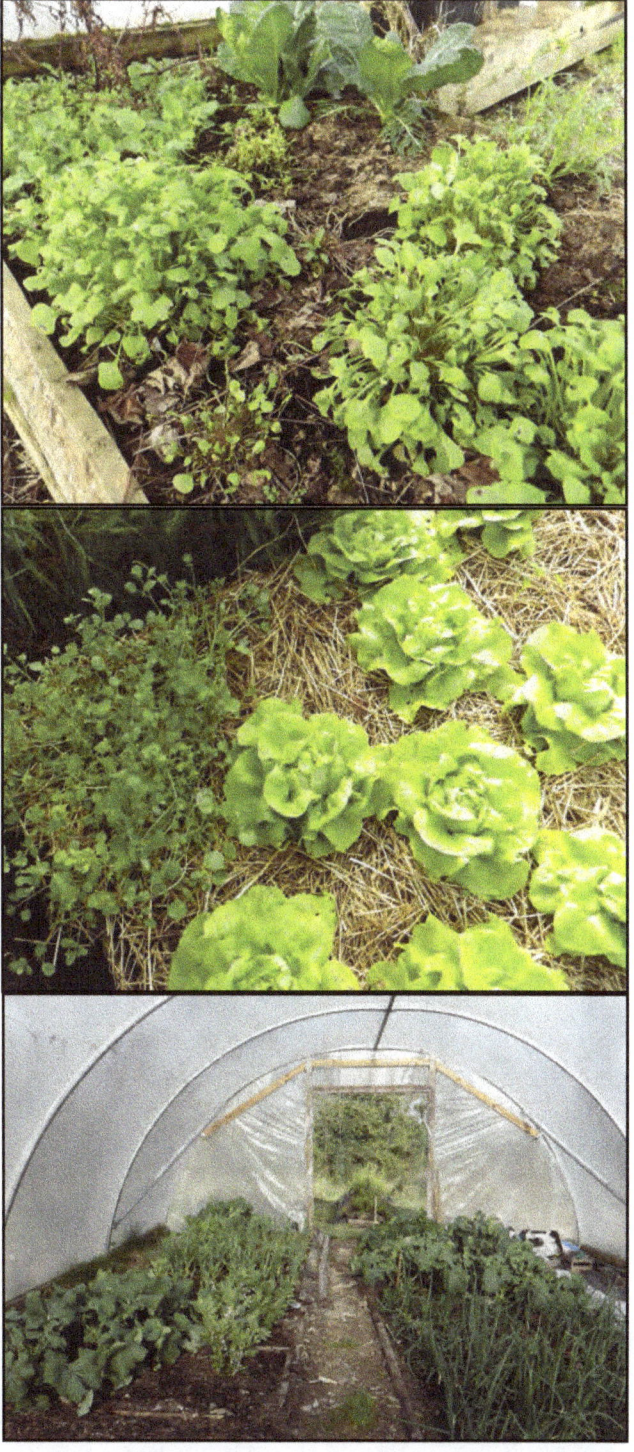

Photos of polytunnel crops in April: top - Claytonia and Japanese greens Hayachinena in background; middle - Lettuce and Watercress; bottom - mixed Brassicas, Onions and Garlic.

EDIBLE SPRING GARDEN FLOWERS

Borage
Broccoli
Chamomile
Garlic
Marigold
Primrose

SPRING CROP STAPLES

Broad beans
Peas
Potatoes, earlies

SPRING FRUIT

Strawberries
Eleagnus species

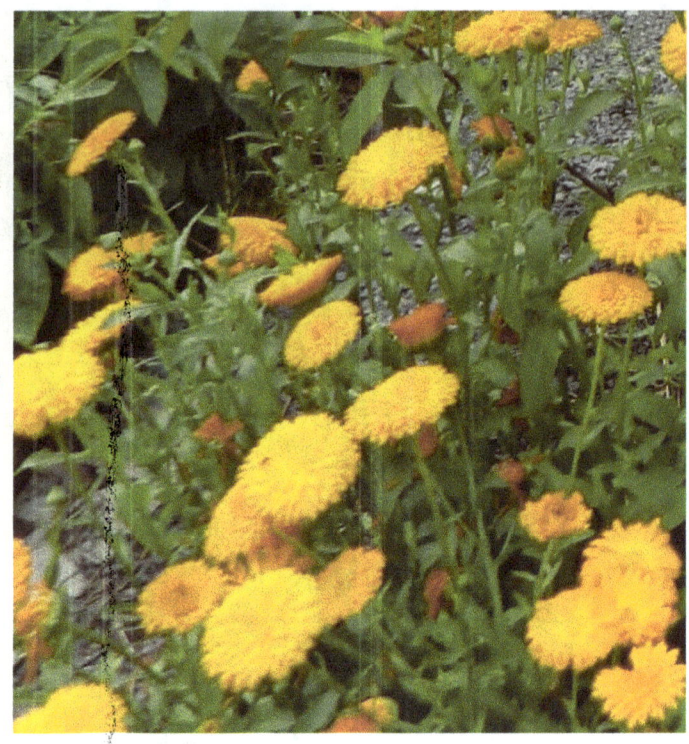

SPRING RECIPES

ANGELICA, CANDIED AND STEWED

The flavour of this beautiful wild herb is strong, so only small amounts are needed. It's an aromatic bitter that needs sourness, such as Lemon juice, to balance out the flavour. When stewed together with tart fruits like Rhubarb or Gooseberries, the young stems of Angelica can improve them by reducing acidity and adding a sweeter flavour, with less added sweetener necessary. Stew Rhubarb with Angelica stems in about a 3:1 ratio.

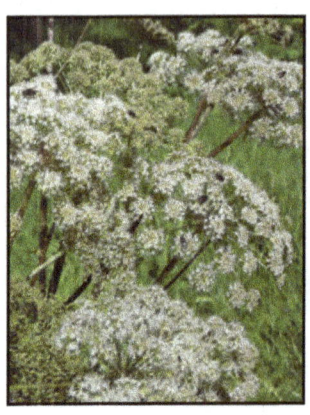

Harvest leaves before flowering starts in the second year in late spring. They have a Liquorice like flavour and can be added raw to salads. Young leaves are made into tea for indigestion, tension, headaches and respiratory problems. But avoid large doses, especially pregnant women and diabetics.[1]

Candied Angelica is a deep green coloured aromatic confectionary for decorating cakes, made from tender young springtime shoots chopped into short lengths and simmered in water until tender. It's then candied in an equal weight of sugar that it soaks in for two days, then boiled until the liquid becomes clear. It's strained off and the green stems dried for storing.

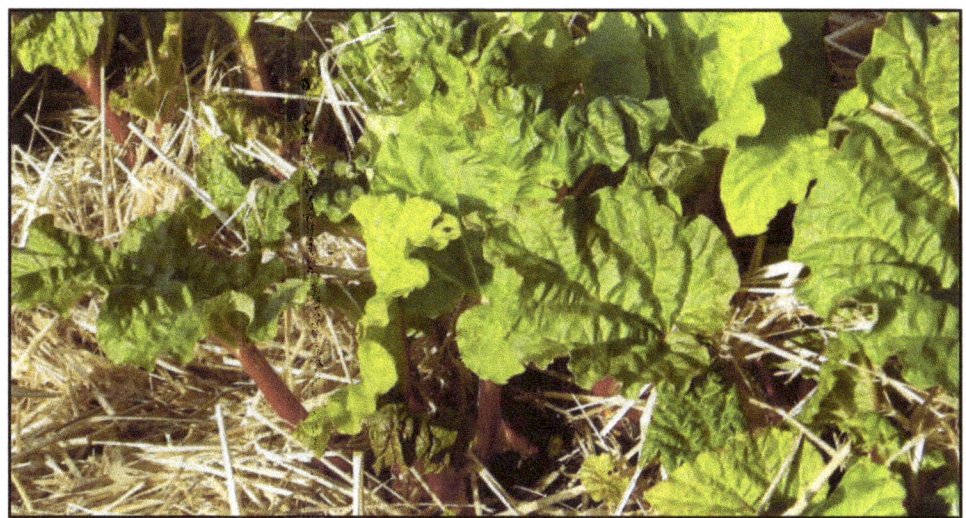

Above - Timperley Early Rhubarb variety powering in February sunshine.

BROAD BEAN AND POTATO MASH

Mash lightly steamed fresh Broad Beans and cooked Potatoes together with an added dash of Olive oil, salt, Pepper and finely chopped fresh herbs - Rosemary, Thyme, Sage, Summer/Winter Savoury, Lovage, etc, to taste.

GARLIC PICKLES

First prepare a 2% brine solution with two tablespoons of good, unrefined salt (I use Celtic grey or pink Himalayan salt) per litre of warm water. The water should have no Chlorine or Fluoride, as this kills good bacteria. Stir the solution until all the salt has dissolved and allow it to cool. Remove skin from Garlic cloves. A friend gave me a good tip about doing this - if you have a lot of Garlic to peel, put them into a bowl of hot water for a few minutes and the skins will then come off much more easily. Pack a sterilised jar nearly to the top with the peeled cloves. Then add the brine to the jar to fill almost to the top. All Garlic must be covered, but leave a space of 2cm or so at the top. Close the jar and put in a warm spot at room temperature. Shake the jar gently and 'burp it' daily.

After a few days you'll see little bubbles of air coming up, it means the good bacteria are starting to work. Some of the liquid may evaporate out of the jar and it will need to be topped up. After a week or so of bubbling, you can close the jars tight and they will keep for a long time, stored it in a cool spot. You can also start eating it, adding it raw to dishes, like salads, pestos, mayonnaise etc; or adding it to dishes at the end of cooking. Some people simply swallow a clove whole. You don't want to cook it, as this destroys the extra vitamins and probiotics. You might also experiment with adding grated fresh Ginger and Tumeric or other spices to the jar during preparation. Don't worry if the brine and Garlic turns dark or blue at some point, as this is perfectly normal. [2]

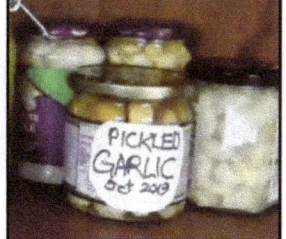

MINT CHUTNEY

This is based on an Indian recipe. [3]

Mint leaves & tender stalks, 50 gms
Grated Ginger
Chopped Garlic
Minced fresh Chilli
Lemon juice
1 tsp salt
2 tsp sugar
Water
optional: nuts, seeds,
Coriander leaves, Tamarind etc.

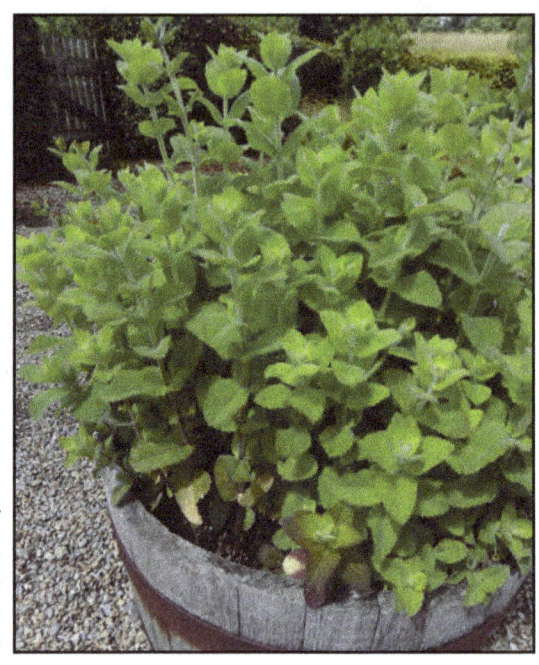

Put in the blender with just enough water to make a paste. Small quantities go with any meal, Mint being a good digestive stimulant. I look forwards to trying this recipe with more local ingredients to substitute for the imported stuff. If my Sumac seedlings grow, I'll use some for Lemon flavour; and if I dig up some Shepherd's Purse roots, I could try them as a Ginger substitute. I might add Lovage or Sweet Cicely leaves and perhaps use marinated Blackcurrants, as a substitute for Tamarind fruit.

MINT PESTO

Use Mint as the dominant leaf in a pesto or dip.

Mint leaves, a big handful
Other greens - e.g. spicy Mustard leaves
Zucchinis, optional
Garlic, to taste
Olive oil
Salt and Pepper
Optional - nuts, grated Parmesan cheese, tahini.

Combine and blend until smooth. Put into sterilised jars and cover with a layer of Olive oil to keep the air out and it will keep for a short time.

MINT AND PARSLEY TABOULI SALAD

This traditional Greek recipe I've made gluten free.

Quinoa, 1 cup cooked and cooled
Olive oil, 1/3 cup, or less
Lemon juice, 1/4 cup fresh
Garlic, to taste

Mint, 1 cup fresh leaves
Parsley, big bunch
Pepper freshly ground and salt, 1/2 tsp each.

Blend Olive oil, Lemon juice, and Garlic in a blender.
Add half of the Mint leaves, Salt and Pepper. Whizz until smooth.
Chop the remaining leaves. Pour dressing over the Quinoa and toss well.
Add remaining leaves and toss more before serving.

MINT YOGURT SALAD DRESSING

Yogurt, 1/2 cup
Lemon juice, 2 tsp.
Garlic, minced
Mint, 1/4 cup finely chopped leaves
Salt and freshly ground black Pepper

Combine all ingredients. Add additional Lemon juice to thin, as you like.
Serve with salad or as a dip.

NETTLES AND POTATOES, SAG ALOO STYLE

Based on the classic Indian recipe Sag Aloo, this combines Potatoes and Onions with tasty spices and young spring Nettle tops, or you can use Spinach, Chard, Kale etc.

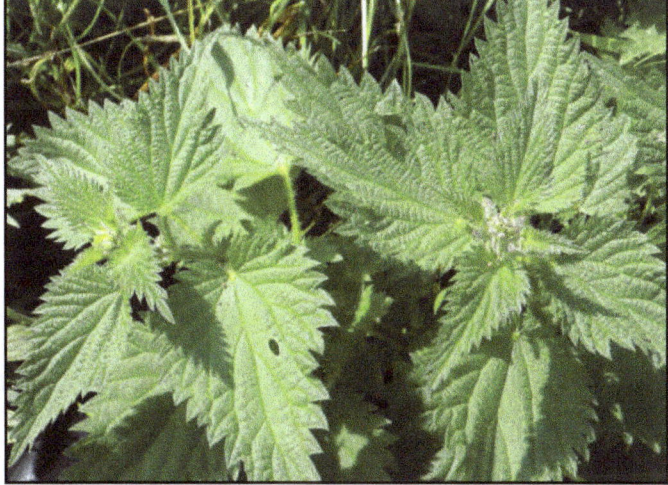

Potatoes, diced
Onions, chopped
Young Nettles, big bunch, or other greens that are briefly pre-steamed.
Garlic cloves,
Knob of Ginger, peeled and grated
Salt and spices - Chilli, Tumeric, Cummin, Curry leaf, Asafoetida, Mustard seeds etc

Lightly fry Onions, Ginger and Garlic. Add salt and spices and fry briefly, then add Potatoes and stir fry briefly. Half cover the mix with water and simmer in a covered pan for 15 minutes or so. When cooked, switch off, add steamed leaves on top and let it sit to soak up the liquid.

With Nettles, first chop roughly, then heat leaves in another pot with only the water left on them after washing. Stir continuously a few minutes, then add a few drops of oil to finish. This ensures that the sting is gone! Put them on top at the end of cooking the dish.

NETTLE PIE

Not a baked pie, this is a quickly made, nutritious dish that I created.

Nettle tops, a saucepan full, washed and shaken dry
Semolina or Polenta, half a cup
Coconut cream - half a cup or so
Salt, Pepper, other flavourings
Toasted seeds for topping, a small handful
Coconut oil, 1 tbsp
Optional - cheese or fried Tofu for topping,

Heat oil in heavy bottomed saucepan. Add Nettles and stir fry constantly for two minutes Add 1.5 cups of boiling water plus coconut cream. When boiling again, constantly stir while slowly drizzling in the semolina/polenta and simmer until thick. Pour into a shallow dish and top with dry toasted seeds. Allow to cool and set hard. Serve slices cold or warmed up under grill.

Optional - heat up under grill with cheese or Tofu on top and serve with a splash of Fermented Tomato Sauce (see page 213).

WATERCRESS AND SEAWEED SOUP

Watercress, a bunch chopped roughly
Milk or Coconut milk, 1 can
Potatoes, chopped into small chunks
Onions, finely chopped
Oil
Carrageen / Irish Moss, a handful
Stock (optional)
Spices - Chilli, Nutmeg, Salt, etc.
Yoghurt or Coconut cream (optional) for serving.

First soak a handful of Carrageen for ten minutes, then drain and remove tough bits. Fry Onions until soft. Add Potatoes and fry for a few minutes more. Add in Coconut milk and Carrageen. Add stock and spices and simmer ten minutes or so. Add Watercress and simmer another ten minutes. Liquidise and reheat, or just lightly mash by hand.

WILD GARLIC AND SEED/NUT PESTO

Toasted Hazelnuts or Sunflower seeds, a handful
Olive oil, half a cupful or less
Wild Garlic, a bunch of leaves
Salt and Pepper
Parmesan cheese, grated (optional)
Lemon juice, or young leaves of Lemonbalm
Water.

Blend nuts with a small amount of the Olive oil and water first, until smooth, then add Wild Garlic leaves and seasoning. Blend again. Gradually add more Olive oil to the desired consistency. Add cheese, if using, and Lemon juice to taste. Pour into sterilised jars and seal with a thin layer of Olive oil on top.

SPRING RECIPES REFERENCES

1. Jekka's Complete Herb Book, Jekka McVicar, Kyle Books, 2007, UK.
2. Recipe courtesy of Betta O'Connor.
3. The Hare Krishna Book of Vegetarian Cooking, The Bhaktivedanta Book Trust, 1984.

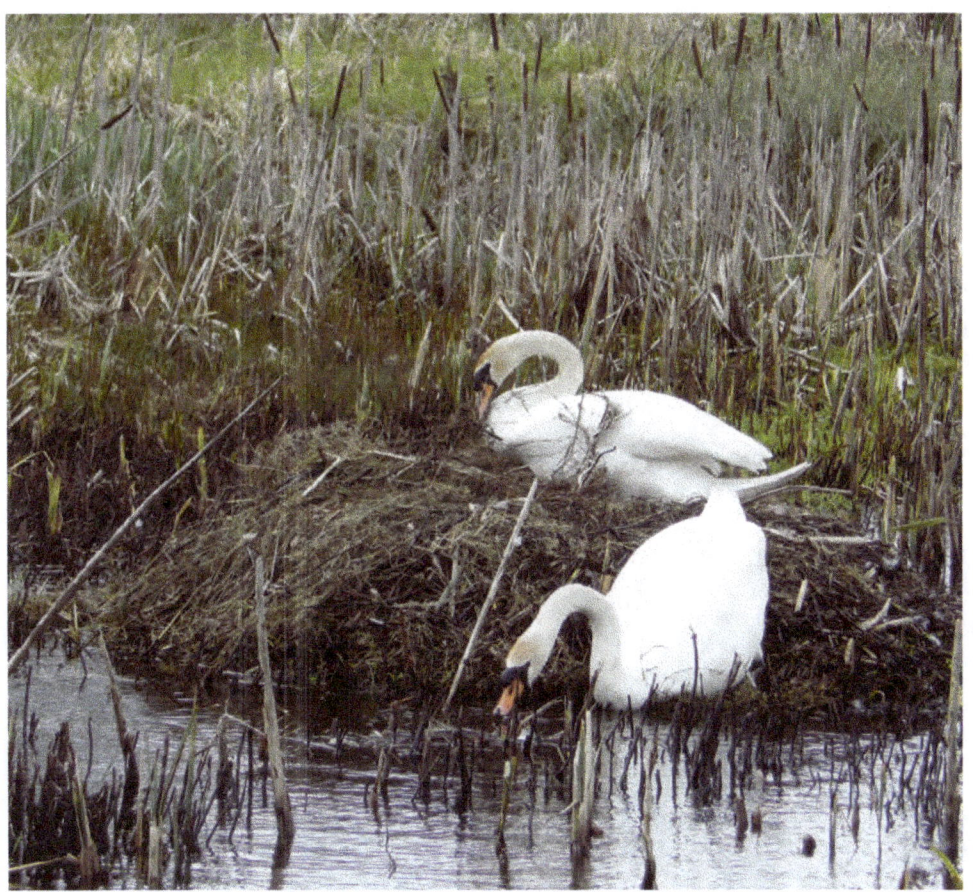

Above - Spring is also time to make a nest.

PEASANT IN PARADISE

CHAPTER SEVEN

SUMMERTIME

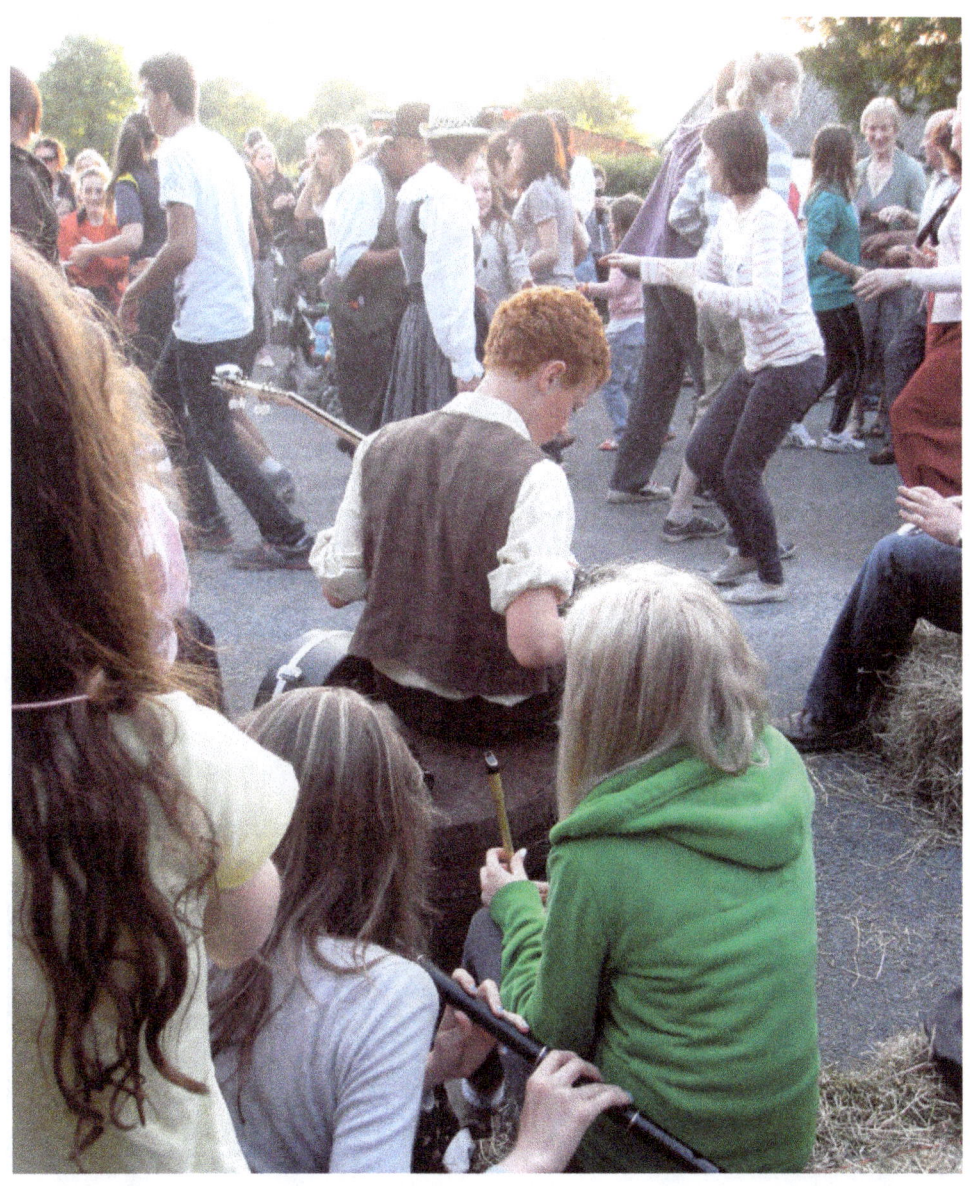

SUMMERTIME

Beltane, the Celtic start of summer celebration on May 1st, heralded a time of reduced farm work, giving peasants more time to frolic in the long, balmy days. Crops were growing strongly and apart from the gathering of turf from the bog, it was an easy, joyful time. July, the final month of summer, was even called the 'lazy month'. Around then, larders were getting near to empty and frugality was the order of the day. Not much energy to do things. But dieticians today say that a bit of hunger does wonders for longevity and health, so there's a positive in it!

At the height of the summer Sun, around the midsummer solstice of June 21st, it's maximum energy time. The stimulation of the light on these long days (with sunshine from 5am to 10pm, if you're lucky) gives us boundless energy and I might be out late working in the garden. In Christian times June 23rd is celebrated as St John's Eve, apparently John the Baptist was beheaded this day. Whatever! In County Leitrim, it's the night for the bonfire, or "bone fire" as the old ones call it, that must hark back to ancient practises of Sun worship. People have been building up their bonfire stacks for weeks for this night.

MIDSUMMER DANCING AT THE CROSSROADS

In recent years the old tradition of dancing at the crossroads has been revived in my locality. If it isn't raining, the local crossroads at Effrinagh will host hundreds of keen dancers, musicians and their families on St John's Eve. Traffic has to wait until the dancing set is finished to get through! It's near the site of 'Jimmy's Hall', the subject of a film by Ken Loach of the same name. This was followed by a fabulous play by the Abbey Theatre. Since then there's been some memorable public dance events with a 1920s theme, as seen in the photos.

On June 23rd 1921 Jimmy Gralton returned from working in America to help on the family farm in Effrinagh, arriving in time to attend the crossroads dance. The locals had no sheltered place to gather, so afterwards they got together and built a hall on the edge of the Gralton family farm. This gave them an independent venue where they held educational classes and had meetings about evictions, and of course, there was dancing. The latest American styles too. The landlord class was not happy and because people were having too much fun, the church pressured the government to put a stop to it. The hall was burned down and Gralton was deported (he had an American passport) - the only Irishman deported from his homeland - and was never allowed to return.

Today, a stone monument stands proudly on the site and there are occasional gatherings there. It's a reminder of the idealism of the hatchling new Irish Free State, that promised an end to landlordism and repression of the peasantry. Unfortunately the church replaced the exiting colonial power with it's own domination, repression and undermining of self-determination, as the Jimmy's Hall story shows us.

But Jimmy's joyful legacy lives on.

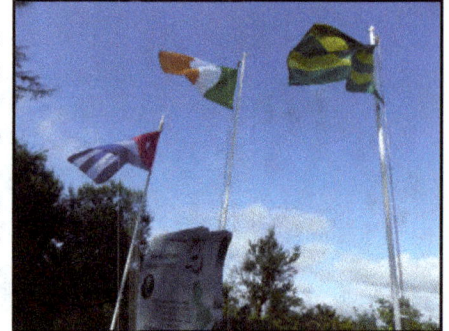

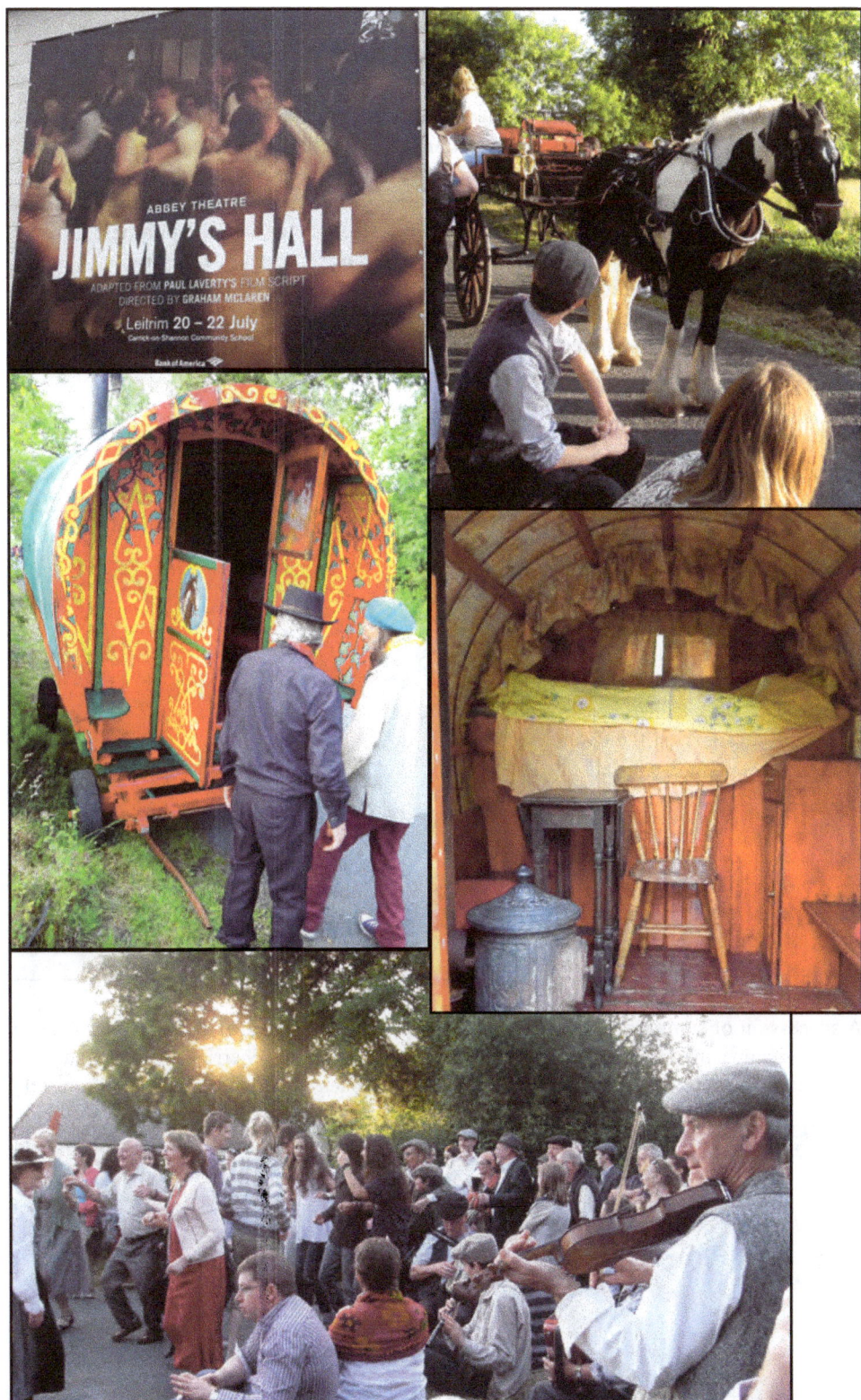

SUMMER ACTIVITIES

* Maintaining gardens and watering in dry spells.
* Sowing seeds on a regular basis, fortnightly is ideal.
* Harvesting greens, peas, beans, herbs, Rhubarb, berries, early Potatoes.
* Harvesting and storing seeds for next year's crops and sprouting.
* Pruning Apricots, Figs, Peaches, Nectarines, Plums and Tomatoes.
* Thinning fruit and protecting it from birds when nearly ripe.
* Planting Courgettes, Squash, Sweetcorn, beans and root crops.
* Preserving Green beans, (recipe page 212), and making berry preserves.
* Selling surplus produce at a roadside honesty stall.
* Frolicking in the warm sunshine!

SUMMER FRUITS

My summer gardens are a real jungle now and abundance is the fruit of my labours. The milk of Mother Earth's kindness flows steadily and conjures up for me the image of the beautiful Cow Goddess of southern India, Kamadenhu, who watches benelovently over cash registers on the counters of many a southern Indian restaurant. True to its Indo-European cultural origins, Ireland has Bo-ann, the white Cow Goddess, tutelary deity of the River Boyne, who also traversed the heavens to create the Milky Way. Perhaps the 'milk of human kindness' is the Cow Goddess's benelovent legacy?

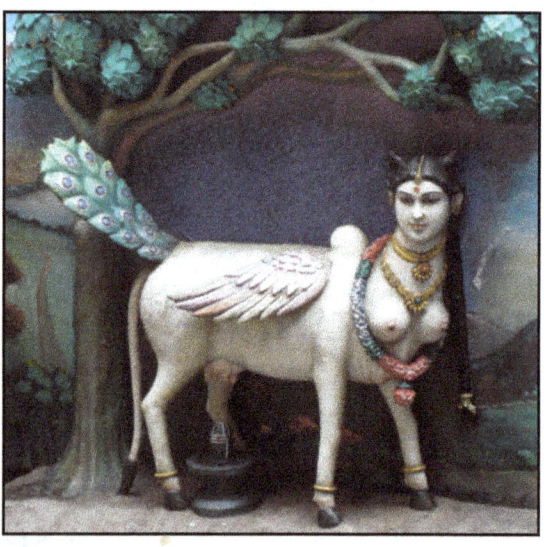

A succession of summer fruits start after Beltane - firstly Rhubarb, then early Strawberry varieties come in, followed by Siberian Honeyberries, Gooseberries, Alpine and Wild Strawberries; while Tomatoes, Currants, Cherries, Peaches and other berries ripen from July.

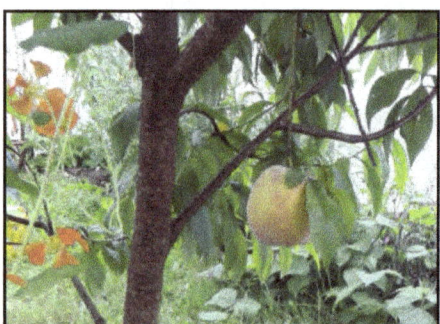
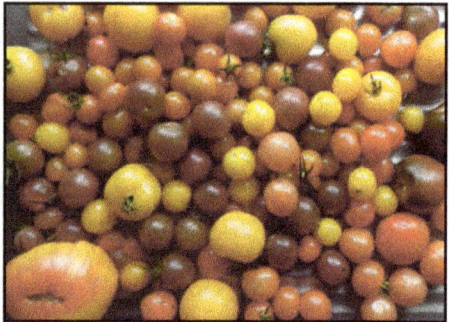

SUMMER FLOWERS

Top left - Purple Potatoes, right - Quinoa; bottom left - Jerusalem Artichoke, right - Meadowsweet.

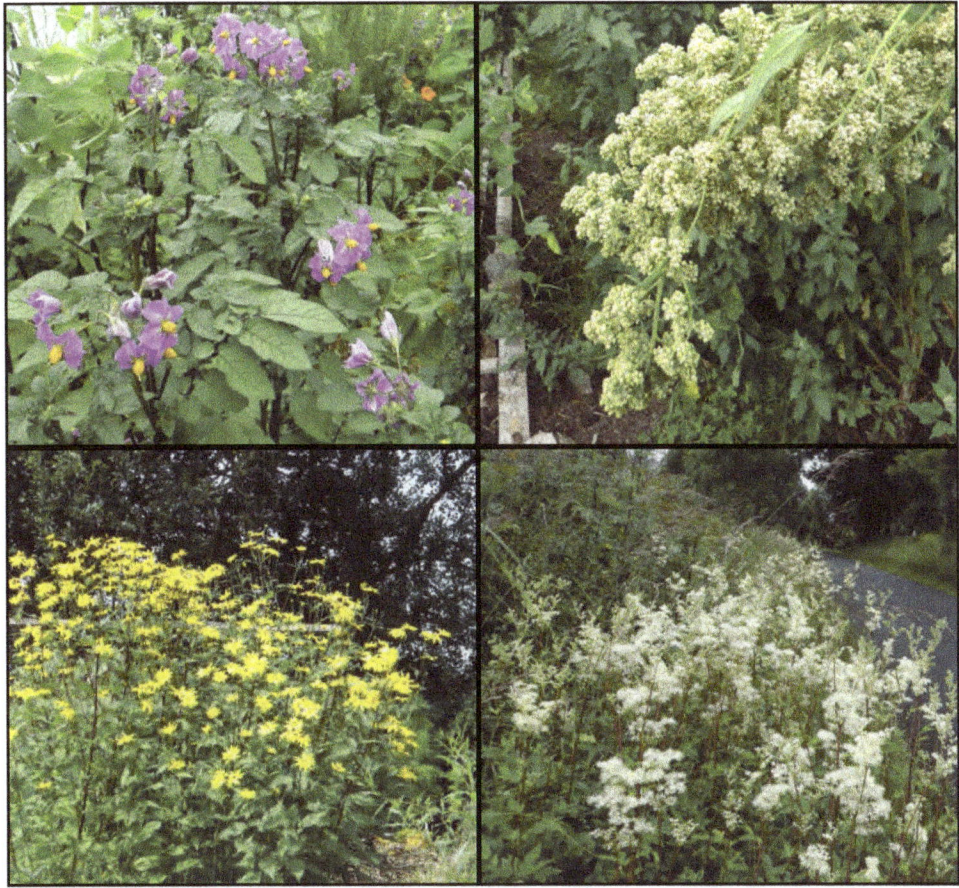

SUMMER WILDFLOWER RECIPES

MEADOWSWEET

The flowers and leaves are very sweet and are traditionally used for flavouring food and alcoholic drinks. Fresh new leaves, flower heads and roots all make tasty tea, although with a diuretic effect, so don't overdo it. Young leaves are also good for soups and sauces. Young leaves can be dried for use as a sweetener as well. Rhubarb can be cooked with eight or nine flower heads added to 1kg of Rhubarb stalks and thus less extra sweetener will be needed. [1]

LIME / LINDEN

The flowers of the Small Leaved Lime tree (Tilia cordata) are eaten in salads, sandwiches and soups. Tea is also made from the flowers and is very popular in France. Gather the flowers and lay them on trays or sheets of paper in a warm, well ventilated room and they should be dry in two weeks or so. One teaspoon of the dried flowers makes a cup of tea that's drunk for its sedative effect, having a strong honey aroma and helpful for colds and other ailments. It's recommended to only use young unopened flowers, older ones have narcotic properties.

You can also grind young unopened Linden flowers with the immature fruit into a paste that's used as a Chocolate substitute (but does not keep).[2]

ELDERFLOWER FRITTERS

Elderflower heads should be carefully picked over for dirt or insects, rather than washed, and the short stalks retained as a handle. They can then be for dipped into a batter of flour, egg and water[3] (or Gram/Chickpea flour and water for a vegan batter) and fried in oil.

TRADITIONAL ELDERFLOWER CORDIAL

7 big Elderflowers
2 or 3 sliced Lemons, rinds grated
1kg or so sugar or honey
1lt water

Dissolve sweetener in the hot water, then add the Lemon and Elderflowers and leave it soaking for one day, stirring occasionally. It's then strained through muslin/cheesecloth and poured into sterilised bottles and sealed. (Other recipes call for boiling it and also adding Tartaric Acid or Citric Acid.)

DANDELION FLOWER BUD SALAD

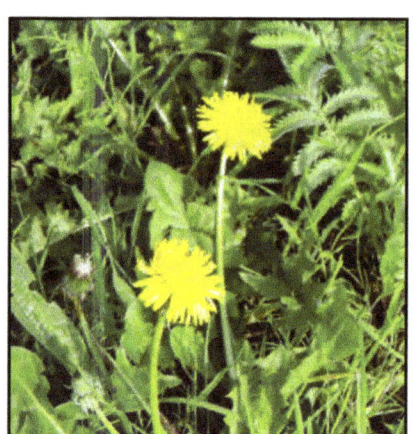

A 19th century French recipe calls for equal quantities of unopened flower buds with a few surrounding leaves, plus chopped (or grated) Beetroot. The bitterness of the Dandelion is offset by the sweet Beetroot.[3]

DANDELION FLOWER TEMPURA / BHAJIS

Gather lots of flowers and remove the stalks
Onions, finely chopped
Batter of flour, beaten eggs and water
Or vegan batter - Gram (Chickpea) flour and water
Coconut oil
Salt

Mix flowers and Onion, then dip in batter and fry large spoonfuls in oil.
Drain on kitchen paper [4]

SUMMER'S EDIBLE GARDEN FLOWERS

- **Artichoke**
- **Borage**
- **Broccoli**
- **Cardoon**
- **Chamomile**
- **Chicory**
- **Chives**
- **Clovers**
- **Cowslip**
- **Currants**
- **Dandelion**
- **Day Lilly**
- **Elder tree**
- **Evening Primrose**
- **Garlic**
- **Honeysuckle**
- **Hops**
- **Huazontle**
- **Hyssops**
- **Mallows**
- **Marigold**
- **Meadowsweet**
- **Nasturtium**
- **Reed Mace**
- **Rose petals**
- **Shungiku**

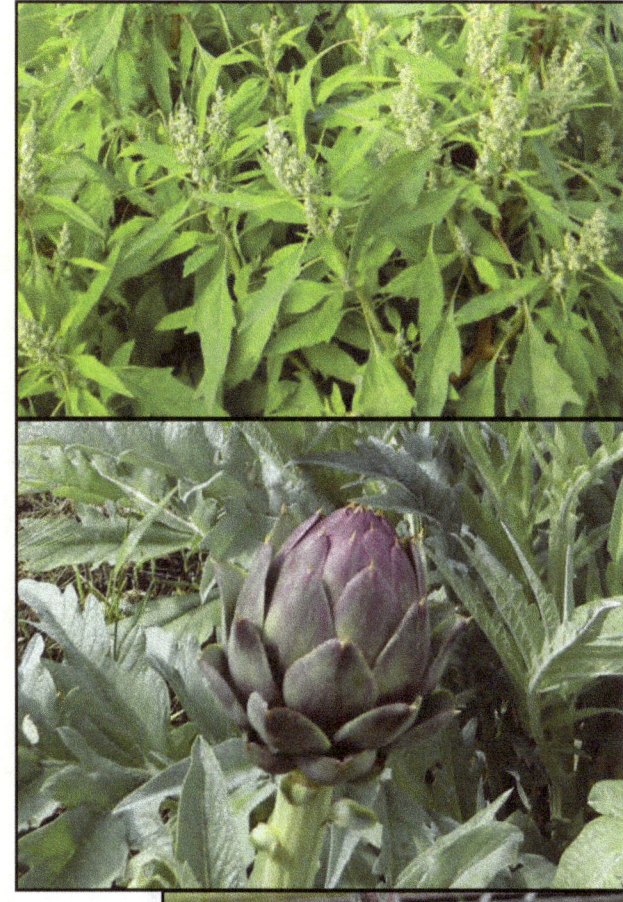

Top - Huazontle flower shoots are edible, this 'Aztec Broccoli' is in the Chenopodium family.
Middle - Sicilian Purple Artichoke ready to eat.

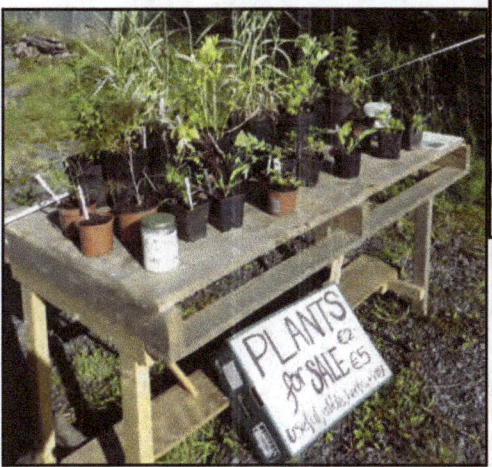

Above - Borage flowering.
Left - My pandemic plant stall proved a hit for the many local road walkers and cyclists in the lockdowns of 2020. I got to meet some neighbours for the first time because of it too!

SUMMER'S EDIBLE LEAVES AND SHOOTS

- **Angelica**
- **Amaranths**
- **Asparagus**
- **Beetroot**
- **Bergamot**
- **Blackcurrant**
- **Borage**
- **Cabbage**
- **Cardoon**
- **Celery**
- **Celery Leaf**
- **Chickweed**
- **Comfrey**
- **Cowslip**
- **Dandelion**
- **Fennel**
- **Hops**
- **Hyssops**
- **Kale**
- **Lady's Mantle**
- **Lemonbalm**
- **Mallow**
- **Marigold**
- **Mints**
- **Mugwort**
- **Nasturtium**
- **Orach**
- **Parsley**
- **Raspberry**
- **Shepherd's Purse**
- **Sorrel**
- **Spinach**
- **Yarrow**

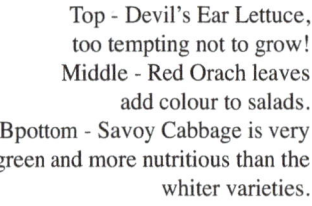

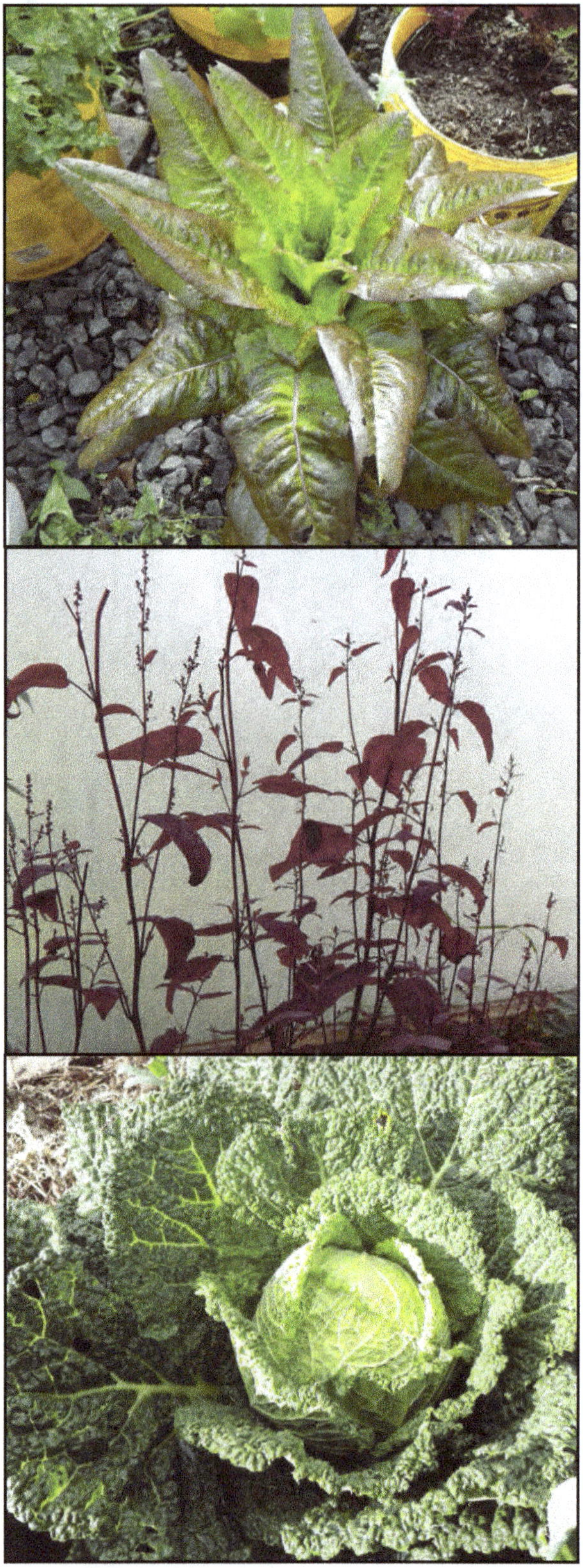

Top - Devil's Ear Lettuce, too tempting not to grow!
Middle - Red Orach leaves add colour to salads.
Bpottom - Savoy Cabbage is very green and more nutritious than the whiter varieties.

SUMMER HARVEST
IN THE POLYTUNNEL

Apricot
Basil
Blueberry
Broad Bean
Cherry
Courgette
Cucumber
French Beans
Herbs
Kohl Rabi
Mangetout Peas
Nectarine
Peach
Potatoes, earlies
Salad greens
Strawberry
Sweet Corn
Tomato

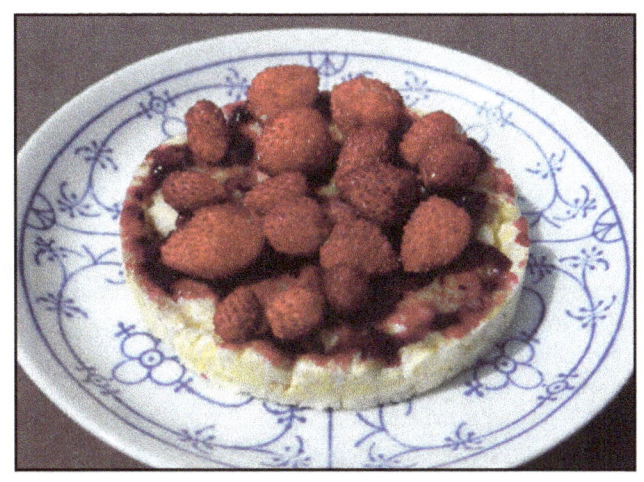

Below - At a Summer Solstice ritual, I give thanks to the land for all the wonderful abundance.

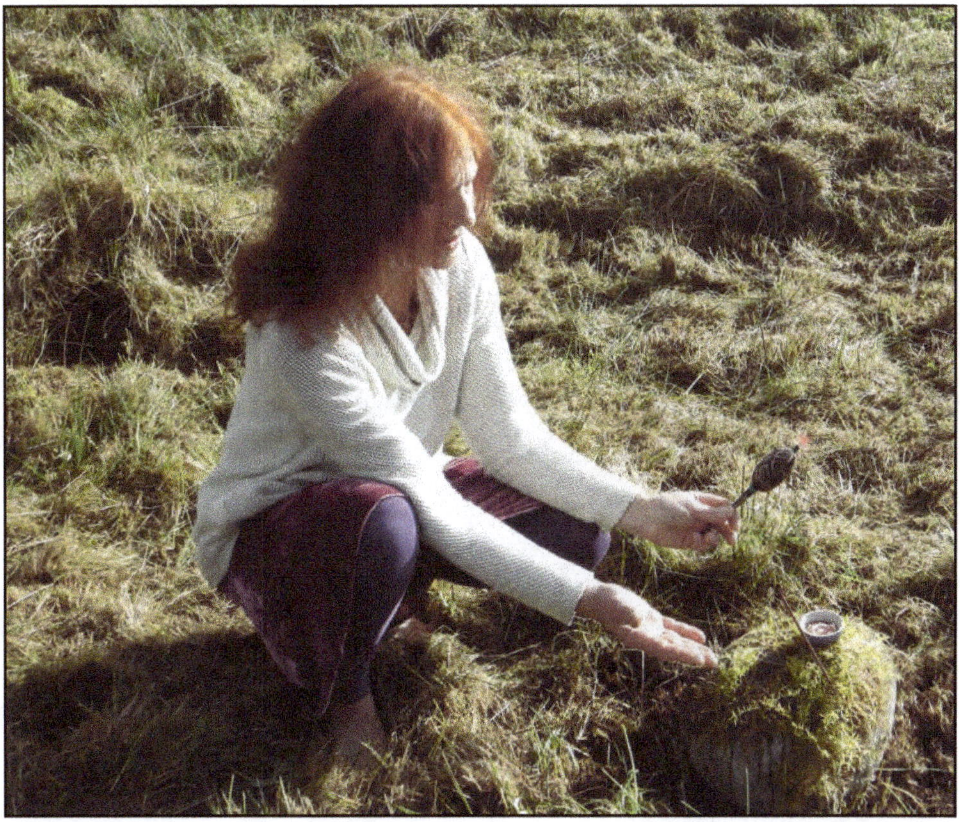

SUMMER RECIPES

FERMENTED GREEN BEANS

Green or Runner Beans
Brine (2 tbs salt dissolved in 1lt hot
      non-tap water, cooled)
Spices - Peppercorns, Garlic, Chilli, Coriander etc

Fill a tall clean jar with upright fresh beans, their tops removed and tightly packed together, plus spices. Pour in the cooled brine to completely cover them. Cover the jar over with a clean cloth so it can breathe. Keep in a warm place for a couple of weeks, allowing it to out-gas (otherwise close the jar and 'burp' it regularly). Then seal the jar tight and store it in a cool, dark place. They keep very well and can be chopped into salads (going well with Potatoes), or added to cooked meals at the end, but try to avoid boiling them. [5]

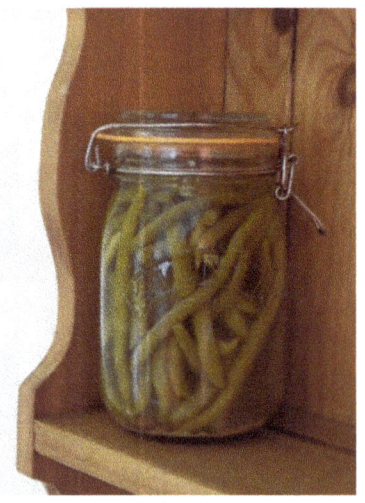

BLACKCURRANT AND HONEY SPREAD

This is an old traditional French recipe, it's absolutely delicious and one of my favourite home products. You pick the berries when they start to drop off. Currants can be snipped from their clusters with scissors, or else cut the whole laden branch, if the bush has attained a good size, and take branches indoors for picking the currants later. Stripping them off with a fork is easiest. (I've taken cuttings from the harvested branches and, though not meant to be the correct time of year for this, they've all rooted nicely, so this gives me new plants as well.)

Clean, wash, drain and weigh the Currants. Put them into a non-metal saucepan (enamel, ceramic or glass) and cook rapidly with no added water, stirring fairly constantly for 35 minutes. Use a wooden spoon. Then, after taking it off the heat, add in the same weight of honey, or a bit less, and stir well. Do not cook the honey. Pour the mix into sterilised jars and close tight. Some people cover the mix with beeswax or paraffin to keep it airtight. Mine didn't get that and some have a little mould growing on the top, but it's easily removed and they are still good after a year in storage.[6]

BLACKCURRANT SYRUP

Despite sugar being neither affordable nor available to the peasantry in Norway in the past, they were able to preserve Currants, by making a syrup with just the natural sweetness. Whole berries (the stalks are ok too) are put into a big pot with boiling water poured over them. This is left to ferment for a couple of days. Any fungus on the surface is removed. It's then strained and the liquid brought to a fast boil. The scum is removed as it boils fast for five minutes. The syrup is then poured into sterilised bottles and stored in a cool dark place. Diluted with water this makes a refreshing drink, hot or cold. It can be also added to fruit soups or used in sauces for winter puddings.[7]

POTATO CAKES

Some of the popular Potato Cakes made around the world include Potato Bhajis in India, Jewish Latkes, French Polpettes (mashed Potato plus Fetta cheese), as well as Boxty, a dish dear to the people of northern Ireland. These are variations on a pancake or rissole made from Potatoes that are either grated raw, or cooked and mashed.

There are many tedious ways to make Potato Cakes, some that take hours of boiling. Raw Potato can also be rather messy and formidable to deal with. Fear not, this recipe[8], that I've based on the Indian approach, is the easiest and with the lowest Carbon footprint.

Potatoes - 500 gm, grated just before cooking
(or use half Jerusalem Artichokes)
One Onion, grated just before cooking
2 tblsp flour (Gram flour is good)
2 beaten eggs, or do it vegan by increasing Gram flour to about half a cup
Salt, Pepper, spices - e.g. Garam Masala
Optional additives - e.g. chopped leaves of Chives, Spring Onions, Garlic, Wild Garlic or Lovage; Sesame Seeds sprinkled on top, etc
Oil for frying
Heavy bottomed fry pan

Potatoes are around 75% water and the bulk of this has to be removed, to make the rissoles work. The easiest is the Indian way. Wash your hands well, then pick up a big lump of grated Potato and Onion mix and squeeze out the water between your hands. It's messy yes, but fast and efficient. When the mix is much drier, put it in a bowl, add in the other ingredients, and mix them well together. Cook the rissoles by putting large spoonfuls into the hot oil in the pan and squashing them down flat. I like to sprinkle Sesame seeds over the top of them. Fry the rissoles both sides, then drain the oil off and serve them with yoghurt, sour cream, chutney, relish etc.

TOMATO SAUCE, FERMENTED

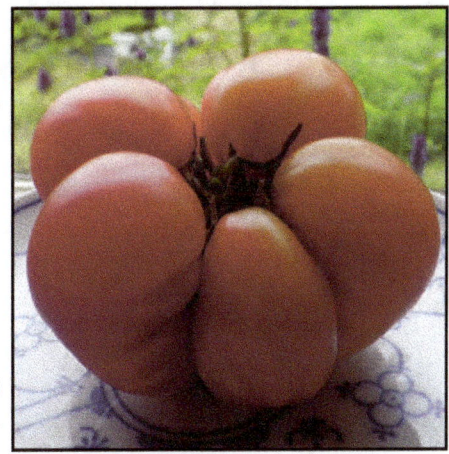

This ancient Italian peasant recipe is brilliant in its simplicity, stores well, has enhanced nutrition and is delicious!

Tomatoes
Olive oil
Salt, 2 tbsp per litre
Whey, half cupful (optional)
Pepper or Chilli flakes / powder
Sterilised bottles
Non-metallic fermenting bucket or stoneware pot
(my Sauerkraut pot with its water seal is perfect).

Fill the bucket or pot up to 10cm from the top with Tomatoes. Mash and squish them up by hand. I use a Potato masher. Add whey and cover, allowing it to breathe. Stir vigorously twice daily.

When bubbling stops, after a week or so, put it all through a sieve to remove skin and seeds. Add spices and salt, then pour into bottles and cover the top over with a dash of Olive oil. Only have caps on loosely, to release gases. Store in a cool place. It will keep for a year or so. [6]

SUMMERTIME REFERENCES

1. Wild Foods for Free, Jonathan Hilton, Hamlyn, UK, 2007.
2. Plants for a Future, Ken Fern, Permanent Publications, UK, 2000.
3. Food for Free, Richard Mabey, Collins, Ireland, 1972.
4. Favourite Wild Food Recipes, by Simon Haseltine, Salmon Ltd, UK.
5. Fermenting - recipes and preparation, Daphne Lambert, Flame Tree, UK, 2016.
6. Preserving without Canning of Freezing, Terre Vivante,
7. European Peasant Cookery, Elisabeth Luard, Grub St, London, 2004.
8. Potato - the definitive guide to Potatoes and Potato cooking, Alex Barker and Sally Mansfield, Anness Publishing, 2002, UK.

CHAPTER EIGHT

AUTUMN

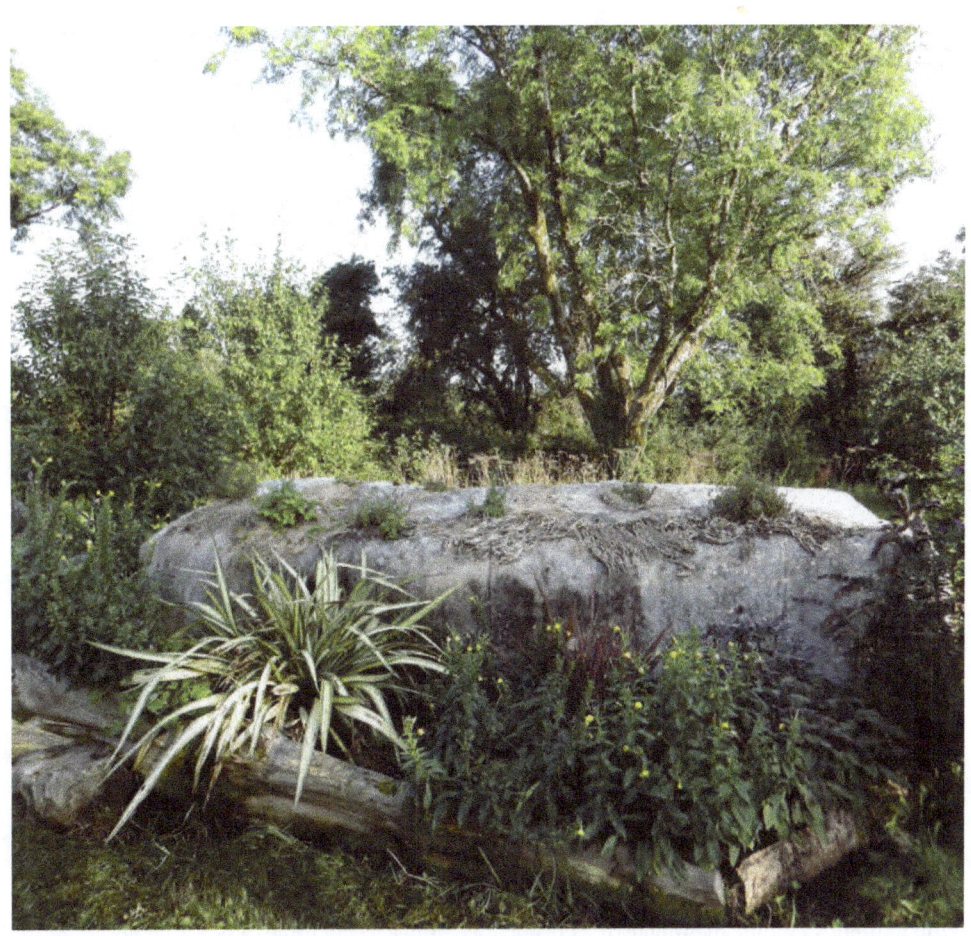
A living sculpture in the backyard, it's also a clamp for storing root vegetables in.

AUTUMN HARVEST

In Celtic tradition the season of harvest and abundance starts on August 1st with the first fruits festival, called Lammas by the English and Lughnasa in Europe. In ancient Ireland it was Bron Trogain, the festival of Crom Dubh and Aine, and this was the most fun-filled event of the year. Great excitement grew with the prospect of this festive time and the hungry month of July was a great appetiser.

Sadly now largely forgotten in Ireland, it was severely suppressed by the church, no doubt for its original honouring of favourite underworld god Crom Dubh and goddess Aine, who were not easily Christianised. Dubh means dark, with evil connotations. However to the peasantry Crom Dubh was sometimes mythologised in disguise as a generous landlord. (I've written about this festival in my other books and I was so charmed by accounts of it that I wrote a musical on the subject too. 'Lammas Fair' was performed to a full house at a fringe festival in Castlemaine, Australia in 2011.)

In the great Irish harvest myth of Lough Gur in County Limerick, Ethne, the Corn Child, was annually taken down into the Earth, to the underworld of the gods, at this time. Ethne personified the seeds of next year's crops. Likewise, farmers sowed seeds for next year's crops in the autumn. And in our plant nurseries we also sow some seeds then, ones that need to be stratified, to experience the cold through winter in order to germinate in the spring.

Ancient Irish harvest festival lore also mentions the symbolic giving of tithes, in the form of flower garlands taken up hilltops and left as a token of gratitude to the deities.[1] The practical eco-peasant also gives back in order to to sustain the cycles of life, by gathering plant and animal waste and making compost with it over the cold months, returning the nutrients back to the Good Earth and kindling new life.

Harvesting times saw strengthened social bonding, before the machine age ended the need for it. Neighbours and friends rallied together to bring in the corn crops or hay. After a long day's work at meitheals, a hearty meal was provided, then the music and dancing began. A good harvest meant that many more happy days could be expected. Spirits were high!

October 31st was the traditional end of autumn, end of year festival, and another reason for feasting. This was the time to cull unwanted cattle so they wouldn't be a burden to feed over winter. Bull fights were a feature and the losers were eaten. Piles of cattle bones found at megalithic ritual centres, such as Croms Dubh's stone circle near Lough Gur, attest to this annual feast.[2]

Todays crops are more diverse and ripening times are spread over several months. The concept of a communal celebration of harvest, a thanksgiving to Mother Earth for our sustenance, was stamped out. The new Christian view held firm that the land is our servant and the sacred is above us and out of personal reach. It was a very unpopular doctrine to impose on the peasantry and not well received. For them, the Otherworld and the sacred were everywhere.

With autumn's bounty, the image of a cornucopia comes to my mind, a whirling vortex of the fruits of the Earth pouring its goodness over us. Or the 'cauldrons of plenty' of various deities, including ancient Irish underworld god and agriculture influencer The Dagda, the 'Good God', whose cauldron is constantly replenished and never fails to satisfy.

Right - An Earth goddess with her 'horn of plenty', in the British Museum.
Below - The Amaranth "Love Lies Bleeding' has edible seed.

1. The Festival of Lughnasa, Maire MacNeill, Oxford University Press, London, 1962.
2. Mythic Ireland', Michael Dames, Thames & Hudson, London, 1992.

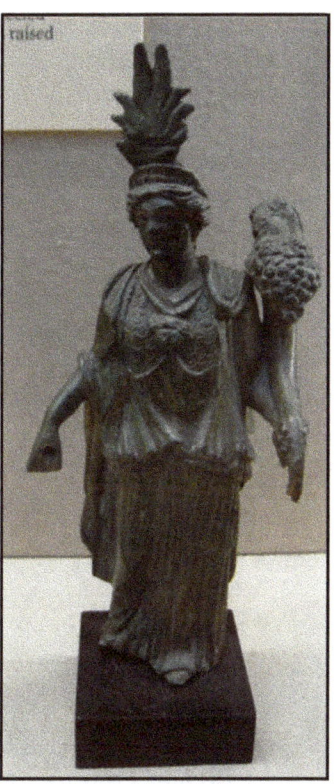

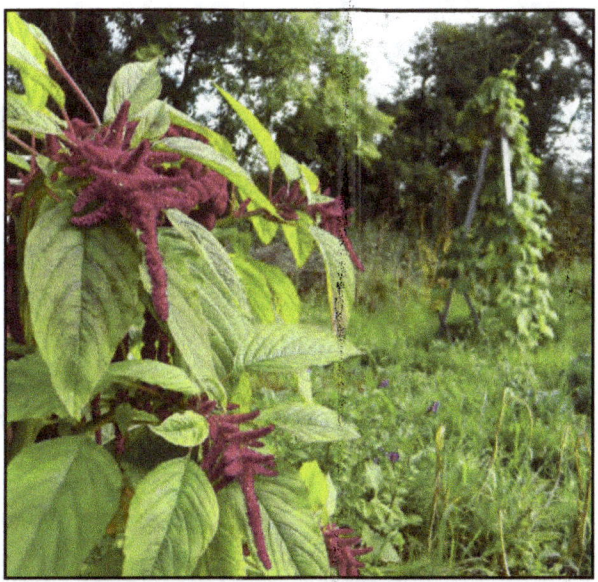

AUTUMN ACTIVITIES

* Protecting fruit from birds when nearly ripe.
* Harvesting and preserving fruit, veggies, herbs and grains.
* Harvesting and storing seeds for next year's crops and sprouting.
* Drying and curing before the harvest goes into storage.
* Regular sowing of salad greens and veggies for winter and spring, including overwintering Garlic, Onions and cereal crops.
* Feasting on the harvest!

AUTUMN'S ABUNDANCE

In this season, the wealth of the Good Earth is ours for the plucking. All types of herbs, vegetables, grains and fruit are available in this season. There are a host of lesser-known edible plants also available, including the following.

AUTUMN'S EDIBLE LEAVES AND SHOOTS

- Amaranth
- Celery Leaf
- Chard (right)
- Chicory
- Endive
- Grape
- Kale
- Mallow
- Mashua
- Spinach
- Watercress

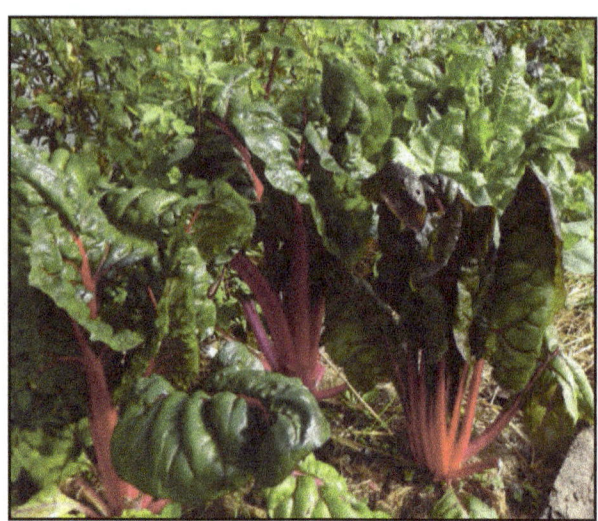

AUTUMN'S EDIBLE FLOWERS

- Broccoli
- Clover
- Day Lilly
- Evening Primrose
- Nasturtium (right)
- Mallow
- Marigold
- Rose
- Shungiku

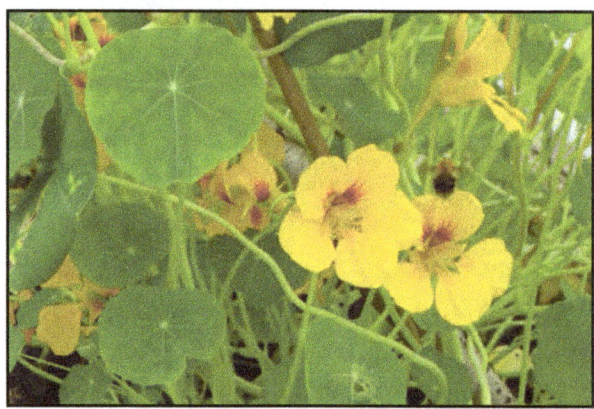

AUTUMN'S EDIBLE BERRIES, SEEDS & NUTS

- Amaranth
- Aronia
- Beech nut
- Dock
- Elder
- Fennel
- Hazelnut
- Hawthorn
- Monkey Puzzle
- Nettle
- Oak
- Plantain
- Rowan
- Sloe

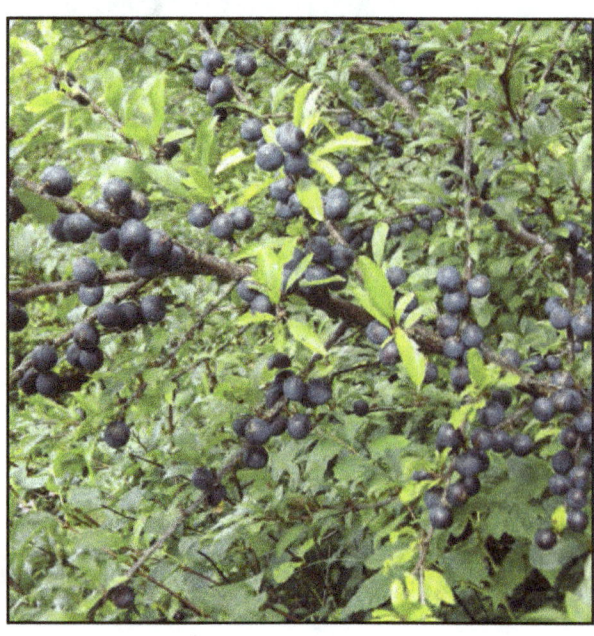

AUTUMN'S EDIBLE ROOTS

Angelica
Celeriac
Celery Leaf
Cowslip
Dandelion
Day Lilly
Dock
Horseradish
Marshmallow
Mashua
Meadowsweet
Nettles
Oca
Shepherd's Purse
Swede
Sweet Cicely
Turnip

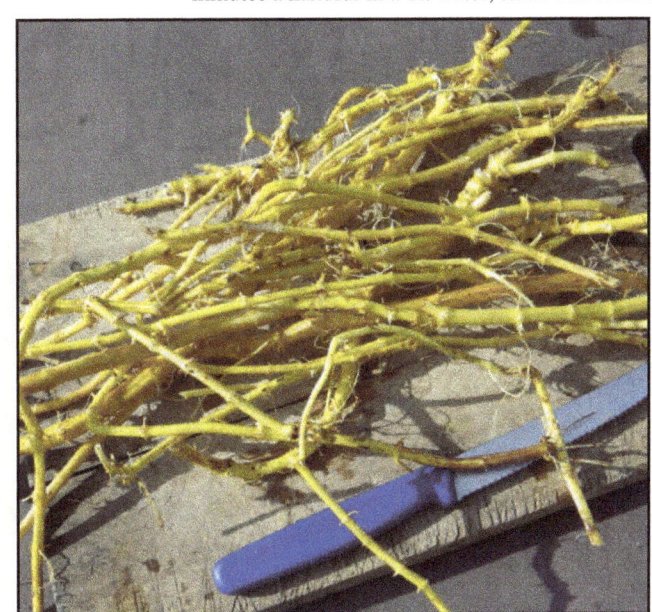

Below - Nettle roots are a tonic for prostrate enlargement, inflammation and infections, says Kress. Simmer for 20 minutes a handful in a 1lt water, strain and drink.

DITCHING THE REFRIGERATOR

I focus on growing as much of my food as possible and select varieties that can be dried easily, or otherwise stored without using much power. I don't rely on a refrigerator, only using a small 12 volt chest fridge in hot spells, if they happen. There are several important reasons to stop relying on refrigeration. What most people don't realise is that between 25 and 30% of the world's electricity is used for refrigeration, as reported by the Australian Broadcasting Commission in 2019. And there's planet-unfriendly and toxic aspects too.

"When your fridge is finished, the gas that is contained in the fridge is released to the atmosphere. It is estimated that one kilogram of refrigerant contributes as much to the greenhouse effect as two tonnes of Carbon dioxide — the equivalent of running a car uninterrupted for six months…Also [the gases] are toxic. If someone gets in contact with them they can have some health problems," Dr Cazorla said in the report.[1]

Another thing to consider about refrigeration are its affects on the quality of the food. The cold is meant to suppress bacteria. But does that make old food good to eat, or is the fridge just a 'food mausoleum'? Do we consider the effect of eating food that has been exposed to electro-magnetic fields? It has been warned about. Energetically, the food's quality is disturbed by electricity and so I never use it to boil water for tea, let alone cook food with it! It's healthier to use gas or wood for cooking and probably a gas fridge is better than an electric one.

1. https://www.abc.net.au/news/science/2019-03-28/plastic-crystals-could-keep-us-and-the-planet-cool-in-the-future/10943796

TRADITIONAL WAYS TO PRESERVE FOOD

Since the dawn of human civilisations, people have developed ways to preserve foodstuffs naturally, to prevent them from spoiling and to tide them over lean times and winter. Before the era of refrigeration, the three basic techniques of food preservation were as follows.

CELLARS AND CLAMPS

These cool, humid and dark places are perfect for storing tubers like Potatoes, plus Apples and Pears. But if you live in County Leitrim they might become seasonal swimming pools also, so here it was traditional to make a clamp, by piling up the Potatoes, or whatever root crop, on the surface of the ground and covering it over with soil or a nice thatched straw roof.

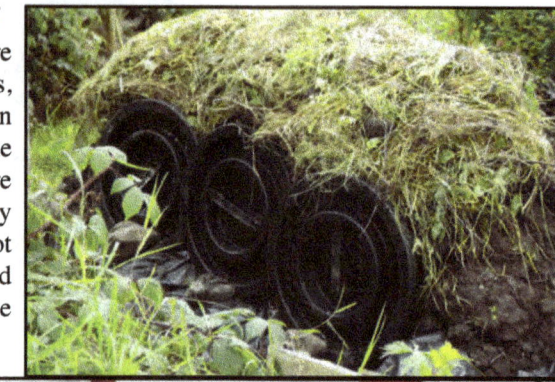

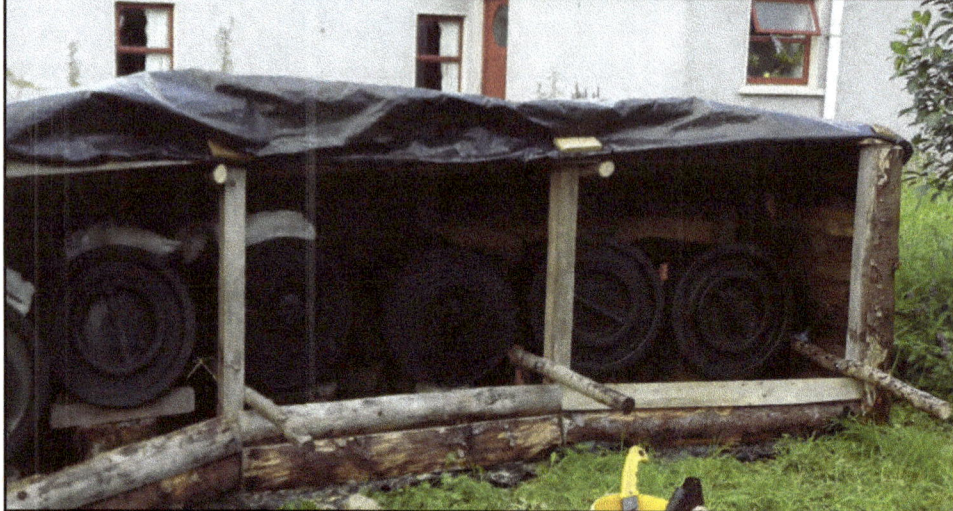

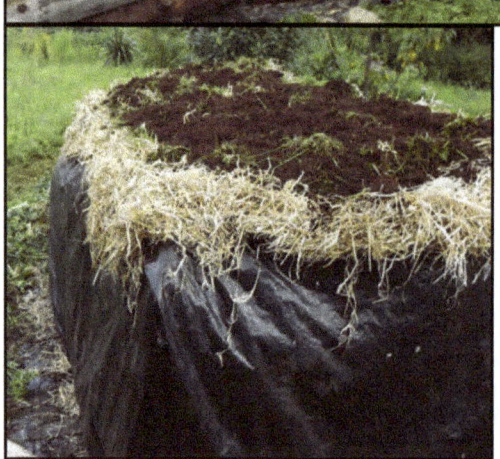

I have been experimenting with making clamps from bins laid on their side on the ground (slightly elevated) and covered over with straw, soil and mulch, as in the top photo, which resulted in a roof garden. Inside the bins the root crops are nestled into a pile of damp sand. Later I made a clamp with a timber structure covering it. This developed into a living sculpture, as seen above and left, and as it looked one year later on page 215.

DEHYDRATION

This works best for fruit, rather than vegetables, however Tomatoes and Rhubarb, due to their higher acid and sugar content, can also be dried. My dehydrator does use a bit of electricity, so a solar one would be better, if the sun comes out.

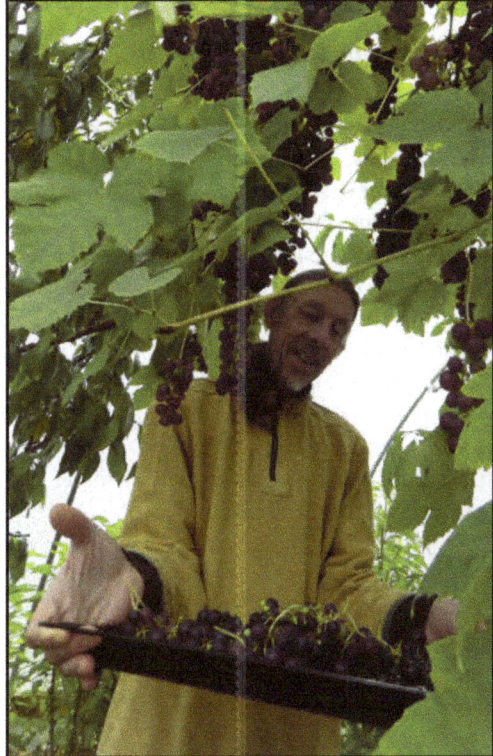

We delight in Strawberry slices that are dried in the dehydrator, but my favourite dried food are the Raisins that we make from the Black Hamberg Grapes. They are very versatile - eaten as snack food, or added to desserts and muesli etc.

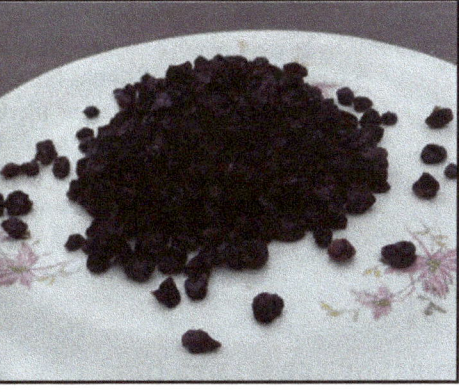

FERMENTING

Since ancient times, foods have been fermented to preserve them. The art of fermenting food, using salt, vinegar, alcohol, oil, honey, yeast, bacteria and the like, was a vibrant living food culture. People in Sudan, for example, traditionally make around ninety different fermented foods, using grains, milk, bones, locusts etc.[1] But in modern times we have been instilled with a fear of microbes, so-called 'germs', and are told to lead sterile lives, when quite the opposite should be the case. The advent of refrigeration hastened the decline of the art of fermenting.

But now the pendulum is swinging back, as we rediscover the wisdom of harnessing the power of beneficial micro-organisms for enhanced living. Knowledge of the benefits has greatly increased these days. The wisdom of the peasantry is vindicated yet again!

Fermenting is a form of pre-digestion, making foods easier for us to digest and increasing levels of more bio-available nutrients, while reducing some toxins. It can taste more delicious too. One of the simplest methods is to soak grains overnight, or for a few hours, in water with some whey added (optional), before they are cooked. This short ferment reduces levels of phytates /phytic acid, the anti-nutritional factor, and thus increases digestibility.

Fermenting fosters healthy guts and feeds essential gut microbiota - the population weighing some 2kg!- that is fundamental to our health and wellbeing. These beneficial microbes help us to synthesise and absorb vitamins and minerals, as well as regulate our immune system. They are disturbed by the taking of antibiotics and also by stress, pollution, chemicals, etc.

BENEFITS OF HOME MADE PRESERVES

* Extends the storage life of foods without need for refrigeration.
* Uses up crop surpluses in times of plenty, or damaged foods
(the bad bits being removed of course).
* Pre-digests food for us, breaking down proteins, fats and carbohydrates.
* Help maintain a proper balance of micro-organisms in our guts and
these help us to absorb minerals, synthesise vitamins and regulate immunity.
* Removes anti-nutritional factors in grains, legumes and other foods,
such as phytic acid in grain.
* They can taste delicious and bring more variety to one's diet.
* Commercially made preserves tend to be pasteurised, which kills microbes,
and are often loaded with undesirables, such as sugar and Palm Oil,
as well as having a higher Carbon footprint. Your own preserves will be alive.
* Home made preserves make lovely, special gifts.

TYPES OF FERMENTATION

Fermenting involves various bacteria, fungi, yeasts and moulds that culture foodstuffs into more nutritious forms. There are four different types of fermentation.

LACTIC ACID FERMENTATION

Lacto-fermentation was originally the main technique used, with veggies fermenting naturally in their own juices and wild lacto-bacillus feeding off the food's nutrients and converting starches and sugar into lactic acid. It suits most vegetables, but generally not fruit. (The only fruit I know of that are pickled this way are Plums and Tomatoes.) It usually involves using a brine (salty water) to immerse them in. Lacto-fermentation also transforms milk products into yoghurt, cheese and the like. Other lacto-ferments need special cultures to be introduced.

YEAST FERMENTING

Yeasts of the Saccharomyces genus (that produce ethyl alcohol from carbohydrates) are used for bread rising and alcoholic drinks.

VINEGAR BASED PICKLES

Acetic acid, produced by Acetobacteria, is used for these pickles. Preserving fruit and veggies in vinegar is easy and fairly fool-proof, but it doesn't generate as much nutritional benefits as lacto-fermenting does.

MOULDS

Moulds are used in other fermentation practises, such as cheese making that uses moulds from the genus Penicillium. Moulds from the genus Rhizopus are used to inoculate cooked

Soyabeans to make Tempeh in Indonesia; while the mould Aspergillus oryzae is the starter culture used with Rice for Miso making in Japan. Elsewhere, Kombucha, Kefir, Kvas, as well as Coffee, Tea and Ginger Beer are traditional fermented drinks involving various different microorganisms. Vanilla, Chocolate and Olives are other foods that must be fermented to become edible.

Lacto-bacillus are probiotic, which means a health promoting bacteria culture that can handle living in our acid guts. Prebiotic is the term for their favourite foods, soluble fibre being particularly good for them. Excellent sources of prebiotics are the Allium family (Garlic, Onions, Leeks), Asparagus, Jerusalem Artichokes, Plums and Bananas. Heat destroys the goodness of probiotics, so it's best to mostly use them raw. Prebiotics, however, are not destroyed by heat, so they can be cooked. By optimising the amount of probiotics and probiotics in our diet we help to balance our microbiome, which protects our wellbeing and happiness. Because not just physical health, but also our emotions are positively affected by our guts.[1]

Below - Onions, Garlic and Potatoes drying in the Bath House.

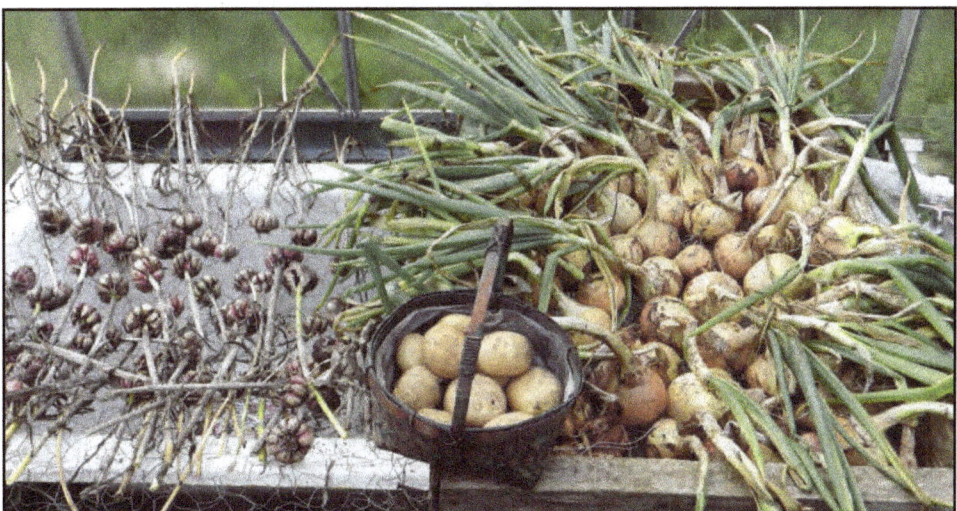

THE ONE PICKLE JAR REVOLUTION!
If you had asked me twenty years ago if I made pickles, I would have said "No, I don't have time!" Actually, I had a resistance to doing it, despite all the benefits that the food gurus tell us about. Logically, I should be making delicious, sugar free, unpasteurised pickles for a super nutritional supplement to my diet. So, why wasn't I? Well all the books did make it look a bit complicated and daunting, with giant pots bubbling in ample kitchens, and special equipment for the job. It looked a bit technical and I never had the space nor time, I told myself.

But eventually it dawned on me that pickle making doesn't have to be a major industrial operation. It doesn't have to happen all at once. A jar or two at a time, or more if there's a helper, makes it achievable. So I stopped resisting and got stuck in, and the more I practised, the quicker and better it got. I harvest small amounts of fruit and veg as they ripen, and pickle them as I go. It only takes a little bit of the day. And this way I have been steadily developing my pickle making skills.

I re-use old jars for my preserves. I avoid using ones with metal lids for vinegar pickles, as they corrode quickly. I've found that large jars are not the best, because without a 'fridge, the contents might go off after opening if not eaten quickly enough. So now I favour smaller jars. When the jars are past their prime for pickles, I can still store dried foods in them.

ROOT VEGGIES PICKLED IN VINEGAR

Jerusalem and Chinese Artichokes, Ocas, Fennel bulbs, Turnips, Carrots, Beetroot, Daikon radish and the like are perfect for this.

Below - Making a jar of Sunroot pickles.

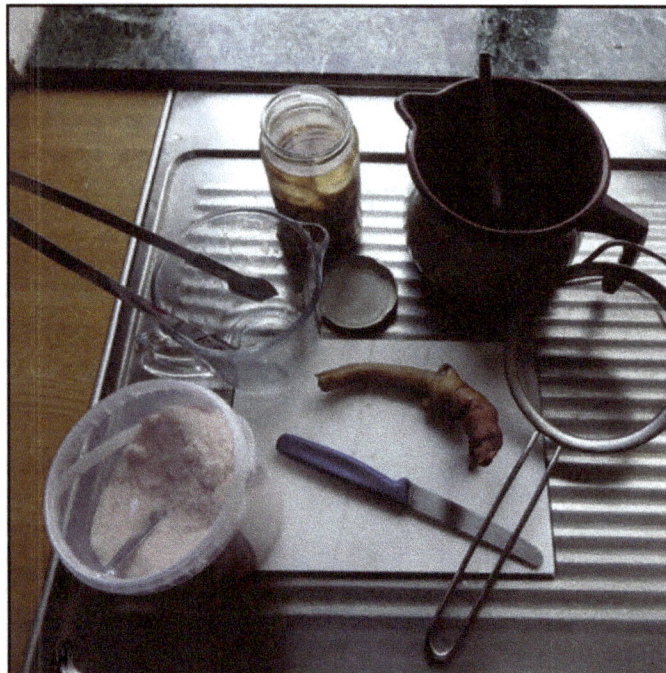

For a vinegar pickle, the first stage is brining. I soak the clean, thinly sliced roots overnight in a salt solution. Each book I've consulted gives different ratios, from a 2% - 10% salt to water solution, so take your pick! The 2% solution, that is most often advocated, is equivalent to two tablespoons of salt per litre of water.

Twenty four hours later I drain them, put them in sterilised jars (boiling one or two glass jars at a time for a few minutes, but only dipping lids and tongs into the pot after boiling stops), then cover them with the following vinegar mixture.

To Apple cider vinegar I add one sixth of its quantity of pure water, plus a mix of spices, such as Peppercorns, Bay leaves, grated or thinly sliced Ginger and Garlic, plus some brown sugar. This can be carefully heated in a double pot of simmering water for a while, but don't let it boil. When cooled down, you pour it over the sliced roots in the sterilised jars, making sure there is more than enough liquid to cover them, because there may be a little evaporation over time. They'll keep for ages, with no need for refrigeration. The vinegar can be re-used in salad dressings too.

This method is surely better than the recommended brief boiling of vinegar and spices, as you are just warming it enough for the spices to release their flavours and the sugar to dissolve.

Joy Larkom, in explaining the Asian approach, says that pickling vinegar can be used either hot or cold. "Hot vinegar is considered better for soft pickles and cold for vegetables you wish to remain crisp," she wrote. [2]

Fermenting food needs a warm place to develop, so my Irish kitchen is the best spot, but not always. Recipes talk about fermenting at 'room temperature' and don't specify what temperature that means. In summertime my unheated Irish kitchen tends to be too cold to make Sauerkraut, but in winter the wood heater corner is more consistently warm.

A modern consideration for pickle making is that microorganisms are badly affected by electro-magnetic fields, so it's best not to store them where they'll be affected by wifi, 'smart meters', phone masts etc. A Malaysian friend who makes Tempeh in Penang had to screen the building with Carbon paint and wire mesh on windows, to stop radiation from a phone mast put up in a school ground across the road from spoiling the fermentation process. It's the same problem for our gutbiota, which is no doubt why I tend to vomit after bad exposures. But I've learned that if I wear a protective vest made from Silver, that covers my vital organs and belly, when I'm exposed - I don't get sick. (Women contemplating pregnancy are well advised to also do this.)

1. Fermenting - Recipes and Preparation, by Daphne Lambert, Flame Tree Publishing, 2016, UK.
2. Oriental Vegetables - the complete guide for the gardening cook, Joy Larkom, Frances Lincoln, UK, 2007.

AUTUMN FORAGING

If you are into wild foraging, you may not need a garden at all. The woods and hedgerows are loaded with fruit now!

BEECHNUTS
The nuts are sweet, protein rich and good in salads or soups when roasted. However they are small and fiddly to shell. They contain 50% oil, that tastes a bit like Olive oil. Roasted and ground, Beechnuts can be drunk as a coffee substitute; or dried and ground to add to other flours for baking. But if eaten in large amounts, Beechnuts can be toxic. [1]

ELDERBERRIES
The juicy berries of Elder trees that ripen in early autumn must be properly ripe and cooked before eating them. Pick them when clusters start to turn upside down and before they turn mushy. Wash well and strip them off with a fork. Add Elderberries to Apple pies, Gooseberry jam, or Blackberry or Crabapple jelly, etc.

ELDERBERRY JUICE
For juice, cook berries for a few minutes, then press and strain them. Serve hot with honey. Or add 10% honey, a little alcohol and bottle it, so it can be stored. [2]

ELDERBERRY SYRUP
To one part ripe berries add half a part of water, then simmer and stir for twenty minutes. Cool and press through a jelly bag or muslin. Add sugar, at half the weight of the liquid, plus some Cinnamon, Cloves and Lemon slices to make it tastier. Simmer this for 20 minutes, then strain and pour hot into sterilised bottles. Drink this neat by the teaspoon for colds, or dilute with boiling water for a hot drink. [3]

HAZELNUTS

Nuts are harvested when leaves turn to autumn colours. Good eaten raw, they are quite oily. The extracted oil is good for salad dressings etc. Roasting nuts first enhances the flavour. Nuts can be liquidised to make a milk substitute. Kept in the shell in a dark, dry place, they will store for up to one year.[1]

HAWTHORN BERRIES

Dried berries can be ground and added to flour for baking. But removing the big seed is always tricky.

Fresh berries make good jam, especially when added to Elderberry and Apple; they are also good in chutney. Berries can also be made into wine.

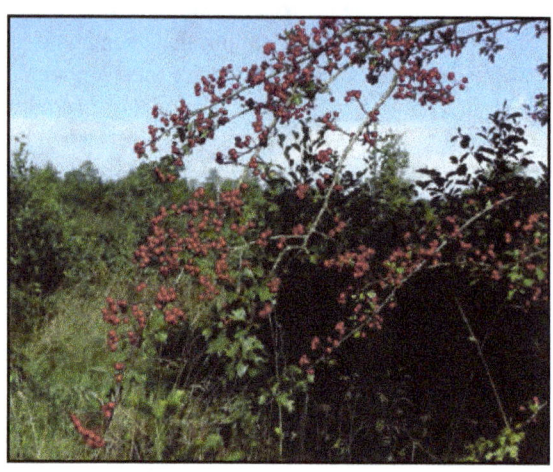

HAWTHORN LEATHER

A medicinal leather can be made by first boiling berries for fifteen minutes, then removing the seeds, which is not easy. I rub them through a sieve. Spread the pulp in a thin layer to dry in the sun or dehydrator. Eating a 2cm^2/one inch square piece of this leather daily is a great tonic for the heart.

HAWTHORN BERRY SYRUP

Put berries in a pot, cover them in water and bring to the boil, then mash them and leave them overnight. The next day bring them back to the boil and simmer until it looses half its volume. Strain through some muslin and add an equal amount of sugar to the liquid. Bring back to the boil rapidly, then pour it warm into sterilised bottles. A teaspoon taken daily helps to maintain a healthy heart and circulation.[3]

OAK ACORNS

Acorns being toxic and bitter due to high tannin levels (which is lowest when they're fully ripe) need to be left to mellow for a couple of weeks after picking before they are processed. For leaching out tannin, the peasantry would then put a sack of shelled acorns into constantly running water (e.g. a stream) and then roast them to remove any remaining. One source suggests soaking them for two to three hours, but Ken Fern says for "a few months".[4] If you don't have a running stream, you can soak shelled acorns in water for eight hours, then change the water and soak them another four hours. When soak water is a light colour, roast them to remove remaining tannins.

Once roasted, acorns will keep for several months. Roast acorn has several uses. As a coffee substitute widely drunk across Europe during World War Two, acorns were leached, then chopped and roasted to a light brown colour. They were then ground and roasted again.[2] This drink is made more tasty and nutritious by adding spices such as Cinnamon.[5] Ground roast acorns can also be used as a flour substitute. Acorn flour mixed 50:50 with other flours gives a rich, nutty flavour to cakes, breads, biscuits etc.

ROSEHIPS

The ripe red fruits of Wild Roses are packed with vitamins A, B and K, while the vitamin C content is twenty to forty times greater than that of Oranges.³ You can eat Rosehips straight off the bush, but only eat the red flesh and avoid the itchy seed hairs inside. Or boil them for ten minutes, then strain carefully through a coffee filter paper for an immune strengthening tea, high in vitamin C.

ROSEHIP VINEGAR

Pack a sterilised jar with clean Rosehips and cover them with Apple cider vinegar. Leave to mature in a sunny spot for a month. Speed up the process by first slitting each Rosehip with a knife. The strained liquid is great for colds and sore throats, taken as a gargle or as a hot drink, with a tablespoonful added to water; or dress salads with it. ³

ROSEHIP SYRUP

Slit skins of clean Rosehips and put layers of them into wide mouthed jars, alternating with thin layers of natural sugar in-between. Leave in a sunny spot for a couple of months or so, until liquefied. Strain through a muslin cloth or jelly bag carefully. Keep this as a delicious medicine, taking teaspoonfuls frequently as a cold preventative. Use it to also flavour puddings or add it to hot drinks.³

Boiled Rosehip Syrup, the better known method, was advocated by Britain's Ministry of Food during World War Two, when imports of citrus fruits stopped. A simple version goes like this. Put Rosehips and half their volume of water into a pot and boil, covered, for twenty minutes. Cool then strain. Then boil the liquid with half its amount of sugar for ten minutes and pour hot into sterilised bottles. It will keep longer than the unboiled version, but will retain less vitamin C.³

FERMENTED ROSEHIP PUREE

An eighteenth century recipe is simple and, if honey is used rather than sugar, very wholesome too. Best of all, it doesn't need boiling, so it retains more vitamins. But it is more work. You cut the hips in half and clean out the prickly seeds. Pack the cleaned hips into an earthenware pot and leave them to mellow down until soft enough for rubbing through a sieve. To the resulting puree is added the same weight (or less) of warm, melted sugar or liquid honey. Mix well, pour into sterilised jars and seal.²

ROWAN BERRIES

The bright red berries of Rowan trees are bitter but very nutritious, with more vitamin C than citrus fruits. It's best to eat only a handful at most when they're raw, as the Parascorbic Acid in seeds can upset your stomach, however cooking destroys it. Pick the whole berry clusters in October, before they turn mushy. The berries can be made into jelly, but you'll need to add a little chopped Crab apple for a good setting. The jelly has a sharp marmalade taste and dark orange colour. Rowan berries can also be made into juice, or brewed into alcoholic drinks.²

They are taken medicinally too, with raw and cooked berries being slightly laxative and diuretic, and also cleansing the kidneys. Eating the dried berries can help gastric problems. For coughs and sore throats, gargling with a tea of berries or flowers is recommended.⁵ The leaves are also used medicinally, being dried and made into tea, at two teaspoons per cup and taken twice daily.

SLOE SYRUP

In a Romanian recipe for Sloe Syrup, good for storing through the winter, the Sloes are each pricked and then soaked, covered in water for three days. You strain them, then add an equal amount of sugar to the liquid, i.e. one litre of juice to one kilo sugar, bring this to the boil, then pour it into sterilised bottles and seal them after it cools.[6]

PICKLED SLOES

Sloe berries can also be preserved by lacto-fermentation. Very salty brine (three tablespoons of salt per litre of water) is poured over the berries that are packed into jars or stoneware pots.[7] Mine are still in the jar, while I ponder what to do with them (right).

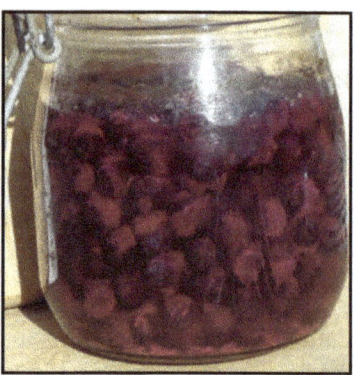

Joy Larkom says that Umemboshi plums, which are a very similar fruit, are pickled in Japan by being sprinkled with salt and weighted down in a barrel, with the resulting juice drained off and used for pickling other things.[8] This method could be worth trying with Sloe berries.

DANDELION DRINK

Roots are sweetest when dug in the autumn at two years of age. Scrub them clean, then roast the roots until brown and brittle, and grind them up for a coffee substitute, which needs to be boiled for a few minutes before drinking.[9]

DANDELION ROOT STIR FRY

Dandelion root is popular as a cooked vegetable in Japanese cuisine. The finely chopped roots are cut into thin rings that are sautéed briefly in vegetable oil, then a little water and a pinch of salt is added, and they are covered with a lid to cook briefly until soft. At the end, a dash of Soya sauce is added.[2]

Below left - Redcurrants. Below right - Seabuckthorn.

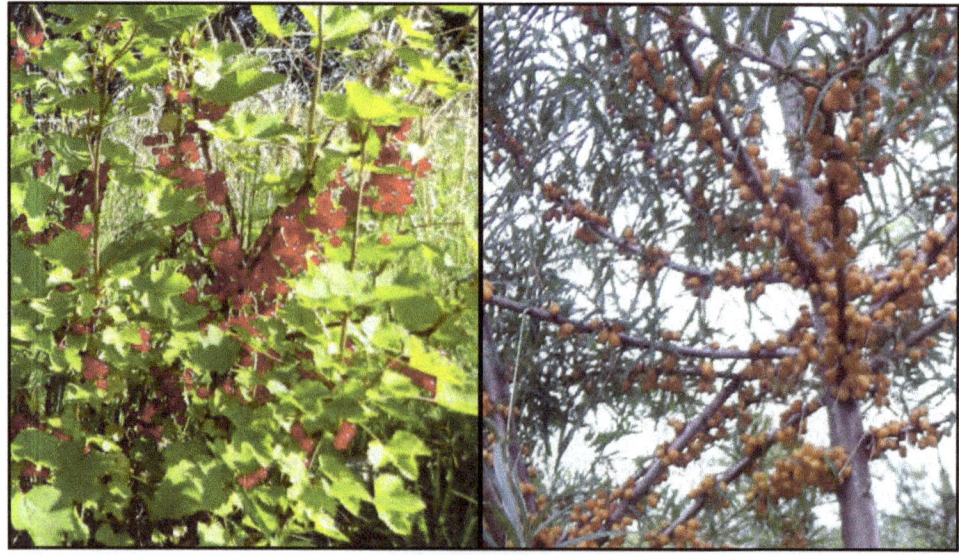

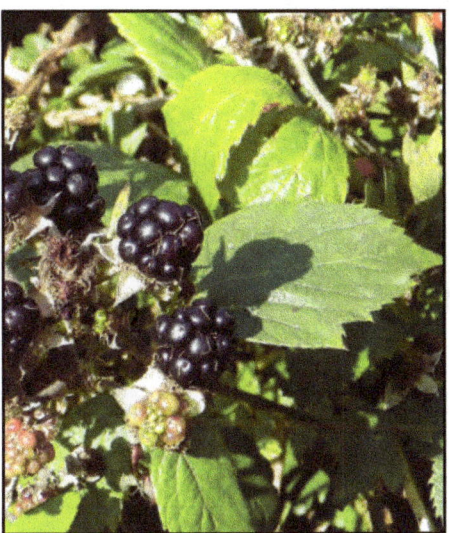

FORAGING REFERENCES

1. Wild Foods for Free, Jonathan Hilton, Hamlyn, UK, 2007.
2. Food for Free, Richard Mabey, Collins, Ireland, 1972.
3. Hedgerow Medicine - harvest and make your own herbal remedies, Julie Bruton-Seal and Matthew Seal, Merlin Unwin, UK, 2008.
4. Plants for a Future, Ken Fern, Permanent Publications, UK, 2000.
5. The Spirit of Trees, Fred Hageneder, Floris Books, UK, 2000.
6. European Peasant Cookery, Elisabeth Luard, Grub St, London, 2004.
7. The Gardeners and Farmers of Terre Vivante, Chelsea Green, Vermont USA, 1999.
8. Oriental Vegetables - the complete guide for the gardening cook, Joy Larkcom, Frances Lincoln Ltd, UK, 2007.
9. Wild and Free cooking from nature, by Cyril and Kit O'Ceirin, Wolf Hill, UK, 2013.

Above - Blackberry.

AUTUMN CROP RECIPES

FRUITY CARRAGEEN FOOL

An easy dessert using Apples, or any fruit really, and Carrageen seaweed (Irish Moss).

Carrageen, a handful
Ginger, a small knob
Apples, cookers, a couple
Raisins, nuts, sweetener, all optional
Creamed coconut, a lump
Polenta, a quarter cup or less, optional
Spices - Cinnamon stick, Cardamon pods, Nutmeg, Cloves, Lemon / Lime zest etc, optional

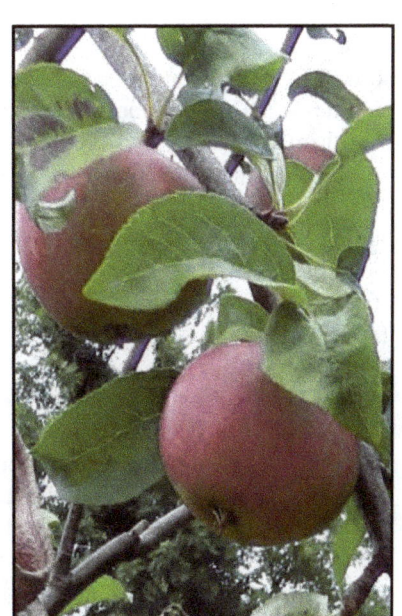

Soak seaweed for ten minutes, then pick off any tough stems or yukky bits. Boil with a few cups of water, plus spices and Coconut cream. Add chopped fruit and stir well as it simmers for a few minutes. Then thicken it up with polenta, by pouring it in slowly as it boils for a few more minutes, stirring constantly. Serve cool or hot, with a dob of yoghurt.

STIR-FRIED BROAD BEAN SPROUTS

This is based on a recipe from northern China - Ching chow tsan do meow.

2 cups sprouted Broad Beans
3 tbsp oil
1 tsp Salt
1 tsp sugar
1.5 cups water
1 tsp Sesame oil

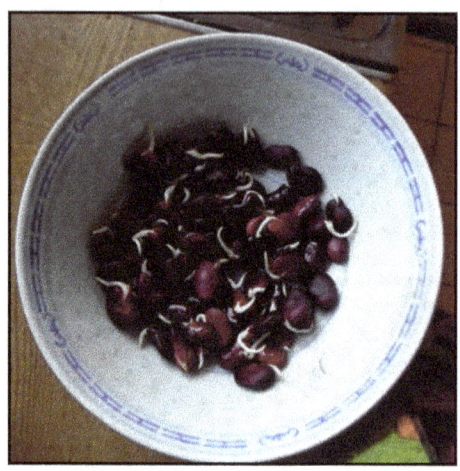

Stir fry the sprouts rapidly on high heat for ten seconds, then add salt, sugar and water, and bring to the boil. Put the lid on and simmer lightly for 25 minutes until the water is almost gone. Remove the lid and keep stirring to evaporate the water fully, then splash on the Sesame oil, stir lightly and serve hot or cold[1].

SWEET SQUASH PIE

I don't bother to make a crust, it's the Squash (or use Pumpkin) that stars in this delicious recipe, which is very fast to put together. I use Winter Squash, the Hokkaido variety that grows so well in the polytunnel that I harvested fifty big ones in 2020. We rubbed a thin coat of oil over them to improve their keeping ability and are still enjoying them almost one year later!

500gm Squash, peeled
3 or 4 eggs
160ml tin of Coconut milk
Tsp salt
4 tbls natural sugar
Spices - Ginger, Cinnamon, Nutmeg etc

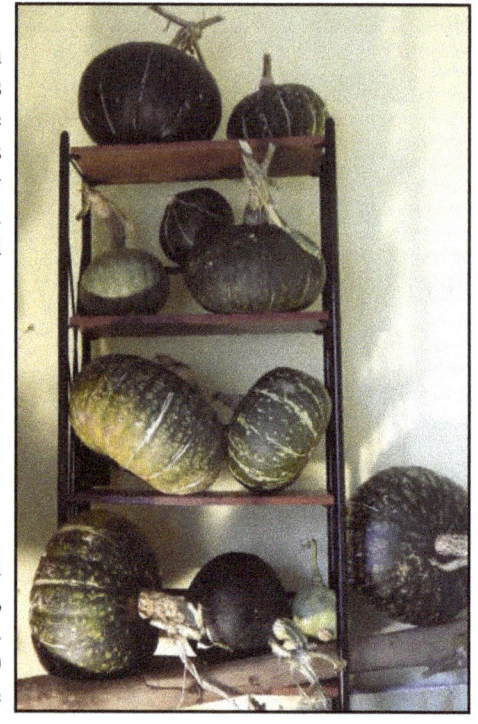

First cut the Squash into small chunks and steam till soft and allow to cool. Beat the eggs, mash or blend the Squash and mix all together. Pre-heat oven at gas mark 4, bake for 60 minutes or so, and when an inserted knife comes out clean, it should be ready.

Another version substitutes a third of the Squash with cooked pudding Rice. This echoes the Russian recipe Zapekanka, that is a mix of Rice, Squash / Pumpkin, eggs, butter, Cinnamon and Nutmeg, and is baked as above.[2]

Above - A bounty of delicious Hokkaido Squash from the polytunnel.
We were still eating the last of the 50 harvested one year later.

QUINOA PATTIES

Apart from the eggs, salt, spices and Sesame seeds, which are optional anyway, this recipe of mine combines the fruits of my garden and so it sure feels good to make it! A vegan version substitutes eggs with a couple of tablespoons of Chickpea (Gram) flour, that's made into a thick paste.

Quinoa, cooked, a cupful
Broad beans, a handful steamed and cooled
Beetroot, small one grated
Potato, medium size, steamed and mashed or chopped
2 eggs, beaten
Onion and Garlic, finely sliced
Black Sesame seeds
Salt, pepper/chilli and spices, optional

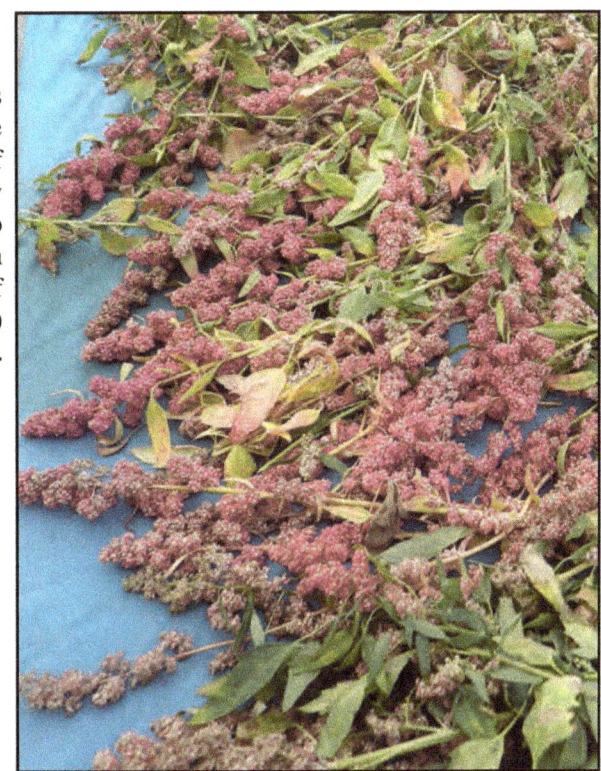

Mix all together, except the Sesame seeds. Leave to soak for an hour or more. Then form the mix into patties and fry in Coconut oil. Sprinkle Sesame seeds on top, before flipping over.

Above - Red Farro Quinoa crop drying in the polytunnel.

HORSERADISH SAUCE

Horseradish roots can be dug or sliced off after the first frost of autumn, in late autumn and throughout winter, once plants are established. Preserve the freshly dug roots in vinegar by putting chopped pieces into a liquidiser with enough Apple cider vinegar to blend them into a paste. Store in sterilised jars with a layer of Olive oil on top to make it last.

HORSERADISH SYRUP

Cough syrup can be made from Horseradish blended with liquid honey and a little Apple cider vinegar. Take a spoonful as needed. Store in jars as above.

BEETROOT, APPLE AND HORSERADISH RELISH

3 cooking Apples
3 Beetroot
4 tbsps Horseradish
1 tbsp fine Salt
1 tbsp Sauerkraut juice - optional.

Grate the Apples, Beetroot and Horseradish, which could make you quite tearful as the volatile oils escape. Maybe wear goggles. Mix well together and pack into a sterilised jar or Sauerkraut pot. Press it down until the emerging liquid covers it. Put a weight on top to ensure that it is submerged (although I didn't find this necessary). Put the lid on very loosely for seven days, leaving it in a warm place to ferment. Then remove any weights and tighten the lid for storage. It's ready to eat from then.[3]

SAUERKRAUT

To get the live juice for the relish above, you need to make the classic lacto-ferment Sauerkraut, as the commercial stuff will probably be pasteurised and dead. I didn't have much luck with making Sauerkraut until I bought special stoneware pots with a water seal, plus a mandoline for speedy Cabbage grating. Now it isn't daunting at all!

I get tight Cabbage heads and good salt, plus peppercorns. I shred the Cabbage with the mandoline and pack it into the pot (pounding it down a bit), putting a sprinkle of salt and some Peppercorns inbetween the layers. I keep adding layers and soon the juices rise up. They need to cover the Cabbage. When nearly full, I put the (sterilised) ceramic weights that come with the pot, on top of the Cabbage, to make sure it's submerged. Better still is to put a large Cabbage leaf on top of the Cabbage and put the weights on top of that. Then I put the pot in a warm corner and fill the groove around the lid rim with water. I enjoy listening to the occasional bubbles, as it 'burps' itself for a week or two. I check occasionally that the Cabbage is covered and when the bubbling stops, it's time to pack it into sterilised jars for storage, or you can start eating it then. The flavour gets stronger the longer you leave it.

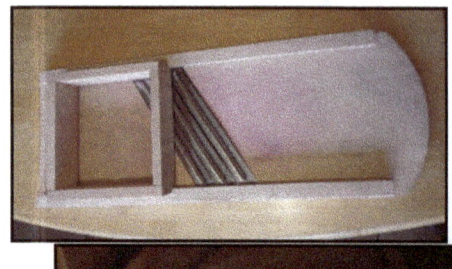

Left - Mandoline for grating Cabbage for Sauerkraut.
Below - Sauerkraut pots wth water seal lids.

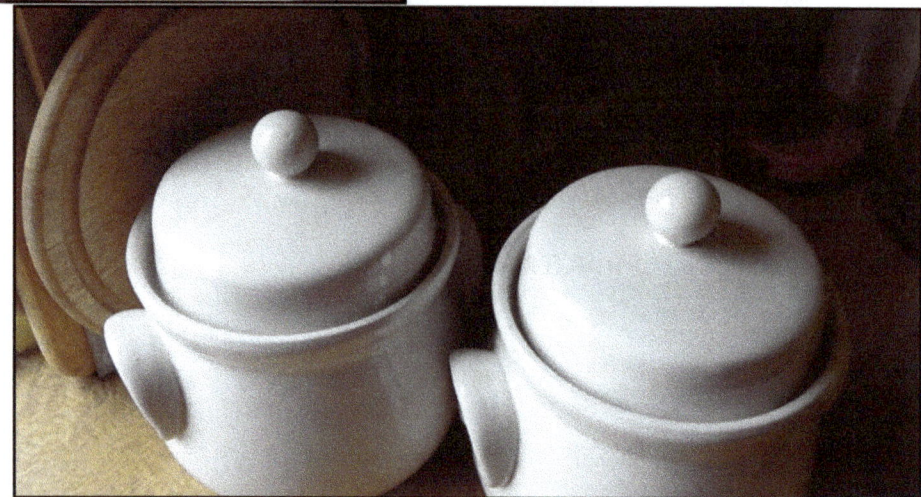

APPLE CIDER VINEGAR

6 sweet Apples, washed and sliced
Pure water to cover them
A dash of Apple Cider Vinegar
1 tbsp organic cane sugar
Sterilised large jar and bottles

Put all into a large jar, cover with a piece of muslin/cheesecloth over the top and leave it in a warm, dark place for a couple of weeks, where it will start to bubble and froth. Make sure that all the Apple bits are submerged and when they have fallen to the bottom, strain them out and put the liquid back into the jar, cover it over and leave it to ferment again for four to six weeks in a warm, dark place. The mat that grows on top is called the 'Mother'. When you are happy with the flavour, bottle it up, store it in a cool, dark place and it should keep a long time.[4]

RECIPE REFERENCES
1. World Vegetarian, more than 650 meatless recipes from around the world, Madhur Jaffrey, 1998, Ebury Press, UK.
2. The Delights of Russian Cuisine, Yvonne Webb, Better Living, Australia.
3. Recipe from Frances Astor.
4. Fermenting - recipes and preparation, Daphne Lambert, Flame Tree, UK, 2016.

Below - My Buddleia shrub lives up to its name of Butterfly Bush.

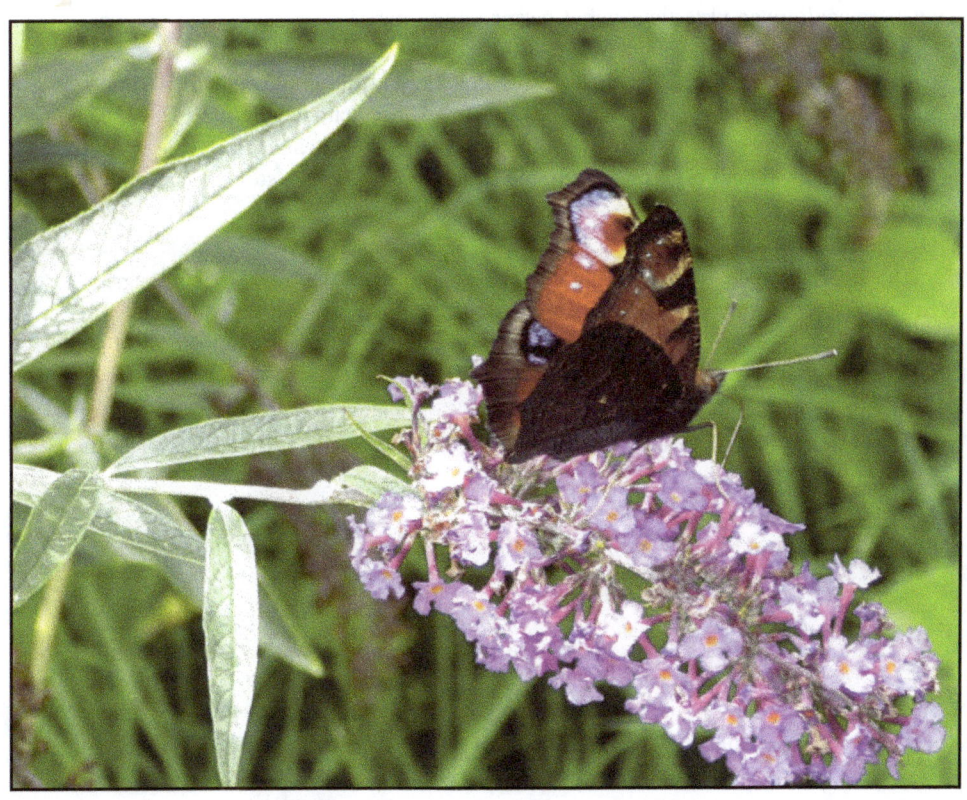

MANY THANKS TO

Peter Cowman, Francis Astor, Heather Colman, Kay Baxter,
Bob Corker, David Holmgren, Su Dennett, Noel Higgins, Shelley Moore,
Colin Austin, Danny Gaffey, Simone ni Chinneide, Peter Russell,
Erica Bear, Peter Schneider and Feidlim Harty
for help, support, inspiration and contributions.

PHOTO CREDITS

All photos by Alanna Moore, except on page 7 - Ulster American Folk Park;
photos by Peter Cowman page 15, 21, 37, 211, 146, 161, 189;
photo by Erica Bear page 163; photos by Heather Colman pages 44 - 45
and photos on pages 105 (Iris) and 108 (Willows) by Féidhlim Harty.

NOTES

CHAPTER TWO - THE NEW PEASANTRY
'Animal, Vegetable, Junk', Mark Bittman, Houghton Mifflin Harcourt, US, 2021.
www.info.fairtrade.net   www.koanga.org.nz
Peter Cowman's site, full of free info, at www.livingarchitecturecentre.com

CHAPTER THREE - ECO-GARDENING
Check out Maddy Harland's explanatory articles about Permaculture, starting here:
www.permaculture.co.uk/articles/what-permaculture-part-1-ethics
'Sensitive Permaculture', Alanna Moore, 2009, Python Press, Ireland.
David Holmgren - www.holmgren.com.au   Pete the Permie - www.petethepermie.com.au
Organic Centre, Rossinver, north Co. Leitrim - www.theorganiccentre.ie
www.pollinators.ie   www.nativewoodlandtrust.ie   www.teagasc.ie
Feidlim Harty's wetland books etc available from www.wetlandsystems.ie/shop.html

CHAPTER FOUR - PLANTS AND ANIMALS
Demeter International - www.demeter.net   BD in Ireland - www.biodynamicagriculture.ie
Wisdom of Bees: Principles of BD Beekeeping, E. Berrevoets, Steiner Books, USA.

CHAPTER SIX - SPRINGTIME
Read about a ritual held at the Shannon Pot with Simone and Alanna in this book:
'Shannon Country - a river journey through time', Paul Clements, Lilliput Press, Dublin, 2020.

CHAPTER - AUTUMN
Daphne Lambert is a founder of the educational trust: www.greencuisinetrust.org

ABOUT THE AUTHOR
Alanna Moore is a gardener, poet, geomancer, teacher, author of nine books,
maker of film documentaries on environmental and esoteric themes,
and a songwriter/singer. She has three Diplomas of Permaculture
from Bill Mollison in the 1990s. See www.geomantica.com

INDEX

Alanna's Peasant Rap - 21

Alder tree - 51, 83, 128

Alfalfa sprouts - 179

Alliums - 113

Almond sprouts - 179

Angelica - 115, 196

Animal feed, homegrown - 156-158

Aronia - 115

Apple cider vinegar - 233

Apple trees - 88 - 89, 114

Ash tree - 89

Autumn harvest - 216-219

Bamboo, leaves - 158

Barberry - 117

Barley - 154

Bean sprouts - 179

Beech tree - 89

Beech leaves - 193

Beech nuts - 225

Bee, Honey - 162-165

Beech tree - 89

Beetroot, Apple, Horseradish Relish - 231

Bergamot - 117

Bill Mollison - 11

Blackcurrant - 117
    and Honey Spread - 212
    Syrup - 212

Blackthorn - 98

Blueberry - 118

Bogs - 101- 102

Bokashi - 67

Borage

Boro, fabric work - 44 - 45

Broad Beans - 112
    and Potato Mash - 197
    Soup, Sicilian - 186
    sprouts stir fried - 229

Bucket gardens - 73 - 78

Buckwheat - 153

Buckwheat pancakes - 32

Buckwheat sprouts - 179

Building Bioloy - 9

Bullace tree - 90

'Bulrush' - 105

Burdock - 118

Cabbage sprouts - 179

Cabbage Tree - 107

Cardoon - 118

Catalan Soup - 183

Celery Leaf - 118

Cherry tree - 90
    Wild and Bird - 90

Chickweed - 119

Chicory - 119

Chinese Artichoke - 119

Chives - 120

Clamps and cellars - 220

Chrysanthemum Greens - 141

Cider Gum - 92

Climate Change - 69

Clovers - 120
    sprouts - 180

Comfrey - 120, 157

Compost, making - 175-176
    systems - 53 - 56
    toilet - 36

Cordyline australis - 107

Cornelian Cherry - 91

Corn - 150-151
    sprouts - 180

Cover crops - 62

Cowslip - 122

Crab Apple - 91

Cress sprouts - 180

Damson Plum - 91

Dancing at the Crossroads - 204-205

Dandelion - 122
    drink - 228
    root stir fry - 228

Day Lilly - 122

Elderberry - 92, 225
    Juice and Syrup - 225

Eleagnus - 122

Elecampane - 123

Eucalyptus gunni - 92

Evening Primrose - 123

Dandelion, flower salad - 208
    flower tempura - 208

Dehydrating - 221

Diet, Conscious - 30
    low Carbon - 29
    Wholefoods - 31

'Dirty Electricity' - 18

Eco living, healthy - 12
    low cost - 17

Electric car - 17

Elderflower, cordial - 208
    fritters - 208

Fennel - 124

Fermented Green Bean Salad - 185

Fermenting food - 221-225

Fire Bath - 39 - 40

Food security - 10

Food Forest, Polytunnel - 71 - 73

Food Forest gardens - 81 - 84

INDEX

plants - 86 - 87
trees - 85

Fruit trees for western Ireland - 100 - 101

Fruity Carageen Fool - 229

Fuchsia - 124

Garbage Enzymes - 69

Garlic - 113, 124
    pickled - 197

Garlic Chives sprouts - 180

Globe Artichoke - 125

Goji Berry - 125

Goldenberry - 125

Good King Henry - 126

Grapes - 126

Grain growing - 147, 157

Green Beans fermented - 212

Greenwash - 9

Guelder Rose - 93

Hawthorn - 93, 193, 226
    leather - 226
    berry syrup - 226

Hazel - 94, 226

Hedgerows - 79 - 81

Holly - 95

Honey Bee - 162-165

Horseradish - 127
    sauce and syrup - 231

Horsetail - 127

Hops - 127

Hummus - 184

Idlis - 33

Iris, Yellow Flag - 105

Irish Idli pancakes - 33

Ivy - 128

Japanese Knotweed - 129

Jerusalem Artichoke - 129, 157

Kale - 113, 129

Khadi clothing - 43

Kitchen, cookware - 35
    low Carbon - 16

Kohl rabi - 130

Korean Mint - 130

Korean Natural Farming - 68, 158

Kune Kune Pig - 159-161

Lavender - 130

Leaf Beet - 130

Leek, Potato and Sunroot Soup - 184

Lemonbalm - 131

Lettuce sprouts - 180

Lime/Linden tree - 194, 207

Linseed sprouts - 180

Living mulch - 63

Lovage - 131

Mahatma Gandhi - 43

Maize - 150-151

Mallows - 131

Mandi washing - 38

Marigold - 132

Marshmallow - 132

Mashua - 133

Meadowsweet - 133, 207

Meitheals - 51

Micro-greens - 177

Microbes - 67
    Korean - 68

Millet, Foxtail - 151-152
    sprouts - 180

Mint - 133
    and Parsley Salad - 198
    Chutney - 198
    Pesto - 198
    Yoghurt Salad Dressing - 199

Mitsuba - 134
    sprouts - 180

Monkey Puzzle tree - 95

Mugwort - 135

Mustard sprouts - 180

Nasturtium - 135

Nettles, Stinging - 135, 148, 194
    and Potatoes dish - 199
    Pie - 200
    roots - 219

New Zealand Flax - 106

Oak trees - 95
    acorns - 226

Oats - 147-148, 157
    sprouts - 181

Oca - 137

Onions - 113, 137
    sprouts - 181

Pears - 96

Pea sprouts - 181

Peasant bathroom - 36
    clothing - 41
    economy - 22- 24
    kitchen - 26
    rap song - 21
    transport - 46-48

Peat Moss, medicine - 102
    EMR protection - 103

Perilla sprouts - 181

Permaculture - 50

Pig, Kune Kune - 159-161

Phormium tenax - 106

Pine trees - 96

Plantain - 138, 157
    sprouts - 181

Polish Peasant Soup - 185

'Power of Pee' rap song - 37

Potato - 110, 138, 157
    Cakes - 213
    No-dig - 65

INDEX

Pumpkin sprouts - 181

Quinoa - 149
       patties - 231
       sprouts - 181

Rain water drinking - 16

Raised garden beds - 60 - 61

Radish sprouts - 181

Ramsons - 145

Raspberry - 138

Reed, Common - 104

Reed Mace, Greater - 105

Refrigerator ditchng - 219

Remineralising soil - 62

Re-wilding - 78 - 80

Rhubarb - 139

Rice sprouts - 181

Rockdust - 62

Rose - 140

Rosehip vinegar, syrup, puree - 227

Rosemary - 140

Rowan berries - 227

Rye - 154
       sprouts - 181

Rowan tree - 97

Sacred hearth - 171

Salad Burnett - 140

Sauerkraut - 232

Seabuckthorn - 140

Seed, sowing - 189-190
       sprouting - 171

Shepherd's Purse - 141

Shungiku - 141
       sprouts - 182

Silver Birch - 97, 193

Sloes - 98
       fermented - 228
       Syrup - 228

Slugs - 64

Soapwort - 142

Soil making - 53 - 55

Sorrel - 142

Spring, foraging - 192-194
       harvest - 195-196

Springtime - 188

Spruce trees - 99, 194

Squash, Pie - 230
       sprouts - 181

Staple crops - 110

Strawberry - 142
       Wild - 142
       Alpine - 143

Strawberry tree - 99

Sugar-free Fruit 'Jams' - 28

Sumac - 143

Summer - 204
    flower recipes - 207-209
    fruits - 206
    harvest - 210-211

Sunflower - 143, 157
    Maximillian - 144
    sprouts - 182

Sunroot - 129, 157

Sweet Cicely - 144

Sweet Woodruff - 144

Tetragonia - 144

Thyme - 144

Tomato Sauce, fermented - 213-214

Tree mounds - 189

Vinegar pickles - 222-224

Violet - 145

Wastewater treatment - 103 - 104
    plants - 104 - 108

Watercress - 106, 145
    and Seaweed Soup - 200
    sprouts - 182

Water Mint - 105

'Weeds' - 63

Wetlands - 101- 102

Wheat sprouts - 182

Whitethorn - 93

Wild Garlic - 145, 194
    Pesto - 200

Wine Dark Sea Soup - 185

Winter - 168
    harvest - 173

Winter Savory - 146

Wholegrain pancakes - 32

Wicking Gardens - 73 - 78

Willow trees - 108

Windbreaks - 51

WWOOFers - 52

Yellow Flag Iris - 105

Yeast - 222

Yoghurt making - 34

Alanna Moore's books, plus DVDs, CDs, courses and services are available at her website:

www.geomantica.com

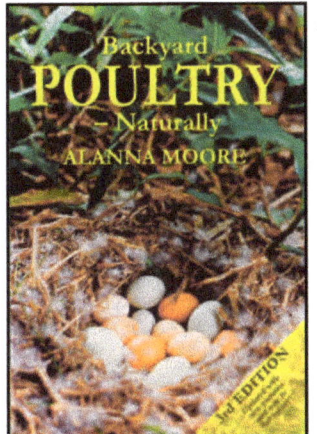

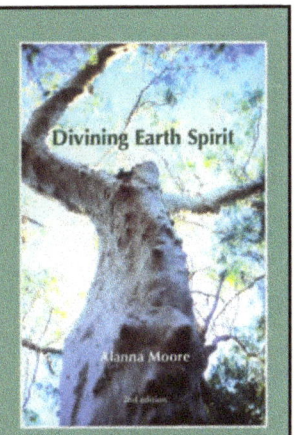

Backyard Poultry - Naturally has been Australia's best selling and most widely acclaimed 'chook' book since 1998.

Divining Earth Spirit looks at the Earth's subtle energies and their effects on us - in folklore (especially in Australia and New Zealand), in current geomantic practice and in scientific understandings.

Stone Age Farming - tapping nature's energies for your farm or garden, is a book that has been inspiring gardeners for 20 years now. From energetic rock dust to modern Power Towers, find out how to get a buzz from your own backyard.

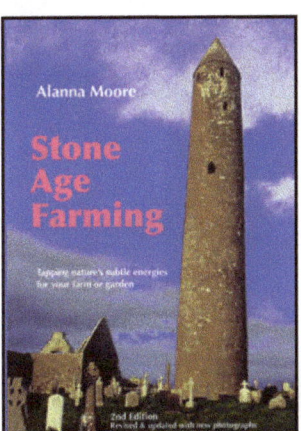

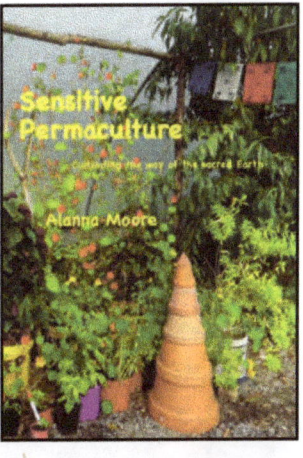

Sensitive Permaculture - Cultivating the Way of the Sacred Earth, is a new take on this sustainable design system, that embraces the 4th Ethic of Permaculture - Care of Spirit.

Plant Spirit Gardener is a practical book for the sensitive gardener that looks at the invisible realms in your backyard and how to connect with plant spirits.

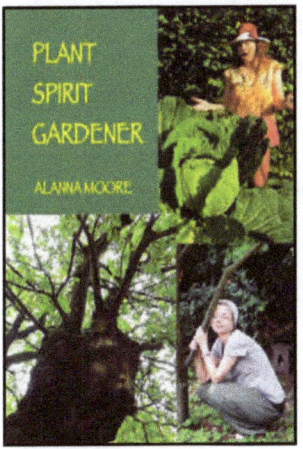

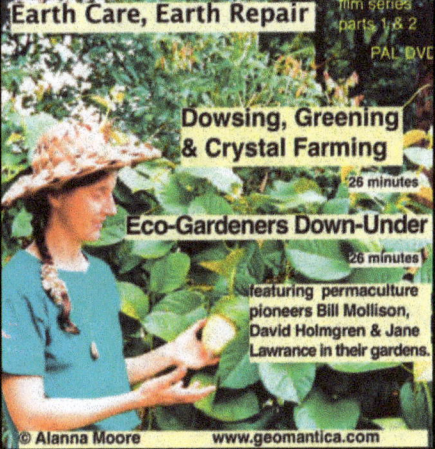

Alanna's 21 fims are on DVD only.

www.ingramcontent.com/pod-product-compliance
Lightning Source LLC
Chambersburg PA
CBHW080357030426
42334CB00024B/2911